Advice to the people in general, with regard to their health: but more particularly calculated for those, who, by their distance from regular physicians, or other very experienced practitioners

S. A. D. Tissot

Advice to the people in general, with regard to their health: but more particularly calculated for those, who, by their distance from regular physicians, or other very experienced practitioners, are the most unlikely to be seasonably provided with the bes
Tissot, S. A. D. (Samuel Auguste David)
ESTCID: T076081
Reproduction from British Library
The last two leaves contain the chapter contents.
London : printed for T. Becket and P.A. de Hondt, 1765.
xxxii,608,[4]p. ; 8°

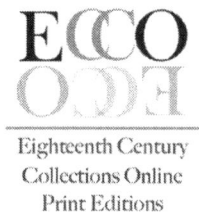

Eighteenth Century
Collections Online
Print Editions

Gale ECCO Print Editions

Relive history with *Eighteenth Century Collections Online*, now available in print for the independent historian and collector. This series includes the most significant English-language and foreign-language works printed in Great Britain during the eighteenth century, and is organized in seven different subject areas including literature and language; medicine, science, and technology; and religion and philosophy. The collection also includes thousands of important works from the Americas.

The eighteenth century has been called "The Age of Enlightenment." It was a period of rapid advance in print culture and publishing, in world exploration, and in the rapid growth of science and technology – all of which had a profound impact on the political and cultural landscape. At the end of the century the American Revolution, French Revolution and Industrial Revolution, perhaps three of the most significant events in modern history, set in motion developments that eventually dominated world political, economic, and social life.

In a groundbreaking effort, Gale initiated a revolution of its own: digitization of epic proportions to preserve these invaluable works in the largest online archive of its kind. Contributions from major world libraries constitute over 175,000 original printed works. Scanned images of the actual pages, rather than transcriptions, recreate the works *as they first appeared.*

Now for the first time, these high-quality digital scans of original works are available via print-on-demand, making them readily accessible to libraries, students, independent scholars, and readers of all ages.

For our initial release we have created seven robust collections to form one the world's most comprehensive catalogs of 18th century works.

Initial Gale ECCO Print Editions collections include:

History and Geography
Rich in titles on English life and social history, this collection spans the world as it was known to eighteenth-century historians and explorers. Titles include a wealth of travel accounts and diaries, histories of nations from throughout the world, and maps and charts of a world that was still being discovered. Students of the War of American Independence will find fascinating accounts from the British side of conflict.

Social Science
Delve into what it was like to live during the eighteenth century by reading the first-hand accounts of everyday people, including city dwellers and farmers, businessmen and bankers, artisans and merchants, artists and their patrons, politicians and their constituents. Original texts make the American, French, and Industrial revolutions vividly contemporary.

Medicine, Science and Technology
Medical theory and practice of the 1700s developed rapidly, as is evidenced by the extensive collection, which includes descriptions of diseases, their conditions, and treatments. Books on science and technology, agriculture, military technology, natural philosophy, even cookbooks, are all contained here.

Literature and Language
Western literary study flows out of eighteenth-century works by Alexander Pope, Daniel Defoe, Henry Fielding, Frances Burney, Denis Diderot, Johann Gottfried Herder, Johann Wolfgang von Goethe, and others. Experience the birth of the modern novel, or compare the development of language using dictionaries and grammar discourses.

Religion and Philosophy
The Age of Enlightenment profoundly enriched religious and philosophical understanding and continues to influence present-day thinking. Works collected here include masterpieces by David Hume, Immanuel Kant, and Jean-Jacques Rousseau, as well as religious sermons and moral debates on the issues of the day, such as the slave trade. The Age of Reason saw conflict between Protestantism and Catholicism transformed into one between faith and logic -- a debate that continues in the twenty-first century.

Law and Reference
This collection reveals the history of English common law and Empire law in a vastly changing world of British expansion. Dominating the legal field is the *Commentaries of the Law of England* by Sir William Blackstone, which first appeared in 1765. Reference works such as almanacs and catalogues continue to educate us by revealing the day-to-day workings of society.

Fine Arts
The eighteenth-century fascination with Greek and Roman antiquity followed the systematic excavation of the ruins at Pompeii and Herculaneum in southern Italy; and after 1750 a neoclassical style dominated all artistic fields. The titles here trace developments in mostly English-language works on painting, sculpture, architecture, music, theater, and other disciplines. Instructional works on musical instruments, catalogs of art objects, comic operas, and more are also included.

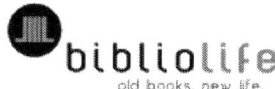

The BiblioLife Network

This project was made possible in part by the BiblioLife Network (BLN), a project aimed at addressing some of the huge challenges facing book preservationists around the world. The BLN includes libraries, library networks, archives, subject matter experts, online communities and library service providers. We believe every book ever published should be available as a high-quality print reproduction; printed on-demand anywhere in the world. This insures the ongoing accessibility of the content and helps generate sustainable revenue for the libraries and organizations that work to preserve these important materials.

The following book is in the "public domain" and represents an authentic reproduction of the text as printed by the original publisher. While we have attempted to accurately maintain the integrity of the original work, there are sometimes problems with the original work or the micro-film from which the books were digitized. This can result in minor errors in reproduction. Possible imperfections include missing and blurred pages, poor pictures, markings and other reproduction issues beyond our control. Because this work is culturally important, we have made it available as part of our commitment to protecting, preserving, and promoting the world's literature.

GUIDE TO FOLD-OUTS MAPS and OVERSIZED IMAGES

The book you are reading was digitized from microfilm captured over the past thirty to forty years. Years after the creation of the original microfilm, the book was converted to digital files and made available in an online database.

In an online database, page images do not need to conform to the size restrictions found in a printed book. When converting these images back into a printed bound book, the page sizes are standardized in ways that maintain the detail of the original. For large images, such as fold-out maps, the original page image is split into two or more pages

Guidelines used to determine how to split the page image follows:

• Some images are split vertically; large images require vertical and horizontal splits.
• For horizontal splits, the content is split left to right.
• For vertical splits, the content is split from top to bottom.
• For both vertical and horizontal splits, the image is processed from top left to bottom right.

ADVICE
TO THE
PEOPLE in GENERAL,
WITH
Regard to their HEALTH:

But more particularly calculated for those, who, by their Distance from regular Physicians, or other very experienced Practitioners, are the most unlikely to be seasonably provided with the best Advice and Assistance, in acute Diseases, or upon any sudden inward or outward Accident.

WITH

A Table of the most cheap, yet effectual Remedies, and the plainest Directions for preparing them readily.

Translated from the FRENCH Edition of

Dr. TISSOT's *Avis au Peuple*, &c.

Printed at *Lyons*; with all his own Notes; a few of his medical Editor's at *Lyons*; and several occasional Notes, adapted to this *English* Translation,

By J. KIRKPATRICK, M.D.

In the Multitude of the People is the Honour of a King; and for the Want of People cometh the Destruction of the Prince.
Proverbs xiv, 28.

LONDON:
Printed for T. BECKET and P. A. DE HONDT, at *Tully*'s Head, near *Surry-Street*, in the *Strand*.
MDCCLXV.

THE TRANSLATOR'S PREFACE.

THOUGH the great Utility of those medical Directions, with which the following Treatise is thoroughly replenished, will be sufficiently evident to every plain and sensible Peruser of it; and the extraordinary Reception of it on the Continent is recited in the very worthy Author's Preface; yet something, it should seem, may be pertinently added, with Regard to this Translation of it, by a Person who has been strictly attentive to the Original. a Work, whose Purpose was truly necessary and benevolent; as the Execution of it, altogether, is very happily accomplished.

It will be self evident, I apprehend, to every excellent Physician, that a radical Knowledge of the Principles, and much Experience in the Exercise, of their Profession, were necessary to accommodate such a Work to the Comprehension of those, for whom it was more particularly calculated. Such Gentlemen must observe, that the certain Axiom of *Nature's curing Diseases*, which is equally true in our Day, as it was in that of HIPPOCRATES, so habitually animates this Treatise, as not to require the least particular Reference. This *Hippocratic* Truth as certain (though much less subject to general Observation) as that Disease, or Age, is finally prevalent over all sublunary Life, the most attentive Physicians discern the soonest, the most ingenuous readily confess: and hence springs that wholesome Zeal and Severity, with which Dr. TISSOT encounters such Prejudices of poor illiterate Persons, as either oppose, or very ignorantly precipitate, her Operations, in her Attainment of Health. These Prejudices indeed may seem, from this Work, to be still greater, and perhaps grosser too, in *Switzerland* than among ourselves; though it is certain there is but too much Room for the Application of his salutary Cautions and Directions, even in this Capital, and doubtless abundantly more at great Distances from it. It may be very justly supposed, for *one* Instance, that in most of those Cases in the Small Pocks, in which the Mother undertakes the Cure of her Child, or confides it to a Nurse, that Saffron, in a greater or less Quantity, and Sack or Mountain Whey, are generally still used in the Sickening before Eruption, to accelerate that very Eruption, whose gradual Appearance, about the fourth Day, from that of Seizure inclusive, is so favourable and promising to the Patient, and the Precipitation of which is often so highly pernicious to them. Most of, or rather all, his other Cautions and Corrections seem equally necessary here,

The Translator's Preface.

here, as often as the Sick are similarly circumstanced, under the different acute Diseases in which he enjoins them.

Without the least Detraction however from this excellent Physician, it may be admitted that a few others, in many other Countries, might have sufficient Abilities and Experience for the Production of a like Work, on the same good Plan. This, we find, Dr. HIRZEL, principal Physician of *Zurich*, had in Meditation, when the present Treatise appeared, which he thought had so thoroughly fulfilled his own Intention, that it prevented his attempting to execute it. But the great Difficulty consisted in discovering a Physician, who, with equal Abilities, Reputation and Practice, should be qualified with that *much rarer* Qualification of caring so much more for the Health of those, who cou'd never pay him for it, than for his own Profit or Ease, as to determine him to project and to accomplish so necessary, and yet so self-denying, a Work. For as the Simplicity he proposed in the Style and Manner of it, by condescending, in the plainest Terms, to the humblest Capacities, obliged him to depress himself, by writing rather beneath the former Treatises, which had acquired him the Reputation of medical Erudition, Reasoning and Elegance; we find that the Love of Fame itself, so stimulating even to many ingenuous Minds, was as impotent as that of Wealth, to seduce him from so benign, so generous a Purpose. Though, upon Reflection, it is by no Means strange

strange to see wise Men found their Happiness, which all [however variously and even oppositely] pursue, rather in Conscience, than on Applause, and this naturally reminds us of that celebrated Expression of CATO, or some other excellent Ancient, "that he had rather *be* good, than *be reputed* so."

However singular such a Determination may now appear, the Number of reputable medical Translators into different Languages, which this original Work has employed on the Continent, makes it evident, that real Merit will, sooner or later, have a pretty general Influence, and induce many to imitate that Example, which they either could not, or did not, propose. As the truly modest Author has professedly disclaimed all Applause on the Performance, and contented himself with hoping an Exemption from Censure through his Readers' Reflection on the peculiar Circumstances and Address of it, well may his best, his faithfullest Translators, whose Merit and Pains must be of a very secondary Degree to his own, be satisfied with a similar Exemption especially when joined to the Pleasure, that must result from a Consciousness of having endeavoured to extend the Benefits of their Author's Treatise to Multitudes of their own Country and Language.

For my own Particular, when after reading the Introduction to the Work, and much of the Sequel, I had determined to translate it, to be as just as possible to the Author, and to his *English*

glish Readers, I determined not to interpolate any Sentiment of my own into the Text, nor to omit one Sentence of the Original, which, besides its being *Detraction* in its literal Sense, I thought might imply it in its worst, its figurative one; for which there was no Room. To conform as fully as possible to the Plainness and Perspicuity he proposed, I have been pretty often obliged in the anatomical Names of some Parts, and sometimes of the Symptoms, as well as in some pretty familiar, though not entirely popular Words, to explain all such by the most common Words I have heard used for them; as after mentioning the *Diaphragm*, to add, or *Midriff* — the *Trachæa* — or *Windpipe* — *acrimonious*, or *very sharp*, and so of many others. This may a little, though but a little, have extended the Translation beyond the Original; as the great Affinity between the *French* and *Latin*, and between the former and many *Latin* Words borrowed from the *Greek*, generally makes the same anatomical or medical Term, that is technical with us, vernacular or common with them. But this unavoidable Tautology, which may be irksome to many Ears, those medical Readers, for whom it was not intended, will readily forgive, from a Consideration of the general Address of the Work. while they reflect that meer Style, if thoroughly intelligible, is least essential to those Books, which wholly consist of very useful, and generally interesting, Matter.

As many of the Notes of the Editor of *Lyons*, as I have retained in this Version (having translated from the Edition of *Lyons*) are subscribed *E. L.* I have dispensed with several, some, as evidently less within Dr. Tissot's Plan, from tending to theorize, however justly or practically, where he must have had his own Reasons for omitting to theorize: a few others, as manifestly needless, from what the Author had either premised, or speedily subjoined, on the very same Circumstance: besides a very few, from their local Confinement to the Practice at *Lyons*, which lies in a Climate somewhat more different from our own than that of *Lausanne*. It is probable nevertheless, I have retained a few more than were necessary in a professed Translation of the original Work: but wherever I have done this, I have generally subjoined my Motive for it, of whatever Consequence that may appear to the Reader. I have retained all the Author's own Notes, with his Name annexed to them, or if ever the Annotator was uncertain to me, I have declared whose Note I supposed it to be.

Such as I have added from my own Experience or Observation are subscribed *K*, to distinguish them from the others; and that the Demerit of any of them may neither be imputed to the learned Author, nor to his Editor. Their principal Recommendation, or Apology is, that whatever Facts I have mentioned are certainly true. I have endeavoured to be temperate in their Number and Length, and to imitate that strict

strict Pertinence, which prevails throughout the Author's Work. If any may have ever condescended to consider my Way of writing, they will conceive this Restraint has cost me at least as much Pains, as a further Indulgence of my own Conceptions could have done. The few Prescriptions I have included in some of them, have been so conducted, as not to give the Reader the least Confusion with Respect to those, which the Author has given in his Table of Remedies, and which are referred to by numerical Figures, throughout the Course of his Book.

The moderate Number of Dr. Tissot's Prescriptions, in his Table of Remedies, amounting but to seventy-one, and the apparent Simplicity of many of them, may possibly disgust some Admirers of pompous and compound Prescription. But his Reserve, in this important Respect, has been thoroughly consistent with his Notion of Nature's curing Diseases; which suggested to him the first, the essential Necessity of cautioning his Readers against doing, giving, or applying any thing, that might oppose her healing Operations (a most capital Purpose of his Work) which important Point being gained, the mildest, simplest and least hazardous Remedies would often prove sufficient Assistants to her. Nevertheless, under more severe and tedious Conflicts, he is not wanting to direct the most potent and efficacious ones. The Circumstances of the poor Subjects of his medical Consideration, became also a very natural Object to him, and

was

was in no wise unworthy the Regard of the humane Translator of BILGUER ON AMPUTATIONS, or rather *against* the crying Abuse of them; an excellent Work, that does real Honour to them both; and which can be disapproved by none, who do not prefer the frequently unnecessary Mutilation of the afflicted, to the Consumption of their own Time, or the Contraction of their Employment.

Some Persons may imagine that a Treatise of this Kind, composed for the Benefit of labouring People in *Swisserland*, may be little applicable to those of the *British* Islands: and this, in a very few Particulars, and in a small Degree, may reasonably be admitted. But as we find their common Prejudices are often the very same; as the *Swifs* are the Inhabitants of a colder Climate than *France*, and generally, as Dr TISSOT often observes, accustomed to drink (like ourselves) more strong Drink than the *French* Peasantry; and to indulge more in eating Flesh too, which the Religion of *Berne*, like our own, does not restrain, the Application of his Advice to them will pretty generally hold good here. Where he forbids them Wine and Flesh, all Butchers Meat, and in most Cases all Flesh, and all strong Drink should be prohibited here especially when we consider, that all his Directions are confined to the Treatment of acute Diseases, of which the very young, the youthful, and frequently even the robust are more generally the Subjects. Besides, in some few of the *English* Translator's Notes,

The Translator's Preface.

Notes, he has taken the Liberty of moderating the Coolers, or the Quantities of them (which may be well adapted to the great Heats and violent *Swiſs* Summers he talks of) according to the Temperature of our own Climate, and the general Habitudes of our own People. It may be obſerved too, that from the ſame Motive, I have ſometimes aſſumed the Liberty of diſſenting from the Text in a very few Notes, as for Inſtance, on the Article of Paſtry, which perhaps is generally better here than in *Swiſſerland* (where it may be no better than the coarſe vile Traſh that is hawked about and ſold to meer Children) as I have frequently, in preparing for Inoculation, admitted the beſt Paſtry (but not of Meat) into the limited Diet of the Subjects of Inoculation, and conſtantly without the leaſt ill Conſequence. Thus alſo in Note * Page 287, 288, I have preſumed to affirm the Fact, that a ſtrong ſpirituous Infuſion of the Bark has ſucceeded more ſpeedily in ſome Intermittents, in particular Habits, than the Bark in Subſtance. This I humbly conceive may be owing to ſuch a *Menſtruum's* extracting the Reſin of the Bark more effectually (and ſo conveying it into the Blood) than the Juices of the Stomach and of the alimentary Canal did, or could. For it is very conceivable that the *Craſis*, the Conſiſtence, of the fibrous Blood may ſometimes be affected with a morbid Laxity or Weakneſs, as well as the general Syſtem of the muſcular Fibres.

Theſe

These and any other like Freedoms, I am certain the Author's Candour will abundantly pardon; since I have never diffented for Diffention's Sake, to the beft of my Recollection; and have the Honour of harmonizing very generally in Judgment with him. If *one* ufeful Hint or Obfervation occurs throughout my Notes, his Benevolence will exult in that effential Adherence to his Plan, which fuggefted it to me: While an invariable ecchoing Affentation throughout fuch Notes, when there really was any falutary Room for doubting, or for adding (with Refpect to ourfelves) would difcover a Servility, that muft have difgufted a liberal manly Writer. One common good Purpofe certainly fprings from the generous Source, and replenifhes the many Canals into which it is derived, all the Variety and little Deviations of which may be confidered as more expanfive Diftributions of its Benefits.

Since the natural Feelings of Humanity generally difpofe us, but efpecially the more tender and compaffionate Sex, to advife Remedies to the poor Sick, fuch a Knowledge of their real Difeafe, as would prevent their Patrons, Neighbours and Affiftants from advifing a wrong Regimen, or an improper or ill-timed Medicine, is truly effential to relieving them: and fuch we ferioufly think the prefent Work is capable of imparting, to all commonly fenfible and confiderate Perufers of it. A Vein of unaffected Probity, of manly Senfe, and of great Philanthropy, concur to fuftain the Work. And whenever the

Prejudices

Prejudices of the Ignorant require a forcible Eradication; or the crude Temerity and Impudence of Knaves and Impostors cry out for their own Extermination, a happy Mixture of strong Argument, just Ridicule, and honest Severity, give a poignant and pleasant Seasoning to the Work, which renders it occasionally entertaining, as it is continually instructive.

A general Reader may be sometimes diverted with such Customs and Notions of the *Swiss* Peasants, as are occasionally mentioned here: and possibly our meerest Rustics may laugh at the brave simple *Swiss*, on his introducing a Sheep into the Chamber of a very sick Person, to save the Life of the Patient, by catching its own Death. But the humblest Peasantry of both Nations are agreed in such a Number of their absurd unhealthy Prejudices, in the Treatment of Diseases, that it really seemed necessary to offer our own the Cautions and Counsels of this principal Physician, in a very respectable Protestant Republick, in Order to prevent their Continuance. Nor is it unreasonable to presume, that under such a Form of Government, if honestly administered upon its justest Principles, the People may be rather more tenderly regarded, than under the Pomp and Rage of Despotism, or the Oppression of some Aristocracies.

Besides the different Conditions of * Persons, to whom our Author recommends the Patronage and

---

* Of all these the Schoolmasters, *with us*, may seem the most reasonably exempted from this Duty

and Execution of his Scheme, in his Introduction; it is conceived this Book must be serviceable to many young Country Practitioners, and to great Numbers of Apothecaries, by furnishing them with such exact and striking Descriptions of each acute Disease and its Symptoms, as may prevent their mistaking it for any other; a Deception which has certainly often been injurious, and sometimes even fatal: for it is dreadful but to contemplate the Destruction or Misery, with which Temerity and Ignorance, so frequently combined, overwhelm the Sick. Thus more Success and Reputation, with the Enjoyment of a better Conscience, would crown their Endeavours, by a more general Recovery of, or Relief to, their Patients. To effect this, to improve every Opportunity of eschewing medical Evil, and of doing medical Good, was the Author's avowed Intention; which he informs us in his Preface, he has heard, from some intelligent and charitable Persons, his Treatise had effected, even in some violent Diseases. That the same good Consequences may every where attend the numerous Translations of it, must be the fervent Wish of all, except the Quacks and Impostors he so justly characterizes in his thirty-third Chapter; and particularly of all, who may be distinguishably qualified, like himself, to,

—*Look through Nature up to Nature's GOD!*

The

The AUTHOR's DEDICATION.

To the most Illustrious, the most Noble and Magnificent Lords, the Lords President and Counsellors of the Chamber of Health, of the City and Republick of Berne.

Most honourable Lords,

When I first published the following Work, my utmost Partiality to it was not sufficient to allow me the Confidence of addressing

dressing it to Your Lordships. But Your continual Attention to all the Objects, which have any Relation to that important Part of the Administration of the State, which has been so wisely committed to Your Care, has induced You to take Notice of it. You have been pleased to judge it might prove useful, and that an Attempt must be laudable, which tends to the Extermination of erroneous and inveterate Prejudices, those cruel Tyrants, that are continually opposing the Happiness of the People, even under that Form and Constitution of Government, which is the best adapted to establish and to increase it.

Your

Your Lordships Approbation, and the splendid Marks of * Benevolence, with which You have honoured me, have afforded me a juster Discernment of the Importance of this Treatise, and have inclined me to hope, MOST ILLUSTRIOUS, MOST NOBLE, AND MAGNIFICENT LORDS, that You will permit this new Edition of it to appear under the Sanction of your Auspices; that while the Publick is assured of Your general Goodness and Beneficence, it may also be informed of my profoundly grateful Sense of them, on the same Occasion.

May the present Endeavour then, in fully corresponding to my Wishes,

---

* See the Author's Preface, immediately following this Dedication.

The Author's, &c.

Wishes, effectually realize Your Lordships utmost Expectations from it; while You condescend to accept this small Oblation, as a very unequal Expression of that profound Respect, with which I have the Honour to be,

MOST ILLUSTRIOUS, MOST NOBLE, AND MAGNIFICENT LORDS,

Your most humble

And most

Obedient Servant,

LAUSANNE,   TISSOT.
Dec. 3, 1762.

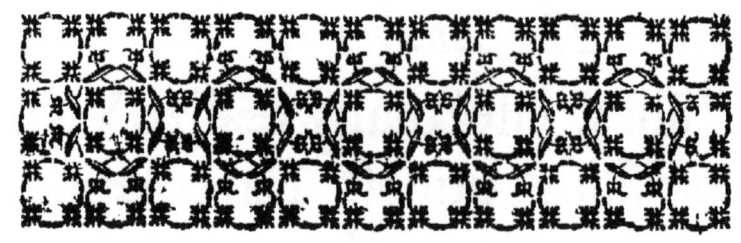

THE AUTHOR's PREFACE.

IF *Vanity too often disposes many to speak of themselves, there are some Occasions, on which a total Silence might be supposed to result from a still higher Degree of it: And the very general Reception of the* Advice to the People *has been such, that there would be Room to suspect me of that most shocking Kind of Pride, which receives Applause with Indifference (as deeming its own Merit superior to the greatest) if I did not appear to be strongly impressed with a just Sense of that great Favour of the Publick, which has been so very obliging, and is so highly agreable, to me.*

Unfeignedly affected with the unhappy Situation of the poor Sick in Country Places in Swisserland,

Swisserland, where they are lost from a Scarcity of the best Assistance, and from a fatal Superfluity of the worst, my sole Purpose in writing this Treatise has been to serve, and to comfort them. I had intended it only for a small Extent of Country, with a moderate Number of Inhabitants, and was greatly surprized to find, that within five or six Months after its Publication, it was become one of the most extensively published Books in Europe; and one of those Treatises, on a scientific Subject, which has been perused by the greatest Number of Readers of all Ranks and Conditions. To consider such Success with Indifference, were to have been unworthy of it, which Demerit, at least on this Account, I cannot justly be charged with, since Indifference has not been my Case, who have felt, as I ought, this Gratification of Self-love; and which, under just and prudent Restrictions, may perhaps be even politically cherished; as the Delight naturally arising from having been approved, is a Source of that laudable Emulation, which has sometimes produced the most essential good Consequences to Society itself. For my own particular, I can truly aver, that my Satisfaction has been exquisitely heightened on this Occasion, as a Lover of my Species; since judging from the Success of this Work (a Success which has exceeded my utmost Expectations) of the Effects that may reasonably be expected from it, I am happily conscious of that Satisfaction, or

even

even Joy, which every truly honest Man must receive, from rendering essential good Offices to others. Besides which, I have enjoyed, in its utmost Extent, that Satisfaction which every grateful Man must receive from the Approbation and Beneficence of his Sovereign, when I was distinguished with the precious Medal, which the illustrious Chamber of Health of the Republick of Berne honoured me with, a few Months after the Publication of this Treatise; together with a Letter still more estimable, as it assured me of the extraordinary Satisfaction the Republick had testified on the Impression of it; a Circumstance, which I could not avoid this publick Acknowledgement of, without the greatest Vanity and Ingratitude. This has also been a very influencing Motive with me, to exert my utmost Abilities in perfecting this new Edition, in which I have made many Alterations, that render it greatly preferable to the first; and of which Amendments I shall give a brief Account, after saying somewhat of the Editions, which have appeared elsewhere.

The first is that, which Messrs Heidegger, the Booksellers published in the German Language at Zurich, about a Year since. I should have been highly delighted with the meer Approbation of M. HIRZEL, first Physician of the Canton of Zurich, &c whose superior and universal Talents, whose profound Knowledge in the Theory of Physick, and the Extent and Success of whose Practice have justly elevated him among the small Number of extraordinary Men of our own Times, he having lately obtained the Esteem and the Thanks of all Europe, *for the History of one of her* * *Sages*. But I little expected the Honour this Gentleman has done me, in translating the Advice to the People into his own Language. Highly sensible nevertheless as I am of this Honour, I must always reflect with Regret, that he has consumed that important Time, in rendering my Directions intelligible to his Countrymen, which he might have employed much more usefully, in obliging the World with his own.

He has enriched his Translation with an excellent Preface, which is chiefly employed in a just and beautiful Portrait and Contrast of the true, and of the false Physician, with which I should have done myself the Pleasure to have adorned the present † Edition; if the Size of this Volume, already too large, had not proved an Obstacle to so considerable an Addition, and if the Manner, in which Mr. HIRZEL speaks of its Author, had permitted me with Decency to publish his Preface. I have been informed by some Letters, that there have been two other

---

* *Le Socrate rustic,* a Work, which every Person should read.

† This Preface is indeed premised to this *French* Edition, but a Translation of it was omitted to avoid extending the Bulk and Price of the Work. Dr. Tissot must then have been ignorant of an Addition when printed at Lyons.

other German *Translation of it; but I am not informed by whom. However,* M. Hirzel's *Preface, his own Notes, and some Additions with which I have furnished him, renders his Edition preferable to the first in* French, *and to the other German Translations already made.*

The second Edition is that, which the younger Didot, *the Bookseller, published towards the End of the Winter at* Paris. *He had requested me to furnish him with some Additions to it, which I could not readily comply with.*

The Third Edition is a Dutch *Translation of it, which will be very speedily published by* M. Renier Aremberg, *Bookseller at* Rotterdam. *He had begun the Translation from my first Edition, but having wrote to know whether I had not some Additions to make, I desired him to wait for the Publication of this. I have the good Fortune to be very happy in my Translators, it being* M. Bikker, *a celebrated Physician at* Rotterdam *(so very advantagiously known in other Countries, by his beautiful* Dissertation on Human Nature, *throughout which Genius and Knowledge proceed Hand in Hand) who will present his Countrymen with the* Advice to the People, *in their own Language: and who will improve it with such Notes, as are necessary for a safe and proper Application of its Contents, in a Climate, different from that in which it was wrote. I have also heard, there has been an* Italian *Translation of it.*

After this Account of the foreign Editions, I return to the present one, which is the second of the original French Treatise. I shall not affirm it is greatly corrected, with Respect to fundamental Points: for as I had advanced nothing in the first, that was not established on Truth and Demonstration, there was no Room for Correction, with Regard to any essential Matters. Nevertheless, in this I have made, 1, a great Number of small Alterations in the Diction, and added several Words, to render the Work still more simple and perspicuous. 2, The typographical Execution of this is considerably improved in the Type, the Paper and Ink, the Spelling, Pointing, and Arrangement of the Work. 3, I have made some considerable Additions, which are of three Kinds. Not a few of them are new Articles on some of the Subjects formerly treated of; such as the Articles concerning Tarts and other Pastry Ware; the Addition concerning the Regimen for Persons, in a State of Recovery from Diseases, the Preparation for the Small Pocks; a long Note on the Jesuits Bark; another on acid Spirits, one on the Extract of Hemlock: besides some new Matter which I have inserted, such as an Article with Regard to proper Drinks, one on the Convulsions of Infants, one on Chilblains, another on Punctures from Thorns, one upon the Reason of the Confidence reposed in Quacks, and the thirty-

first

first Chapter entirely: in which I have extended the Consideration of some former Articles, that seemed to me a little too succinct and short. There are some Alterations of this last, this additional, Kind, interspersed almost throughout the whole Substance of this Edition, but especially in the two Chapters relating to Women and Children.

The Objects of the XXXI Chapter are such as require immediate Assistance, viz. Swoonings, Hæmorrhages, that is, large spontaneous Bleedings, the Attacks of Convulsions, and of Suffocations; the Consequences of Fright and Terror; Disorders occasioned by unwholesome or deadly Vapours; the Effects of Poison, and the sudden Invasions of excessive Pain.

The Omission of this Chapter was a very material Defect in the original Plan of this Work. The Editor of it at Paris was very sensible of this Chasm, or Blank, as it may be called, and has filled it up very properly: and if I have not made Use of his Supplement, instead of enlarging myself upon the Articles of which he has treated, it has only been from a Purpose of rendering the whole Work more uniform; and to avoid that odd Diversity, which seems scarcely to be avoided in a Treatise composed by two Persons. Besides which, that Gentleman has said nothing of the Articles, which employ the greatest Part of that Chapter, viz. the Swoonings, the Con-

Consequences of great Fear, and the noxious Vapours

Before I conclude, I ought to justify myself, as well as possible, to a great Number of very respectable Persons both here and abroad, (to whom I can refuse nothing without great Chagrine and Reluctance) for my not having made such Additions as they desired of me. This however was impossible, as the Objects, in which they concurred, were some chronical Distempers, that are entirely out of the Plan, to which I was strictly attached, for many Reasons. The first is, that it was my original Purpose to oppose the Errors incurred in Country Places, in the Treatment of acute Diseases; and to display the best Method of conducting such, as do not admit of waiting for the Arrival of distant Succour; or of removing the Patients to Cities, or large Towns. It is but too true indeed, that chronical Diseases are also liable to improper Treatment in small Country Places: but then there are both Time and Conveniance to convey the Patients within the Reach of better Advice; or for procuring them the Attendance of the best Advisers, at their own Places of Residence. Besides which, such Distempers are considerably less common than those to which I had restrained my Views: and they will become still less frequent, whenever acute Diseases, of which they are frequently the Consequences, shall be more rationally and safely conducted. The

The second Reason, which, if alone, would have been a sufficient one, is, that it is impossible to subject the Treatment of chronical Distempers to the Capacity and Conduct of Persons, who are not Physicians. Each acute Distemper generally arises from one Cause; and the Treatment of it is simple and uniform; since those Symptoms, which manifest the Malady, point out its Cause and Treatment. But the Case is very differently circumstanced in tedious and languid Diseases, each of which may depend on so many and various Causes (and it is only the real, the true Cause, which ought to determine us in selecting its proper Remedies) that though the Distemper and its Appellation are evidently known, a meer By-stander may be very remote from penetrating into its true Cause; and consequently be incapable of chusing the best Medicines for it. It is this precise and distinguishing Discernment of the real particular Cause [or of the contingent Concurrence of more than one] that necessarily requires the Presence of Persons conversant in the Study and the Practice of all the Parts of Physick, and which Knowledge it is impossible for People, who are Strangers to such Studies, to arrive at. Moreover, their frequent Complexness; the Variety of their Symptoms; the different Stages of these tedious Diseases [not exactly attended to even by many competent Physicians] the Difficulty of ascertaining the different Doses of Medicines, whose Activity may make the smallest Error highly dangerous, &c &c.

&c. are really such trying Circumstances, as render the fittest Treatment of these Diseases sufficiently difficult and embarrassing to the most experienced Physicians, and unattainable by those who are not Physicians.

A third Reason is, that, even supposing all these Circumstances might be made so plain and easy, as to be comprehended by every Reader, they would require a Work of an excessive Length; and thence be disproportioned to the Faculties of those; for whom it was intended. One single chronical Disease might require as large a Volume as the present one.

But finally, were I to acknowledge, that this Compliance was both necessary and practicable, I declare I find it exceeds my Abilities; and that I am also far from having sufficient Leisure for the Execution of it. It is my Wish that others would attempt it, and may succeed in accomplishing it; but I hope these truly worthy Persons, who have honoured me by proposing the Atchievement of it to myself, will perceive the Reasons for my not complying with it, in all their Force, and not ascribe a Refusal, which arises from the very Nature of the thing, either to Obstinacy, or to any Want of an Inclination to oblige them.

I have been informed my Citations, or rather References, have puzzled some Readers. It was difficult to foresee this, but is easy to prevent it for the future. The Work contains Citations only of two Sorts; one, that points to the Remedies prescribed; and the other, which refers to some Passage in the Book itself, that serves to illustrate those Passages in which I cite. Neither of these References could have been omitted. The first is marked thus, N°. with the proper Figure to it, as 1, 2, &c. This signifies, that the Medicine I direct is described in the Table of Remedies, according to the Number annexed to that Character. Thus when we find directed, in any Page of the Book, the warm Infusion N° 1; in some other, the Ptisan N°. 2; or in a third, the Almond Milk, or Emulsion N°. 4, it signifies, that such Prescriptions will be found at the Numbers 1. 2, and 4; and this Table is printed at the End of the Book.

If, instead of forming this Table, and thus referring to the Prescriptions by their Numbers, I had repeated each Prescription as often as I directed it, this Treatise must have been doubled in Bulk, and insufferably tiresome to peruse. I must repeat here, what I have already said in the former Edition, that the * Prices of the Medicines, or of a great Number of them, are those at which the Apothecaries may afford them, without any Loss, to a Peasant in humble Circumstances. But it should be remembered, they are not set down at the full Prices which they may honestly demand; since that would be unjust for some to insist on

them

* The Reasons for omitting the Prices *here*, may be seen Page 23 of this Translation.

them at. Besides, there is no Kind of Tax in Swisserland, and I have no Right to impose one.

The Citations of the second Kind are very plain and simple. The whole Work is divided into numbered Paragraphs distinguished by the Mark §. And not to swell it with needless Repetitions, when in one Place I might have even pertinently repeated something already observed, instead of such Repetition at Length, I have only referred to the Paragraph, where it had been observed. Thus, for Example when we read Page 81, § 50—When the Disease is so circumstanced as we have described, § 46,—this imports that, not to repeat the Description already given, I refer the Reader to that last § for it.

The Use of these Citations is not the least Innovation, and extremely commodious and easy: but were there only a single Reader likely to be puzzled by them, I ought not to omit this Explanation of them, as I can expect to be generally useful, only in Proportion as I am clear: and it must be obvious, that a Desire of being extensively useful is the sole Motive of this Work. I have long since had the Happiness of knowing, that some charitable and intelligent Persons have applied the Directions it contains, with extraordinary Success, even in violent Diseases. And I shall arrive at the Height of my Wishes, if I continue to be informed, that it contributes to alleviate the Sufferings, and to prolong the Days, of my rational Fellow Creatures.

N. B.

N. B. A Small Blank occurring conveniently here in the Impression, the Translator of this Work has employed it to insert the following proper Remark, *viz.*

Whenever the Tea or Infusion of the Lime-tree is directed in the Body of the Book, which it often is, the *Flowers* are always meant, and not the *Leaves*; though by an Error of the Press, or perhaps rather by an Oversight of the Transcribers of this Version, it is printed *Leaves* instead of *Flowers* P. 392, as noted and corrected in the *Errata*. These Flowers are easily procurable here, meerly for gathering, in most Country Places in *July*, as few Walks, Vistas, *&c.* are without these Trees, planted for the pleasant Shade they afford, and to keep off the Dust in Summer, though the Leaf drops rather too early for this Purpose. Their Flowers have an agreeable Flavour, which is communicated to Water by Infusion, and rises with it in Distillation. They were, to the best of my Recollection, an Ingredient in the antiepileptic Water of *Langius*, omitted in our late Dispensatories of the College. They are an Ingredient in the antiepileptic Powder, in the List of Medicines in the present Practice of the *Hotel Dieu* at *Paris*: and we think were in a former Prescription of our *Pulvis de Gutteta*, or Powder against Convulsions. Indeed they are considered, by many medical Writers, as a Specific in all Kinds of Spasms and Pains; and Hoffman affirms, he knew

knew a very tedious Epilepsy cured by the Use of an Infusion of these Flowers.

I also take this Opportunity of adding, that as this Translation is intended for the Attention and the Benefit of the Bulk of the Inhabitants of the *British* Empire, I have been careful not to admit any Gallicisms into it; as such might render it either less intelligible, or less agreeable to its Readers. If but a single one occurs, I either have printed it, or did intend it should be printed, distinguishably in Italics. *K.*

INTRODUCTION.

THE Decrease of the Number of Inhabitants, in most of the States of Europe, is a Fact, which impresses every reflecting Person, and is become such a general Complaint, as is but too well established on plain Calculations. This Decrease is most remarkable in Country Places. It is owing to many Causes; and I shall think myself happy, if I can contribute to remove one of the greatest of them, which is the pernicious Manner of treating sick People in Country Places. This is my sole Object, tho' I may be excused perhaps for pointing out the other concurring Causes, which may be all included within these two general Affirmations; That greater Numbers than usual emigrate from the Country, and that the People increase less every where.

There are many Sorts of Emigration. Some leave their Country to enlist in the Service of different States by Sea and Land; or to be differently

ferently employ'd abroad, some as Traders, others as Domestics, &c.

Military Service, by Land or Sea, prevents Population in various Respects. In the first Place, the Numbers going abroad are always less, often *much* less, than those who return. General Battles, with all the Hazards and Fatigues of War; detached Encounters, bad Provisions, Excess in drinking and eating, Diseases that are the Consequences of Debauches, the Disorders that are peculiar to the Country; epidemical, pestilential or contagious Distempers, caused by the unwholsome Air of Flanders, Holland, Italy and Hungary; long Cruises, Voyages to the East or West Indies, to Guinea, &c. destroy a great Number of Men. The Article of Desertion also, the Consequences of which they dread on returning home, disposes many to abandon their Country for ever. Others, on quitting the Service, take up with such Establishments, as it has occasionally thrown in their Way, and which necessarily prevent their Return. But in the second Place, supposing they were all to come back, their Country suffers equally from their Absence, as this very generally happens during that Period of Life, when they are best adapted for Propagation; since that Qualification on their Return is impaired by Age, by Infirmities and Debauches and even when they do marry, the Children often perish as Victims to the Excesses and Irregularities of their Fathers. they are weak, languishing, distempered, and either die young, or live incapable of being useful to Society. Besides, that the prevailing Habit of Libertinage, which many have contracted, prevents several of them from marrying at all. But notwithstanding all these inconvenient Consequences are real and notorious, yet as the Number of those, who leave their Country on these Accounts, is limited, and indeed rather inconsiderable, if compared with the Number of Inhabitants which must remain at home: as it may be affirmed too, that this relinquishing of their Country, may have been even necessary at some Times, and may become so again, if the Causes of Depopulation should cease, this kind of Emigration is doubtless the least grievous of any, and the last which may require a strict Consideration.

But that abandoning of their Country, or *Expatriation*, as it may be termed, the Object of which is a Change of the Emigrants Condition, is more to be considered, being more numerous. It is attended with many and peculiar Inconveniencies, and is unhappily become an epidemical Evil, the Ravages of which are still increasing; and that from one simple ridiculous Source, which is this; that the Success of one Individual determines a hundred to run the same Risque, ninety and nine of whom may probably be disappointed. They are struck with the apparent Success of one, and are ignorant of the Miscarriage of others. Suppose a hundred Persons might have set out ten Years ago, to *seek their Fortune*, as the saying is, at the End of six Months they are all forgotten, except by their Relations: but if one should return the same Year, with more Money than his own Fortune, more than he set out with; or if one of them has got a moderate Place with little Work, the whole Country rings with it, as a Subject of general Entertainment. A Croud of young People are seduced by this and sally forth, because not one reflects, that of the ninety nine, who set out with the hundredth Person one half has perished, many are miserable, and the Remainder come back, without having gained any thing, but an Incapacity to employ themselves usefully at home, and in their former Occupations. and having deprived their Country of a great many Cultivators, who, from the Produce of the Lands, would have attracted considerable Sums of Money, and many comfortable Advantages to it In short, the very small Proportion who succeed, are continually talked of, the Croud that sink are perpetually forgot. This is a very great and real Evil, and how shall it be prevented? It would be sufficient perhaps to publish the extraordinary Risque, which may be easily demonstrated: It would require nothing more than to keep an exact yearly Register of all these Adventurers, and, at the Expiration of six, eight, or ten Years, to publish the List with the Fate, of every Emigrant I am greatly deceived, or at the End of a certain Number of Years, we should not see such Multitudes forsake their native Soil, in which they might live comfortably by working, to go in Search of Establishments in others, the Uncertainty of which, such Lists would demonstrate to them; and also prove, how preferable their Condition in their own Country would have been, to that they have been reduced to. People would no longer set out, but on almost certain Advantages: fewer would undoubtedly emigrate, more of whom, from that very Circumstance, must succeed. Meeting with fewer of their Country-men abroad, these fortunate few would oftner return. By this Means more Inhabitants would remain in the Country, more would return again, and bring with them more Money to it. The State would be more populous, more rich and happy; as the Happiness of a People, who live on a fruitful Soil, depends essentially on a great Number of Inhabitants, with a moderate Quantity of pecuniary Riches

But the Population of the Country is not only necessarily lessened, in Consequence of the Numbers that leave it, but even those who remain increase less, than an equal Number formerly did Or, which amounts to the same Thing, among the same Number of Persons, there are fewer Marriages than formerly; and the same Number of Marriages produce fewer Christenings I do not enter upon a Detail of the Proofs, since merely looking about us must furnish a sufficient Conviction of the Truth of them. What then are the Causes of this? There are two capital ones, Luxury and Debauchery, which are Enemies to Population on many Accounts.

Luxury compells the wealthy Man, who would make a Figure; and the Man of a moderate Income, but who is his equal in every other Respect, and who *will* imitate him, to be afraid of a numerous Family; the Education of which must greatly contract that Expence he had devoted to Parade and Ostentation: And besides, if he must divide his Estate among a great many Children, each of them would have but a little, and be unable to keep up the State and the Train of the Father's. Since Merit is unjustly estimated by exterior Shew and Expence, one must of Course endeavour to attain for himself, and to leave his Children in, a Situation capable of supporting that Expence. Hence the fewer Marriages of People who are not opulent, and the fewer Children among People who marry.

Luxury is further prejudicial to the Increase of the People, in another Respect. The irregular Manner of Life which it introduces, depresses Health, it ruins the Constitutions, and thus sensibly affects Procreation. The preceding Generation counted some Families with more than twenty Children. the living one less than twenty Cousins. Very unfortunately this Way of thinking and acting, so preventive of Increase, has extended itself even into Villages: and they are no longer convinced there, that the Number of Children makes the Riches of the Countryman. Perhaps the next Generation will scarcely be acquainted with the Relation of Brotherhood.

A

A third Inconvenience of Luxury is, that the Rich retreat from the Country to live in Cities; and by multiplying their Domestics there, they drain the former. This augmented Train is prejudicial to the Country, by depriving it of Cultivaters, and by diminishing Population. These Domestics, being seldom sufficiently employed, contract the Habit of Laziness; and they prove incapable of returning to that Country Labour, for which Nature intended them. Being deprived of this Resource they scarcely ever marry, either from apprehending the Charge of Children, or from their becoming Libertines; and sometimes, because many Masters will not employ married Servants. Or should any of them marry, it is often in the Decline of Life, whence the State must have the fewer Citizens.

Idleness of itself weakens them, and disposes them to those Debauches, which enfeeble them still more. They never have more than a few Children, and these sickly, such as have not Strength to cultivate the Ground, or who, being brought up in Cities, have an Aversion to the Country.

Even those among them who are more prudent, who preserve their Morals, and make some Savings, being accustomed to a City Life, and dreading the Labour of a Country one (of the Regulation of which they are also ignorant) chuse to become little Merchants, or Tradesmen; and this must be a Drawback from Population, as any Number of Labourers beget more Children than an equal Number of Citizens; and also by Reason, that out of any given Number, more Children die in Cities, than in the Country.

The same Evils also prevail, with Regard to female Servants. After ten or twelve Years Servitude, the Maid-Servants in Cities cannot acquit themselves as good Country Servants: and such of them as chuse this Condition, quickly fail under that Kind or Quantity of Work, for which they are no longer constituted. Should we see a Woman married in the Country, a Year after leaving Town, it is easy to observe, how much that Way of living in the Country has broke her. Frequently their first Child-bed, in which Term they have not all the Attendance their Delicacy demands, proves the Loss of their Health; they remain in a State of Languor, of Feebleness, and of Decay: they have no more Children; and this renders their Husbands unuseful towards the Population of the State.

Abortions, Infants carried out of their Country after a concealed Pregnancy, and the Impossibility of their getting Husbands afterwards, are frequently the Effects of their Libertinage.

It is to be apprehended too these bad Effects are rather increasing with us, since, either for want of sufficient Numbers, or from oeconomical Views, it has become a Custom, instead of Women Servants, to employ Children, whose Manners and whose Constitutions are not yet formed, and who are ruined in the same Manner,

per, by their Residence in Town, by their Laziness, by bad Examples, and bad Company.

Doubtless much remains still unsaid on these important Heads, but besides my Intention not to swell this Treatise immoderately, and the many Avocations, which prevent me from launching too far into what may be less within the Bounds of Medicine, I should be fearful of digressing too far from my Subject. What I have hitherto said however, I think cannot be impertinent to it; since in giving Advice to the People, with Regard to their Health, it was necessary to display to them the Causes that impaired it: though what I might be able to add further on this Head, would probably be thought more remote from the Subject.

I shall add then but a single Hint on the Occasion. Is it not practicable, in Order to remedy those Evils which we cannot prevent, to select some particular Part or Canton of the Country, wherein we should endeavour by Rewards, 1*st*. Irremoveably to fix all the Inhabitants. 2*dly*. To encourage them by other Rewards to a plentiful and legitimate Increase. They should not be permitted to go out of it, which must prevent them from being exposed to the Evils I have mentioned. They should by no means intermarry with any Strangers, who might introduce such Disorders among them. Thus very probably this Canton, after a certain Time, would become even overpeopled, and might send out Colonies to the others.

INTRODUCTION.

One Cause, still more considerable than those we have already mention'd, has, to this very Moment, prevented the Increase of the People in France. This is the Decay of Agriculture. The Inhabitants of the Country, to avoid serving in the Militia; to elude the Days-Service impos'd by their Lords, and the Taxes; and being attracted to the City by the Hopes of Interest, by Laziness and Libertinage, have left the Country nearly deserted. Those who remain behind, either not being encouraged to work, or not being sufficient for what there is to do, content themselves with cultivating just as much as is absolutely necessary for their Subsistence. They have either lived single, or married but late; or perhaps, after the Example of the Inhabitants of the Cities, they have refused to fulfil their Duty to Nature, to the State, and to a Wife. The Country deprived of Tillers, by this Expatriation and Inactivity, has yielded nothing, and the Depopulation of the State has daily increased, from the reciprocal and necessary Proportion between Subsistence and Population, and because Agriculture alone can increase Subsistence. A single Comparison will sufficiently evince the Truth and the Importance of these Principles, to those who have not seen them already divulged and demonstrated in the Works of the * Friend of Man.

" An old Roman, who was always ready to
' return to the Cultivation of his Field, subsisted
" himself

---

* The Marquis of Mirabeau

" himself and his Family from one Acre of Land.
" A Savage, who neither sows nor cultivates,
" consumes, in his single Person, as much Game
" as requires fifty Acres to feed them. Conse-
" quently *Tullus Hostilius*, on a thousand Acres,
" might have five thousand Subjects: while a
" Savage Chief, limited to the same Extent of
" Territory, could scarcely have twenty: such
" an immense Disproportion does Agriculture
" furnish, in Favour of Population. Observe
" these two great Extremes. A State becomes
" dispeopled or peopled in that Proportion, by
" which it recedes from one of these Methods,
" and approaches to the other." Indeed it is evident, that wherever there is an Augmentation of Subsistence, an Increase of Population will soon follow; which again will still further facilitate the Increase of Provisions. In a State thus circumstanced Men will abound, who, after they have furnished sufficient Numbers for the Service of War, of Commerce, of Religion, and for Arts and Professions of every kind, will further also furnish a Source for Colonies, who will extend the Name and the Prosperity of their Nation to distant Regions. There will ensue a Plenty of Commodities, the Superfluity of which will be exported to other Countries, to exchange for other Commodities, that are not produced at home; and the Balance, being received in Money, will make the Nation rich, respectable by its Neighbours, and happy. Agriculture, vigorously pursued, is equal to the Production of all these Benefits;

fits; and the present Age will enjoy the Glory of restoring it, by favouring and encouraging Cultivaters, and by forming Societies for the Promotion of Agriculture.

I proceed at length to the fourth Cause of Depopulation, which is the Manner of treating sick People in the Country. This has often affected me with the deepest Concern. I have been a Witness, that Maladies, which, in themselves, would have been gentle, have proved mortal from a pernicious Treatment: I am convinced that this Cause alone makes as great a Havock as the former, and certainly it requires the utmost Attention of Physicians, whose Duty it is to labour for the Preservation of Mankind. While we are employing our assiduous Cares on the more polished and fashionable Part of them in Cities, the larger and more useful Moiety perish in the Country, either by particular, or by highly epidemical, Diseases, which, within a few Years past, have appeared in different Villages, and made no small Ravages. This afflicting Consideration has determined me to publish this little Work, which is solely intended for those Patients, who, by their Distance from Physicians, are deprived of their Assistance. I shall not give a Detail of my Plan, which is very simple, in this Part, but content myself with affirming, I have used my utmost Care to render it the most useful I possibly could; and I dare hope, that if I have not fully displayed its utmost Advantages, I have at least sufficiently shewn those pernicious Methods of

treating

treating Diseases, that should incontestably be avoided. I am thoroughly convinced, the Design might be accomplished more compleatly than I have done it, but those who are so capable of, do not attempt, it: I happen to be less timid; and I hope that thinking Persons will rather take it in good part of me, to have published a Book, the composing of which is rather disagreeable from its very Facility, from the minute Details, which however are indispensable; and from the Impossibility of discussing any Part of it (consistently with the Plan) to the Bottom of the Subject; or of displaying any new and useful Prospect. It may be compared, in some Respects, to the Works of a spiritual Guide, who was to write a Catechism for little Children.

At the same time I am not ignorant there have already been a few Books calculated for Country Patients, who are remote from Succour: but some of these, tho' published with a very good Purpose, produce a bad Effect. Of this kind are all Collections of Receipts or Remedies, without the least Description of the Disease, and of course without just Directions for the Exhibition, or Application, of them. Such, for Example, is the famous Collection of Madam Fouquet, and some more in the same manner. Some others approach towards my Plan; but many of them have taken in too many Distempers, whence they are become too voluminous. Besides, they have not dwelt sufficiently upon the Signs of the Diseases, upon their Causes; the general Regimen in them, and the Mismanagemanagement of them. Their Receipts are not generally as simple, and as easy to prepare, as they ought to be. In short, the greater Part of their Writers seem, as they advanced, to have grown tired of their melancholy Task, and to have hurried them out too expeditiously. There are but two of them, which I must name with Respect, and which being proposed on a Plan very like my own, are executed in a superior Manner, that merits the highest Acknowlegements of the Publick One of these Writers is M. ROSEN, first Physician of the Kingdom of *Sweden*; who, some Years since, employed his just Reputation to render the best Services to his Country Men. He has made them retrench from the Almanacs those ridiculous Tales; those extraordinary Adventures, those pernicious astrological Injunctions, which there, as well as here, answer no End, but that of keeping up Ignorance, Credulity, Superstition, and the falsest Prejudices on the interesting Articles of Health, of Diseases, and of Remedies. He has also taken Care to publish simple plain Treatises on the most popular Distempers, which he has substituted in the Place of the former Heap of Absurdities. These concise Works however, which appear annually in their Almanacs, are not yet translated from the *Swedish*, so that I was unqualified to make any Extracts from them. The other is the Baron VAN SWIETEN, first Physician to their Imperial Majesties, who, about two Years since, has effected for the Use of the Army, what I now attempt

for

for sick People in the Country. Though my Work was greatly advanced, when I first saw his, I have taken some Passages from it: and had our Plans been exactly alike, I should imagine I had done the Publick more Service by endeavouring to extend the Reading of his Book, than by publishing a new one. Nevertheless, as he is silent on many Articles, of which I have treated diffusively; as he has treated of many Distempers, which did not come within my Plan, and has said nothing of some others which I could not omit; our two Works, without entering into the Particulars of the superior Merit of the Baron's, are very different, with Regard to the Subject of the Diseases; tho' in such as we have both considered, I account it an Honour to me to find, we have almost constantly proceeded upon the same Principles.

The present Work is by no means addressed to such Physicians, as are thoroughly accomplished in their Profession; yet possibly, besides my particular medical Friends, some others may read it. I beg the Favour of all such fully to consider the Intention, the Spirit, of the Author, and not to censure him, as a Physician, from the Composition of this Book. I even advise them here rather to forbear perusing it; as a Production, that can teach them nothing. Such as read, in order to criticize, will find a much greater Scope for exercising that Talent on the other Pamphlets I have published. It were certainly unjust that a Performance, whose sole abstracted Object is the

Health

Health and Service of my Countrymen, should subject me to any disagreeable Consequences: and a Writer may fairly plead an Exemption from any Severity of Censure, who has had the Courage to execute a Work, which cannot pretend to a Panegyric.

Having premised thus much in general, I must enter into some Detail of those Means, that seem the most likely to me, to facilitate the beneficial Consequences, which, I hope, may result to others, from my present Endeavours. I shall afterwards give an Explanation of some Terms which I could not avoid using, and which, perhaps, are not generally understood.

The Title of *Advice to the People*, was not suggested to be by an Illusion, which might persuade me, this Book would become a Piece of Furniture, as it were, in the House of every Peasant. Nineteen out of twenty will probably never know of its Existence. Many may be unable to read, and still more unable to understand, it, plain and simple as it is. I have principally calculated it for the Perusal of intelligent and charitable Persons, who live in the Country; and who seem to have, as it were, a Call from Providence, to assist their less intelligent poor Neighbours with their Advice.

It is obvious, that the first Gentlemen I have my Eye upon, are the Clergy. There is not a single Village, a Hamlet, nor even the House of an Alien in the Country, that has not a Right to the good Offices of some one of this Order: And

And I assure myself there are a great Number of them, who, heartily affected with the Distress of their ailing Flocks, have wished many hundred Times, that it were in their Power to give their Parishioners some bodily Help, at the very Time they were disposing them to prepare for Death; or so far to delay the Fatality of the Distemper, that the Sick might have an Opportunity of living more religiously afterwards. I shall think myself happy, if such truly respectable Ecclesiastics shall find any Resources in this Performance, that may conduce to the Accomplishment of their beneficent Intentions. Their Regard, their Love for their People; their frequent Invitations to visit their principal Neighbours; their Duty to root out all unreasonable Prejudices, and Superstition; their Charity, their Learning; the Facility, with which their general Knowlege in Physics, qualifies them to comprehend thoroughly all the medical Truths, and Contents of this Piece, are so many Arguments to convince me, that they will have the greatest Influence to procure that Reformation, in the Administration of Physick to poor Country People, which is so necessary, so desirable, an Object.

In the next Place, I dare assure myself of the Concurrence of Gentlemen of Quality and Opulence, in their different Parishes and Estates, whose Advice is highly regarded by their Inferiors; who are so powerfully adapted to discourage a wrong, and to promote a right Practice, of which they will easily discern all the Advantages The many

Instances I have seen of their entering, with great Facility, into all the Plan and Conduct of a Cure; their Readiness and even Earnestness to comfort the Sick in their Villages; and the Generosity with which they prevent their Necessities, induce me to hope, from judging of these I have not the Pleasure to know, by those whom I have, that they will eagerly embrace an Opportunity of promoting a new Method of doing good in their Neighbourhood. Real Charity will apprehend the great Probability there is of doing Mischief, tho' with the best Intention, for want of a proper Knowledge of material Circumstances, and the very Fear of that Mischief may sometimes suspend the Exercise of such Charity; notwithstanding it must seize, with the most humane Avidity, every Light that can contribute to its own beneficent Exertion.

Thirdly, Persons who are rich, or at least in easy Circumstances, whom their Disposition, their Employments, or the Nature of their Property, fixes in the Country, where they are happy in doing good, must be delighted to have some proper Directions for the Conduct and Effectuation of their charitable Intentions.

In every Village, where there are any Persons, of these three Conditions, they are always readily apprized of the Distempers in it, by their poor Neighbours coming to intreat a little Soup, Venice Treacle, Wine, Biscuits, or any thing they imagine necessary for their sick Folks. In Consequence of some Questions to the Bystanders, or

of

of a Visit to the sick Person, they will judge at least of *what kind* the Disease is; and by their prudent Advice they may be able to prevent a Multitude of Evils. They will give them some Nitre instead of Venice Treacle; Barley, or sweet Whey, in lieu of Soup. They will advise them to have Recourse to Glysters, or Bathings of their Feet, rather than to Wine; and order them Gruel rather than Biscuits. A man would scarcely believe, 'till after the Expiration of a few Years, how much Good might be effected by such proper Regards, so easily comprehended, and often repeated. At first indeed there may be some Difficulty in eradicating old Prejudices, and inveterately bad Customs; but whenever these were removed, good Habits would strike forth full as strong Roots, and I hope that no Person would be inclined to destroy them.

It may be unnecessary to declare, that I have more Expectation from the Care and Goodness of the Ladies, than from those of their Spouses, their Fathers, or Brothers. A more active Charity, a more durable Patience, a more domestic Life; a Sagacity, which I have greatly admired in many Ladies both in Town and Country, that disposes them to observe, with great Exactness; and to unravel, as it were, the secret Causes of the Symptoms, with a Facility that would do Honour to very good Practioners, and with a Talent adapted to engage the Confidence of the Patient: —All these, I say, are so many characteristical Marks of their Vocation in this important and amicable Duty, nor are there a few, who fulfil it with a Zeal, that merits the highest Commendation, and renders them excellent Models for the Imitation of others.

Those who are intrusted with the Education of Youth, may also be supposed sufficiently intelligent to take some Part in this Work; and I am satisfied that much Good might result from their undertaking it. I heartily wish, they would not only study to *distinguish the Distemper* (in which the principal, but by no means an insuperable Difficulty consists, and to which I hope I have considerably put them in the Way) but I would have them learn also the Manner of applying Remedies. Many of them shave; I have known some who bleed, and who have given Glysters very expertly. This however all may easily learn, and perhaps it would not be imprudent, if the Art of bleeding well and safely were reckoned a necessary Qualification, when they are examined for their Employment. These Faculties, that of estimating the Degree of a Fever, and how to apply and to dress Blisters, may be of great Use within the Neighbourhood of their Residence. Their Schools, which are not frequently over-crouded, employ but a few of their ... Hours the greater part of them have no Land to cultivate; and to what better Use can they apply their Leisure, than to the Assistance and Comfort of the Sick? The moderate Price of their Service may be so ascertained, as to incommode no Person, and this little Emolument might

might render their own Situation the more agreeable: besides which, these little Avocations might prevent their being drawn aside sometimes, by Reason of their Facility and frequent Leisure, so as to contract a Habit of drinking too often. Another Benefit would also accrue from accustoming them to this kind of Practice, which is, that being habituated to the Care of sick People, and having frequent Occasions to write, they would be the better qualify'd, in difficult Cases, to advise with those, who were thought further necessary to be consulted.

Doubtless, even among Labourers, there may be many, for some such I have known, who being endued with good natural Sense and Judgment, and abounding with Benevolence, will read this Book with Attention, and eagerly extend the Maxims and the Methods it recommends.

And finally I hope that many Surgeons, who are spread about the Country, and who practice Physic in their Neighbourhood, will peruse it; will carefully enter into the Principles established in it, and will conform to its Directions, tho' a little different perhaps from such as they may have hitherto practised. They will perceive a Man may learn at any Age, and of any Person, and it may be hoped they will not think it too much Trouble to reform some of their Notions in a Science, which is not properly within their Profession (and to the Study of which they were never instituted) by those of a Person, who is solely

solely employed in it, and who has had many Assistances of which they are deprived.

Midwives may also find their Attendance more efficacious, as soon as they are thoroughly disposed to be better informed.

It were heartily to be wished, that the greater Part of them had been better instructed in the Art they profess. The Instances of Mischief that might have been avoided, by their being better qualify'd, are frequent enough to make us wish there may be no Repetition of them, which it may be possible to prevent. Nothing seems impossible, when Persons in Authority are zealously inclined to prevent every such Evil; and it is time they should be properly informed of one so essentially hurtful to Society.

The Prescriptions I have given consist of the most simple Remedies, and I have adjoined the Manner of preparing them so fully, that I hope no Person can be at any Loss in that Respect. At the same time, that no one may imagine they are the less useful and efficacious for their Simplicity, I declare, they are the same I order in the City for the most opulent Patients. This Simplicity is founded in Nature the Mixture, or rather the Confusion, of a Multitude of Drugs is ridiculous. If they have the very same Virtues, for what Purpose are they blended? It were more judicious to confine ourselves to that, which is the most effectual. If their Virtues are different, the Effect of one destroys, or lessens, the Effect of the

the other; and the Medicine ceases to prove a Remedy.

I have given no Direction, which is not very practicable and easy to execute; nevertheless it will be discernible, that some few are not calculated for the Multitude, which I readily grant. However I have given them, because I did not lose Sight of some Persons; who, tho' not strictly of the Multitude, or Peasantry, do live in the Country, and cannot always procure a Physician as soon, or for as long a Time, as they gladly would.

A great Number of the Remedies are entirely of the Country Growth, and may be prepared there, but there are others, which must be had from the Apothecaries. I have set down the Price * at which I am persuaded all the Country Apothecaries will retail them to a Peasant, who is not esteemed a rich one. I have marked the Price, not from any Apprehension of their being imposed

---

* This oeconomical Information was doubtless very proper, where our judicious and humane Author published it, but notwithstanding his excellent Motives for giving it, we think it less necessary here, where many Country Gentlemen furnish themselves with larger or smaller Medicine Chests, for the Benefit of their poor sick Neighbours, and in a Country, where the settled parochial Poor are provided with Medicines, as well as other Necessaries, at a parochial Expence. Besides, tho' we would not suppose our Country Apothecaries less considerate or kind than others, we acknowledge our Apprehension, that such a Valuation of their Druggs (some of which often vary in their Price) might dispose a few of them, rather to discountenance the Extension of a Work, so well intended and executed as Dr. Tissot's, a Work, which may not be wholly unuseful to some of the most judicious among them, and will be really necessary for the rest. *K.*

imposed on in the Purchase, for this I do not apprehend; but, that seeing the Cheapness of the Prescription, they may not be afraid to buy it. The necessary Dose of the Medicine, for each Disease, may generally be purchased for less Money than would be expended on Meat, Wine, Biscuits, and other improper things. But should the Price of the Medicine, however moderate, exceed the Circumstances of the Sick, doubtless the Common Purse, or the Poors-Box will defray it: moreover there are in many Country Places Noblemens Houses, some of whom charitably contribute an annual Sum towards buying of Medicines for poor Patients. Without adding to which Sum, I would only intreat the Favour of each of them to alter the Objects of it, and to allow their sick Neighbours the Remedies and the Regimen directed here, instead of such as they formerly distributed among them.

It may still be objected, that many Country Places are very distant from large Towns; from which Circumstance a poor Peasant is incapable of procuring himself a seasonable and necessary Supply in his Illness. I readily admit, that, in Fact, there are many Villages very remote from such Places as Apothecaries reside in. Yet, if we except a few among the Mountains, there are but very few of them above three or four Leagues from some little Town, where there always lives some Surgeon, or some Vender of Drugs. Perhaps however, even at this Time, indeed, there may not be many thus provided; but they will

will take care to furnish themselves with such Materials, as soon as they have a good Prospect of selling them, which may constitute a small, but new, Branch of Commerce for them. I have carefully set down the Time, for which each Medicine will keep, without spoiling. There is a very frequent Occasion for some particular ones, and of such the School-masters may lay in a Stock. I also imagine, if they heartily enter into my Views, they will furnish themselves with such Implements, as may be necessary in the Course of their Attendance. If any of them were unable to provide themselves with a sufficient Number of good Lancets, an *Apparatus* for Cupping, and a Glyster Syringe (for want of which last a Pipe and Bladder may be occasionally substituted) the Parish might purchase them, and the same Instruments might do for the succeeding School-master. It is hardly to be expected, that all Persons in that Employment would be able, or even inclined, to learn the Way of using them with Address; but one Person who did, might be sufficient for whatever Occasions should occur in this Way in some contiguous Villages, with very little Neglect of their Functions among their Scholars.

Daily Instances of Persons, who come from different Parts to consult me, without being capable of answering the Questions I ask them, and the like Complaints of many other Physicians on the same Account, engaged me to write the last Chapter of this Work. I shall conclude this Introductroduction with some Remarks, necessary to facilitate the Knowledge of a few Terms, which were unavoidable in the Course of it.

The Pulse commonly beats in a Person in good Health, from the Age of eighteen or twenty to about sixty six Years, between sixty and seventy Times in a Minute. It sometimes comes short of this in old Persons, and in very young Children it beats quicker: until the Age of three or four Years the Difference amounts at least to a third, after which it diminishes by Degrees.

An intelligent Person, who shall often touch and attend to his own Pulse, and frequently to other People's, will be able to judge, with sufficient Exactness, of the Degree of a Fever in a sick Person. If the Strokes are but one third above their Number in a healthy State, the Fever is not very violent, which it is, as often as it amounts to half as many more as in Health. It is very highly dangerous, and may be generally pronounced mortal, when there are two Strokes in the Time of one. We must not however judge of the Pulse, solely by its Quickness, but by its Strength or Weakness, its Hardness or Softness, and the Regularity or Irregularity of it.

. There is no Occasion to define the strong and the feeble Pulse. The Strength of it generally affords a good Prognostic, and, supposing it too strong, it may easily be lowered. The weak Pulse is often very menacing

If

If the Pulse, in meeting the Touch, excites the Notion of a dry Stroke, as though the Artery consisted of Wood, or of some Metal, we term it *hard*; the opposite to which is called *soft*, and generally promises better. If it be strong and yet soft, even though it be quick, it may be considered as a very hopeful Circumstance. But if it is strong and hard, that commonly is a Token of an Inflammation, and indicates Bleeding and the cooling Regimen. Should it be, at the same time, small, quick and hard, the Danger is indeed very pressing.

We call that Pulse regular, a continued Succession of whose Strokes are made in equal Intervals of Time, and in which Intervals, not a single Stroke is wanting (since if that is its State, it is called an intermitting Pulse.) The Beats or Pulsations are also supposed to resemble each other so exactly in Quality too, that one is not strong, and the next alternately feeble.

As long as the State of the Pulse is promising; Respiration or Breathing is free; the Brain does not seem to be greatly affected; while the Patient takes his Medicines, and they are attended with the Consequence that was expected; and he both preserves his Strength pretty well, and continues sensible of his Situation, we may reasonably hope for his Cure. As often as all, or the greater Number of these characterizing Circumstances are wanting, he is in very considerable Danger.

The

The Stoppage of Perspiration is often mentioned in the Course of this Work. We call the Discharge of that Fluid which continually passes off through the Pores of the Skin, *Transpiration*; and which, though invisible, is very considerable. For if a Person in Health eats and drinks to the Weight of eight Pounds daily, he does not discharge four of them by Stool and Urine together, the Remainder passing off by insensible Transpiration. It may easily be conceived, that if so considerable a Discharge is stopt, or considerably lessened; and if this Fluid, which ought to transpire through the Skin, should be transfered to any inward Part, it must occasion some dangerous Complaint. In fact this is one of the most frequent Causes of Diseases.

To conclude very briefly—All the Directions in the following Treatise are solely designed for such Patients, as cannot have the Attendance of a Physician. I am far from supposing, they ought to do instead of one, even in those Diseases, of which I have treated in the fullest Manner; and the Moment a Physician arrives, they ought to be laid aside. The Confidence reposed in him should be entire, or there should be none. The Success of the Event is founded in that. It is his Province to judge of the Disease, to select Medicines against it, and it is easy to foresee the Inconveniences that may follow, from proposing to him to consult with any others, preferably to those he may chuse to consult with, only because they have succeeded in the Treatment of

another

another Patient, whose Case they suppose to have been nearly the same with the present Case. This were much the same, as to order a Shoemaker to make a Shoe for one Foot by the Pattern of another Shoe, rather than by the Measure he has just taken.

N. B. Though a great Part of this judicious Introduction is less applicable to the political Circumstances of the British Empire, than to those of the Government for which it was calculated, we think the good Sense and the unaffected Patriotism which animate it, will supersede any Apology for our translating it. The serious Truth is this, that a thorough Attention to Population seems never to have been more expedient for ourselves, than after so bloody and expensive, though such a glorious and successful War, while our enterprizing Neighbours, who will never be our Friends, are so earnest to recruit their Numbers, to increase their Agriculture; and to force a Vent for their Manufactures, which cannot be considerably effected, without a sensible Detriment to our own. Besides which, the unavoidable Drain from the People here, towards an effectual Cultivation, Improvement, and Security of our Conquests, demands a further Consideration. *K*

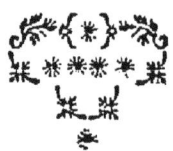

ADVICE

ADVICE TO THE PEOPLE,

With Respect to their HEALTH.

CHAPTER I.

Of the most usual Causes of popular Maladies.

SECT. I.

THE most frequent Causes of Diseases commonly incident to Country People are, 1. Excessive Labour, continued for a very considerable Time. Sometimes they sink down at once in a State of Exhaustion and Faintness, from which they seldom recover: but they are oftener attacked with some inflammatory Disease, as a Quinsey, a Pleurisy, or an Inflammation of the Breast.

There are two Methods of preventing these Evils: one is, to avoid the Cause which produces

duces them; but this is frequently impossible. Another is, when such excessive Labour has been unavoidable, to allay their Fatigue, by a free Use of some temperate refreshing Drink; especially by sweet Whey, by Butter-milk, or by * Water, to a Quart of which a Wine-glass of Vinegar may be added, or, instead of that, the expressed Juice of Grapes not fully ripe, or even of Goosberries or Cherries: which wholesome and agreeable Liquors are refreshing and cordial. I shall treat, a little lower, of inflammatory Disorders. The Inanition or Emptiness, though accompanied with Symptoms different from the former, have yet some Affinity to them with Respect to their Cause, which is a kind of general Exsiccation or Dryness. I have known some cured from this Cause by Whey, succeeded by tepid Baths, and afterwards by Cow's Milk: for in such Cases hot Medicines and high Nourishment are fatal.

§ 2. There is another Kind of Exhaustion or Emptiness, which may be termed real Emptiness,

---

* This supposes they are not greatly heated, as well as fatigued, by their Labour or Exercise, in which Circumstance free and sudden Draughts of cooling Liquors might be very pernicious; and it evidently also supposes these Drinks to be thus given, rather in Summer, than in very cold Weather, as the Juice of the unripe Grapes, and the other fresh Fruits sufficiently ascertain the Season of the Year. We think the Addition of Vinegar to their Water will scarcely ever be necessary in this or the adjoining Island on such Occasions. The Caution recommended in this Note is abundantly enforced by Dr. T. § 2. but considering the Persons, to whom this Work is more particularly addressed, we were willing to prevent every Possibility of a Mistake, in so essential, and sometimes fatal a Point.

ness, and is the Consequence of great Poverty, the Want of sufficient Nourishment, bad Food, unwholesome Drink, and excessive Labour. In Cases thus circumstanced, good Soups and a little Wine are very proper. Such happen however very seldom in this Country: I believe they are frequent in some others, especially in many Provinces of *France*.

§ 3. A second and very common Source of Disorders arises, from Peoples' lying down and reposing, when very hot, in a cold Place. This at once stops Perspiration; the Matter of which being thrown upon some internal Part, proves the Cause of many violent Diseases, particularly of Quinseys, Inflammations of the Breast, Pleurisies, and inflammatory Cholics. These Evils, from this Cause, may always be avoided by avoiding the Cause, which is one of those that destroy a great Number of People. However, when it has occurred, as soon as the first Symptoms of the Malady are perceiveable, which sometimes does not happen till several Days after, the Patient should immediately be bled; his Legs should be put into Water moderately hot, and he should drink plentifully of the tepid Infusion marked No. 1. Such Assistances frequently prevent the Increase of these Disorders; which, on the contrary, are greatly aggravated, if hot Medicines are given to sweat the Patient.

§ 4. A third Cause is drinking cold Water, when a Person is extremely hot. This acts in the same Manner with the second; but its Consequences are commonly more sudden and violent. I have seen most terrible Examples of it, in Quinseys, Inflammations of the Breast, Cholics, Inflammations of the Liver, and all the Parts of the Belly, with prodigious Swellings, Vomitings, Suppressions of Urine, and inexpressible Anguish. The most available Remedies in such Cases, from this Cause, are a plentiful Bleeding at the Onset, a very copious Drinking of warm Water, to which one fifth Part of Whey should be added; or of the Ptisan No. 2, or of an Emulsion of Almonds, all taken warm. Fomentations of warm Water should also be applied to the Throat, the breast and Belly, with Glysters of the same, and a little Milk. In this Case, as well as in the preceding one, (§ 3) a *Semicupium*, or Half-bath of warm Water has sometimes been attended with immediate Relief. It seems really astonishing, that labouring People should so often habituate themselves to this pernicious Custom, which they know to be so very dangerous to their very Beasts. There are none of them, who will not prevent their Horses from drinking while they are hot, especially if they are just going to put them up. Each of them knows, that if he lets them drink in that State, they might possibly burst with it, nevertheless he is not afraid of incurring the like Danger himself. However, this is not the only Case, in which the Peasant seems to have more Attention to the Health of his Cattle, than to his own.

§ 5. The

§ 5. The fourth Cause, which indeed affects every Body, but more particularly the Labourer, is, the Inconstancy of the Weather. We shift all at once, many times a Day, from Hot to Cold, and from Cold to Hot, in a more remarkable Manner, and more suddenly, than in most other Countries. This makes Distempers from Defluxion and Cold so common with us: and it should make us careful to go rather a little more warmly cloathed, than the Season may seem to require; to have Recourse to our Winter-cloathing early in Autumn, and not to part with it too early in the Spring. Prudent Labourers, who strip while they are at Work, take care to put on their Cloaths in the Evening when they return home.* Those, who from Negligence, are satisfied with hanging them upon their Country Tools, frequently experience, on their Return, the very unhappy Effects of it. There are some, tho' not many Places, where the Air itself is unwholsome, more from its particular Quality, than from its Changes of Temperature, as at *Villeneuve*, and still more at *Noville*, and in some other Villages situated among the Marshes which border on the *Rhone*. These Countries

are

---

* This good Advice is enforced in a Note, by the Editor of *Lyons*, who observes, it should be still more closely attended to, in Places, where Rivers, Woods or Mountains retain, as it were, a considerable Humidity, and where the Evenings are, in every Season, cold and moist — It is a very proper Caution too in our own variable Climate, and in many of our Colonies in North *America*. K.

are particularly subject to intermitting Fevers, of which I shall treat briefly hereafter.

§ 6 Such sudden Changes are often attended with great Showers of Rain, and even cold Rain, in the Middle of a very hot Day; when the Labourer who was bathed, as it were, in a hot Sweat, is at once moistened in cold Water; which occasions the same Distempers, as the sudden Transition from Heat to Cold, and requires the same Remedies. If the Sun or a hot Air succeed immediately to such a Shower, the Evil is considerably lighter. but if the Cold continues, many are often greatly incommoded by it.

A Traveller is sometimes thoroughly and unavoidably wet with Mud, the ill Consequence of which is often inconsiderable, provided he changes his Cloaths immediately, when he sets up. I have known fatal Pleurisies ensue from omitting this Caution. Whenever the Body or the Limbs are wet, nothing can be more useful than bathing them in warm Water. If the Legs only have been wet, it may be sufficient to bath them. I have radically, thoroughly, cured Persons subject to violent Cholics, as often as their Feet were wet, by persuading them to pursue this Advice. The Bath proves still more effectual, if a little Soap be dissolved in it.

§ 7 A fifth Cause, which is seldom attended to, probably indeed because it produces less violent Consequences, and yet is certainly hurtful, is the common Custom in all Villages, of having their Ditches or Dunghills directly under their Windows.

Windows. Corrupted Vapours are continually exhaling from them, which in Time cannot fail of being prejudicial, and muſt contribute to produce putrid Diſeaſes. Thoſe who are accuſtomed to the Smell, become inſenſible of it: but the Cauſe, nevertheleſs, does not ceaſe to be unwholeſomly active, and ſuch as are unuſed to it perceive the Impreſſion in all its Force.

§ 8. There are ſome Villages, in which, after the Curtain Lines are eraſed, watery marſhy Places remain in the Room of them. The Effect of this is ſtill more dangerous, becauſe that putrify'd Water, which ſtagnates during the hot Seaſon, ſuffers its Vapours to exhale more eaſily, and more abundantly, than that in the Curtain Lines did. Having ſet out for *Pully le Grand*, in 1759, on Account of an epidemical putrid Fever which raged there, I was ſenſible, on traverſing the Village, of the Infection from thoſe Marſhes; nor could I doubt of their being the Cauſe of this Diſeaſe, as well as of another like it, which had prevailed there five Years before. In other Reſpects the Village is wholeſomly ſituated. It were to be wiſhed ſuch Accidents were obviated by avoiding theſe ſtagnated Places, or, at leaſt, by removing them and the Dunghils, as far as poſſible from the Spot, where we live and lodge.

§ 9 To this Cauſe may alſo be added the Neglect of the Peaſants to air their Lodgings. It is well known that too cloſe an Air occaſions the moſt perplexing malignant Fevers, and the poor Country People reſpire no other in their own

Houses. Their Lodgings, which are very small, and which notwithstanding inclose, (both Day and Night) the Father, Mother, and seven or eight Children, besides some Animals, are never kept open during six Months in the Year, and very seldom during the other six. I have found the Air so bad in many of these Houses, that I am persuaded, if their Inhabitants did not often go out into the free open Air, they must all perish in a little Time. It is easy, however, to prevent all the Evils arising from this Source, by opening the Windows daily: so very practicable a Precaution must be followed with the happiest Consequences.

§ 10. I consider Drunkenness as a sixth Cause, not indeed as producing epidemical Diseases, but which destroys, as it were, by Retail, at all times, and every where. The poor Wretches, who abandon themselves to it, are subject to frequent Inflammations of the Breast, and to Pleurisies, which often carry them off in the Flower of their Age. If they sometimes escape through these violent Maladies, they sink, a long Time before the ordinary Approach of old Age, into all its Infirmities and especially into an Asthma, which terminates in a Dropsy of the Breast. Their Bodies, worn out by Excess, do not comply and concur, as they ought, with the Force or Operation of Remedies; and Diseases of Weakness, resulting from this Cause, are almost always incurable. It seems happy enough, that society loses nothing in parting with these Subjects,

Subjects, who are a Dishonour to it; and whose brutal Souls are, in some Measure, dead, long before their Carcases.

§ 11. The Provisions of the common People are also frequently one Cause of popular Maladies. This happens 1st, whenever the Corn, not well ripened, or not well got in, in bad * *Harvests*, has contracted an unwholesome Quality. Fortunately however this is seldom the Case, and the Danger attending the Use of it, may be lessened by some Precautions, such as those of washing and drying the Grain compleatly; of mixing a little Wine with the Dough, in kneading it; by allowing it a little more Time to swell or rise, and by baking it a little more. 2dly, The fairer and better saved Part of the Wheat is sometimes damaged in the Farmers House; either because he does not take due Care of it, or because he has no convenient Place to preserve it, only from one Summer to the next. It has often happened to me, on entering one of these bad Houses, to be struck with the Smell of Wheat that has been spoiled. Nevertheless, there are known and easy Methods to provide against this by a little Care, though I shall not enter into a Detail of them. It is sufficient to make the People sensible, that since their chief Sustenance consists of Corn, their Health must necessarily be

impaired

---

* Thus I have ventured to translate *Fies (Summers)* to apply it to this and the neighbouring Islands. Their Harvests in *Switzerland* perhaps are earlier, and may occur in *August*; that of some particular Grain, probably still earlier.

inpaired by what is bad. 3dly, That Wheat, which is good, is often made into bad Bread, by not letting it rise sufficiently; by baking it too little, and by keeping it too long. All these Errors have their troublesome Consequences on those who eat it; but in a greater Degree on Children and Valetudinarians, or weakly People.

Tarts or Cakes may be considered as an Abuse of Bread, and this in some Villages is increased to a very pernicious Height. The Dough is almost constantly bad, and often unleavened, ill baked, greasy, and stuffed with either fat or sour Ingredients, which compound one of the most indigestible Aliments imaginable. Women and Children consume the most of this Food, and are the very Subjects for whom it is the most improper: little Children especially, who live sometimes for many successive Days on these Tarts, are, for the greater Part, unable to digest them perfectly. Hence they receive a * Source of

---

* The Abuse just mentioned can scarcely be intended to forbid the moderate Use of good Pastry, the Dough of which is well raised and well baked, the Flower and other Ingredients sound, and the Paste not overcharged with Butter, even though it were sweet and fresh. But the Abuse of Alum and other pernicious Materials introduced by our Bakers, may too justly be considered as one horrible source of those Diseases of Children, which our humane and judicious Author mentions here. What he adds, concerning the Pastries being rendered still more unwholesome by the sour Fruits sometimes baked in it, is true with respect to these Children and others, who are liable to Complaints from Acidities abounding in the Bowels, and for all those who are rickett, or scrophulous, from a cold and viscid State of their Humour. But to healthy sanguine Children

of Obstructions in the Bowels of the Belly, and of a slimy Viscidity or Thickishness, throughout the Mass of Humours, which throws them into various Diseases from Weakness; slow Fevers, a Hectic, the Rickets, the King's Evil, and Feebleness, for the miserable Remainder of their Days. Probably indeed there is nothing more unwholesome than Dough not sufficiently leavened, ill-baked, greasy, and soured by the Addition of Fruits. Besides, if we consider these Tarts in an oeconomical View, they must be found inconvenient also for the Peasant on that Account.

Some other Causes of Maladies may also be referred to the Article of Food, tho' less grievous and less frequent, into a full Detail of which it is very difficult to enter: I shall therefore conclude that Article with this general Remark, that it is the Care which Peasants usually take in eating slowly, and in chewing very well, that very greatly lessens the Dangers from a bad Regimen: and I am convinced they constitute one of the greatest Causes of that Health they enjoy. We may further add indeed the Exercise which the Peasant uses, his long abiding in the open Air, where he passes three fourths of his Life, besides

(which

Children, who are advanced and lively, and others of a sanguine or bilious Temperament, we are not to suppose a moderate Variety of this Food injurious to them, when we consider, that the sharpness and Crudity of the Fruit is considerably corrected by the long Application of Fire, and that they are the Produce of Summer, when bilious Diseases are most frequent. This suggests however no bad Hint against making them immoderately sweet.

(which are also considerable Advantages) his happy Custom of going soon to Bed, and of rising very early. It were to be wished, that in these Respects, and perhaps on many other Accounts, the Inhabitants of the Country were effectually proposed as Models for reforming the Citizens.

§ 12. We should not omit, in enumerating the Causes of Maladies among Country People, the Construction of their Houses, a great many of which either lean, as it were, close to a higher Ground, or are sunk a little in the Earth. Each of these Situations subjects them to considerable Humidity; which is certain greatly to incommode the Inhabitants, and to spoil their Provisions, if they have any Quantity in Store; which, as we have observed, is another, and not the least important, Source of their Diseases. A hardy Labourer is not immediately sensible of the bad Influence of this moist and marshy Habitation; but they operate at the long Run, and I have abundantly observed their most evident bad Effects, especially on Women in Child-bed, on Children, and in Persons recovering of a preceding Disease. It would be easy to prevent this Inconvenience, by raising the Ground on which the House stood, some, or several, Inches above the Level of the adjacent Soil, by a Bed of Gravel, of small Flints, pounded Bricks, Coals, or such other Materials, and by avoiding to build immediately close to, or, as it were, under a much higher Soil. This Object, perhaps,

haps, may well deserve the Attention of the Publick; and I earnestly advise as many as do build, to observe the necessary Precautions on this Head. Another, which would cost still less Trouble, is to give the Front of their Houses an Exposure to the South-East. This Exposure, supposing all other Circumstances of the Building and its Situation to be alike, is both the most wholesome and advantageous. I have seen it, notwithstanding, very often neglected, without the least Reason being assigned for not preferring it.

These Admonitions may possibly be thought of little Consequence by three fourths of the People. I take the Liberty of reminding them, however, that they are more important than they may be supposed; and so many Causes concur to the Destruction of Men, that none of the Means should be neglected, which may contribute to their Preservation.

§ 13. The Country People in *Swisserland* drink, either 1, pure Water, 2. some Wine, 3, Perry, made from wild Pears, or sometimes Cyder from Apples, and, 4, a small Liquor which they call *Piquette*, that is Water, which has fermented with the Cake or Husks of the Grapes, after their Juice has been expressed. Water however is their most general Drink, Wine rarely falling in their Way, but when they are employed by rich Folks; or when they can spare Money enough for a Debauch. Fruit-Wines

Wines and the * *Piquettes* are not used in all Parts of the Country; they are not made in all Years; and keep but for some Months.

Our Waters in general, are pretty good; so that we have little Occasion to trouble ourselves about purifying them; and they are well known in those Provinces where they are chiefly and necessarily used (1) The pernicious Methods taken

---

* This Word's occurring in the plural Number will probably imply, the Swiss make more than one Species of this small Drink, by pouring Water on the Cake or Remainder of their other Fruits, after they have been expressed; as our People in the Cider, and perhaps in the Perry, Counties, make what they call Ciderkin, Perkin, &c. It should seem too from this Section, that the laborious Countrymen in *Swisserland* drink no Malt Liquor, though the Ingredients may be supposed to grow in their Climate. Now Beer, of different Strength, making the greater Part of our most common Drink, it may be proper to observe here, that when it is not strong and heady, but a middling well-brewed Small beer, neither too new, nor hard or sour, it is full as wholesome a Drink for laborious People in Health as any other, and perhaps generally preferable to Water for such, which may be too thin and light for those who are unaccustomed to it, and more dangerous too, when the labouring Man is very hot, as well as thirsty. The holding a Mouthful of any weak cold Liquor in the Mouth without swallowing 'till it becomes warm there, and spurting it out before a Draught is taken down would be prudent, and in Case of great Heat, to take the requisite Quantity rather at two Draughts, with a little Interval between them, than to swallow the Whole precipitately at one, would be more safe, and equally refreshing, though perhaps less grateful. K

(1) The bad Quality of Water is another common Cause of Country Diseases, either where the Waters are unwholesome, from the Soils in which they are found, as when they flow through, or settle, on Banks of Shells, or where they become such, from the Neighbourhood of, or Drainings from Dunghills and Marshes.

When Water is unclear and turbid, it is generally sufficient to let it stand in order to clear itself, by dropping its Sediment.

Of popular Maladies.

taken to improve or meliorate, as it is falsely called, bad Wines, are not as yet sufficiently practiced among us, for me to treat of them here: and as our Wines are not hurtful, of themselves, they become hurtful only from their Quantity. The Consumption of made Wines and *Piquettes* is but inconsiderable, and I have not hitherto known

ment But if that is not effected, or if it be slimy or muddy, it need only be poured into a large Vessel, half filled with fine Sand, or, for want of that, with Chalk; and then to shake and stir it about heartily for some Minutes. When this Agitation is over, the Sand, in falling to the Bottom of the Vessel, will attract some of the Foulness suspended in the Water. Or, which is still better, and very easy to do, two large Vessels may be set near together, one of which should be placed considerably higher than the other. The highest should be half filled with Sand. Into this the turbid, or slimy muddy Water is to be poured, whence it will filter itself through the Body of Sand, and pass off clear by an Opening or Orifice made at the Bottom of the Vessel, and fall from thence into the lower one, which serves as a Reservoir When the Water is impregnated with Particles from the Beds of Selenites, or of any Spar (which Water we call hard, because Soap will not easily dissolve in it, and Puls and other farinaceous Substances grow hard instead of soft, after boiling in it) such Water should be exposed to the Sun, or boiled with the Addition of some Puls, or leguminous Vegetables, or Bread toasted, or untoasted When Water is in its putrid State, it may be kept till it recovers its natural sweet one but if this cannot be waited for, a little Sea Salt should be dissolved in it, or some Vinegar may be added, in which some grateful aromatic Plant has been infused. It frequently happens, that the publick Wells are corrupted by foul Mud at the Bottom, and by different Animals which tumble in and putrify there Drinking Snow-water should be avoided, when the Snow is but lately fallen, as it seems to be the Cause of those swelling wenny Throats in the Inhabitants of some Mountains; and of endemic Cholics in many Persons As Water is so continually used, great Care should be taken to have what is good Bad Water, like bad Air, is one of the most general Causes of Diseases, that which produces the greater Number of them, the most grievous ones, and often produces such as are epidemical *L L i.e the Editor of Lyons.*

known of any ill Effects from them, so that our Liquors cannot be considered as Causes of Distempers in our Country, but in Proportion to our Abuse of them by Excess. The Case is differently circumstanced in some (1) other Countries, and it is the Province of Physicians who reside in them, to point out to their Country-Men the Methods of preserving their Health; as well as the proper and necessary Remedies in their Sickness.

(1) Many Persons, with a Design to preserve their Wines, add Shot to them or Preparations of Lead, Alum, &c. The Government should forbid, under the most severe Penalties, all such Adulterations, as tend to introduce the most painful Cholics, Obstructions, and a long Train of Evils, which it sometimes proves difficult to trace to this peculiar Cause, while they shorten the Lives of, or cruelly torment, such over credulous Customers, as lay in a Stock of bad Wines, or drink of them, without distinction, from every Wine Merchant or Taverner.

Vid. prem. Edit. at Lyons, we have sufficient Reason

CHAPTER

CHAPTER II.

Of the Causes which aggravate the Diseases of the People. General Considerations.

SECT. 14.

THE Causes already enumerated in the first Chapter occasion Diseases; and the bad Regimen, or Conduct of the People, on the Invasion of them, render them still more perplexing, and very often mortal.

There is a prevailing Prejudice among them, which is every Year attended with the Death of some Hundreds in this Country, and it is this—That all Distempers are cured by Sweat, and that to procure Sweat, they must take Abundance of hot and heating things, and keep themselves very hot. This is a Mistake in both Respects, very fatal to the Population of the State; and it cannot be too much inculcated into Country People, that by thus endeavouring to force Sweating, at the very Beginning of a Disease, they are with great Probability, taking Pains to kill themselves. I have seen some Cases, in which the continual Care to provoke this Sweating, has as manifestly killed the Patient, as if a Ball had been shot through his Brains; as such a precipitate and

and untimely Discharge carries off the thinner Part of the Blood, leaving the Mass more dry, more viscid and inflamed. Now as in all acute Diseases (if we except a very few, and those too much less frequent) the Blood is already too thick, such a Discharge must evidently increase the Disorder, by co-operating with its Cause. Instead of forcing out the watery, the thinner Part of the Blood, we should rather endeavour to increase it. There is not a single Peasant perhaps, who does not say, when he has a Pleurisy, or an Inflammation of his Breast, that his Blood is too thick, and that it cannot circulate. On seeing it in the Bason after Bleeding, he finds it *black, dry, burnt*; these are his very Words. How strange is it then, that common Sense should not assure him, that, far from forcing out the *Serum*, the watery Part, of such a Blood by sweating, there is a Necessity to increase it?

§ 15 But supposing it were as certain, as it is erroneous, that Sweating was beneficial at the Beginning of Diseases, the Means which they use to excite it would not prove the less fatal. The first Endeavour is, to stifle the Patient with the Heat of a close Apartment, and a Load of Covering Extraordinary Care is taken to prevent a Breath of fresh Air's squeezing into the Room, from which Circumstance, the Air already in it is speedily and extremely corrupted. and such a Degree of Heat is procured by the Weight of the Patient's Bed-cloaths, that these two Causes alone are sufficient to excite a most ardent Fever, and

an

an Inflammation of the Breast, even in a healthy Man. More than once have I found myself seized with a Difficulty of breathing, on entering such Chambers, from which I have been immediately relieved, on obliging them to open all the Windows. Persons of Education must find a Pleasure, I conceive, in making People understand, on these Occasions, which are so frequent, that the Air being more indispensably necessary to us, if possible, than Water is to a Fish, our Health must immediately suffer, whenever that ceases to be pure; and in assuring them also, that nothing corrupts it sooner than those Vapours, which continually steam from the Bodies of many Persons inclosed within a little Chamber, from which the Air is excluded. The Absurdity of such Conduct is a self-evident Certainty. Let in a little fresh Air on these miserable Patients, and lessen the oppressing Burthen of their Coverings, and you generally see upon the Spot, their Fever and Oppression, their Anguish and Raving, to abate.

§ 16. The second Method taken to raise a Sweat in these Patients is, to give them nothing but hot things, especially Venice Treacle, Wine, or some *Faltranc*, the greater Part of the Ingredients

---

* This Word, which must be of German, not of French Extraction, strictly signifies, *Drink for a Fall*, as we say *Pulvis ad Casum*, &c Powder for a Fall, or a supposed inward Bruise Dr *Tissot* informs me, it is otherwise called the vulnerary Herbs, or the Swiss Tea; and that it is an injudicious *Farrago* or Medley

ents of which are dangerous, whenever there is an evident Fever, besides Saffron, which is still more pernicious. In all feverish Disorders we should gently cool, and keep the Belly moderately open, while the Medicines just mentioned both heat and bind, and hence we may easily judge of their inevitable ill Consequences. A healthy Person wou'd certainly be seized with an inflammatory Fever, on taking the same Quantity of Wine, or Venice Treacle, or of *Faltranc*, which the Peasant takes now and then, when he is attacked by one of these Disorders. How then should a sick Person escape dying by them? Die indeed he *generally* does, and sometimes with astonishing Speed. I have published some dreadful Instances of such Fatality some Years since, in another Treatise. In fact they still daily occur, and unhappily every Person may observe some of them in his own Neighbourhood.

§ 17. But I shall be told perhaps, that Diseases are often carried off by Sweat, and that we ought to be guided by Experience. To this I answer, it is very true, that Sweating cures some particular Disorders, as it were, at their very Onset, for Instance, those Stitches that are called spurious or false Pleurisies, some rheumatic Pains, and some Colds or Defluxions. But this only happens when the Disorders depend solely and simply

ply

ply on ſtopt or abated Perſpiration, to which ſuch Pain inſtantly ſucceeds; and where immediately, before the Fever has thickened the Blood, and inflamed the Humours; and where before any internal Infarction, any Load, is formed, ſome warm Drinks are given, ſuch as *Faltranc* and Honey; and which, by reſtoring Tranſpiration, remove the very Cauſe of the Diſorder. Nevertheleſs, even in ſuch a Caſe, great Care ſhould be had not to raiſe too violent a Commotion in the Blood, which would rather reſtrain, than promote, Sweat, to effect which Elder-flowers are in my Opinion preferable to *Faltranc*. Sweating is alſo of Service in Diſeaſes, when their Cauſes are extinguiſhed, as it were, by plentiful Dilution: then indeed it relieves, by drawing off, with itſelf, ſome Part of the diſtempered Humours; after which their groſſer Parts have paſſed off by Stool and by Urine: beſides which, the Sweat has alſo ſerved to carry off that extraordinary Quantity of Water, we were obliged to convey into the Blood, and which was become ſuperfluous there. Under ſuch Circumſtances, and at ſuch a Juncture, it is of the utmoſt Importance indeed, not to check the Sweat, whether by Choice, or for Want of Care. There might often be as much Danger in doing this, as there would have been in endeavouring to force a Sweat, immediately upon the Invaſion of the Diſorder; ſince the arreſting of this Diſcharge, under the preceding Circumſtances, might frequently occaſion a more dangerous Diſtemper, by repelling

repelling the Humour on some inward vital Part. As much Care therefore should be taken not to check, imprudently, that Evacuation by the Skin, which naturally occurs towards the Conclusion of Diseases, as not to force it at their Beginning, the former being almost constantly beneficial, the latter as constantly pernicious. Besides, were it even necessary, it might be very dangerous to force it violently; since by heating the Patients greatly, a vehement Fever is excited; they become scorched up in a Manner, and the Skin proves extremely dry. Warm Water, in short, is the best of Sudorifics.

If the Sick are sweated very plentifully for a Day or two, which may make them easier for some Hours; these Sweats soon terminate, and cannot be excited again by the same Medicines. The Dose thence is doubled, the Inflammation is increased, and the Patient expires in terrible Anguish, with all the Marks of a general Inflammation. His Death is ascribed to his Want of Sweating; when it really was the Consequence of his Sweating too much at first, and of his taking Wine and hot Sudorifics. An able Swiss Physician had long since assured his Countrymen, that Wine was fatal to them in Fevers, I take leave to repeat it again and again, and wish it may not be with as little Success.

Our Country Folks, who in Health, naturally use red Wine, prefer it when Sick, which is wrong, as it binds them up more than white Wine. It does not promote Urine as well,

but

but increaſes the Force of the circulating Arteries, and the Thickneſs of the Blood, which were already too conſiderable

§ 18. Their Diſeaſes are alſo further aggravated by the Food that is generally given them. They muſt undoubtedly prove weak, in Conſequence of their being ſick, and the ridiculous Fear of the Patients' dying of Weakneſs, diſpoſes their Friends to force them to eat, which, increaſing their Diſorder, renders the Fever mortal This Fear is abſolutely chimerical, never yet did a Perſon in a Fever die merely from Weakneſs. They may be ſupported, even for ſome Weeks, by Water only; and are ſtronger at the End of that Time, than if they had taken more ſolid Nouriſhment, ſince, far from ſtrengthening them, their Food increaſes their Diſeaſe, and thence increaſes their Weakneſs.

§ 19 From the firſt Invaſion of a Fever, Digeſtion ceaſes. Whatever ſolid Food is taken corrupts, and proves a Source of Putridity, which adds nothing to the Strength of the Sick, but greatly to that of the Diſtemper There are in fact a thouſand Examples to prove, that it becomes a real Poiſon: and we may ſenſibly perceive theſe poor Creatures, who are thus compelled to eat, loſe their Strength, and fall into Anxiety and Ravings, in Proportion as they ſwallow.

§ 20. They are alſo further injured by the Quality, as well as the Quantity, of their Food. They are forced to ſup ſtrong Gravey Soups,

Eggs, Biscuits, and even Flesh, if they have but just Strength and Resolution to chew it. It seems absolutely impossible for them to survive all this Trash. Should a Man in perfect Health be compelled to eat stinking Meat, rotten Eggs, stale sour Broth, he is attacked with as violent Symptoms, as if he had taken real Poison, which, in Effect, he has. He is seized with Vomiting, Anguish, a violent Purging, and a Fever, with Raving, and eruptive Spots, which we call the Purple Fever. Now when the very same Articles of Food, in their soundest State, are given to a Person in a Fever, the Heat, and the morbid Matter already in his Stomach, quickly putrify them, and after a few Hours produce all the abovementioned Effects. Let any Man judge then, if the least Service can be expected from them.

§ 21. It is a Truth established by the first of Physicians, above two thousand Years past, and still further ratified by his Successors, that as long as a sick Person has a bad Humour or Ferment in his Stomach, his Weakness increases, in Proportion to the Food he receives. For this being corrupted by the infected Matter it meets there, proves incapable of nourishing, and becomes a certain or additional Cause of the Distemper.

The most observing Persons constantly remark, that whenever a feverish Patient sups, what is commonly called some good Broth, the Fever gathers Strength and the Patient Weakness. The giving such a Soup or Broth, though of the freshest soundest

soundest Meat, to a Man who has a high Fever, or putrid Humours in his Stomach, is to do him exactly the same Service, as if you had given him, two or three Hours later, stale putrid Soup.

§ 22. I must also affirm, that this fatal Prejudice, of keeping up the Patients' Strength by Food, is still too much propagated, even among those very Persons, whose Talents and whose Education might be expected to exempt them from any such gross Error. It were happy for Mankind, and the Duration of their Lives would generally be more extended, if they could be thoroughly persuaded of this medical, and so very demonstrable, Truth;—That the only things which can strengthen sick Persons are those, which are able to weaken their Disease, but their Obstinacy in this Respect is inconceivable. it is another Evil superadded to that of the Disease, and sometimes the more grievous one. Out of twenty sick Persons, who are left in the Country, more than two Thirds might often have been cured, if being only lodged in a Place defended from the Injuries of the Air, they were supplied with Abundance of good Water. But that most mistaken Care and Regimen I have been treating of, scarcely suffers one of the twenty to survive them.

§ 23. What further increases our Horrour at this enormous Propensity to heat, dry up, and cram the sick is, that it is totally opposite to what Nature herself indicates in such Circumstances. The burning Heat of which they complain, the

Dryness

Dryness of the Lips, Tongue and Throat; the flaming high Colour of their Urine; the great Longing they have for cooling things; the Pleasure and sensible Benefit they enjoy from fresh Air, are so many Signs, or rather Proofs, which cry out with a loud Voice, that we ought to attemperate and cool them moderately, by all means. Their foul Tongues, which shew the Stomach to be in the like Condition, their Loathing, their Propensity to vomit, their utter Aversion to all solid Food, and especially to Flesh, the disagreeable Stench of their Breath; their Discharge of fetid Wind upwards and downwards, and frequently the extraordinary Offensiveness of their Excrements, demonstrate, that their Bowels are full of putrid Contents, which must corrupt all the Aliments superadded to them; and that the only thing, which can prudently be done, is to dilute and attemper them by plentiful Draughts of refreshing cooling Drinks, which may promote an easy Discharge of them. I affirm it again, and I heartily wish it may be thoroughly attended to, that as long as there is any Taste of bitterness, or of Putrescence, as long as there is a *Nausea* or Loathing, a bad Breath, Heat and Feverishness with fetid Stools, and little and high-coloured Urine, so long all Flesh, and Flesh-Soup, Eggs, and all kind of Food composed of them, or of any of them, and all Venice Treacle, Wine, and all heating things are so many absolute Poisons.

§ 22. I may possibly be censured as extravagant and excessive on these Heads by the Publick

lick, and even by some Physicians: but the true and enlightened Physicians, those who attend to the Effects of every Particular, will find on the contrary, that far from exceeding in this Respect, I have rather feebly expressed their own Judgment, in which they agree with that of all the good ones, who have existed within more than two thousand Years; that very Judgment which Reason approves, and continual Experience confirms. The Prejudices I have been contending against have cost *Europe* some Millions of Lives.

§ 25. Neither should it be omitted, that even when a Patient has very fortunately escaped Death, notwithstanding all this Care to obtain it, the Mischief is not ended; the Consequences of the high Aliments and heating Medicines being, to leave behind the Seed, the Principle, of some low and chronical Disease, which increasing insensibly, bursts out at length, and finally procures him the Death he has even wished for, to put an End to his tedious Sufferings.

§ 26. I must also take Notice of another dangerous common Practice, which is that of purging, or vomiting a Patient, at the very Beginning of a Distemper. Infinite Mischiefs are occasioned by it. There are some Cases indeed, in which evacuating Medicines, at the Beginning of a Disease, are convenient and even necessary. Such Cases shall be particularly mentioned in some other Chapters: but as long as we are unacquainted with them, it should be considered as a general Rule, that they are hurtful at the Beginning, this being

being true very often; and always, when the Diseases are strictly inflammatory.

§ 27. It is hoped by their Assistance, at that Time, to remove the Load and Oppression of the Stomach, the Cause of a Disposition to vomit, of a dry Mouth, of Thirst, and of much Uneasiness; and to lessen the Leaven or Ferment of the Fever. But in this Hope they are very often deceived; since the Causes of these Symptoms are seldom of a Nature to yield to these Evacuations. By the extraordinary Viscidity or Thickness of the Humours, that foul the Tongue, we should form our Notions of those, which line the Stomach and the Bowels. It may be washed, gargled and even scraped to very little good Purpose. It does not happen, until the Patient has drank for many Days, and the Heat, the Fever and the great Sizeness of the Humours are abated, that this Filth can be thoroughly removed, which by Degrees separates of itself. The State of the Stomach being conformable to that of the Tongue, no Method can effectually scour and clean it at the Beginning; but by giving refreshing and diluting Remedies plentifully, it gradually frees itself; and the Propensity to vomit, with its other Effects and Uneasinesses, go off naturally, and without Purges.

§ 28. Neither are these Evacuations only negatively wrong, merely from doing no Good; for considerable Evil positively arises from the Application of these acid irritating Medicines, which increase the Pain and Inflammation, draw-

ing

ing the Humours upon those Parts that were already overloaded with them; which by no means expel the Cause of the Disease, that not being at this time fitted for Expulsion, as not sufficiently concocted or ripe. and yet which, at the same Time, discharge the thinnest Part of the Blood, whence the Remainder becomes more thick; in short which carry off the useful, and leave the hurtful Humours behind.

§ 29. The Vomit especially, being given in an inflammatory Disease, and even without any Distinction in all acute ones, before the Humours have been diminished by Bleeding, and diluted by plentiful small Drinks, is productive of the greatest Evils, of Inflammations of the Stomach, of the Lungs and Liver, of Suffocations and Frenzies. Purges sometimes occasion a general Inflammation of the Guts, which * terminates in Death. Some Instances of each of these terrible Conse-

---

* It is pretty common to *hear* of Persons recovering from Inflammations of the Bowels, or Guts, which our Author more justly and ingenuously considers as general Passports to Death: for it is difficult to conceive, that a real and *considerable* Inflammation of such thin, membranous, irritable Parts, lined with such putrescent Humours and Contents, and in so hot and close a Situation, could be restored to a sound and healthy State *so often* as Rumour affirms it. This makes it so important a Point, to avert every Tendency to an Inflammation of these feculent Parts, as to justify a Bleeding directed, solely, from this Precaution, and which might have been no otherwise indicated by a Disease, attended with any Symptom, that threatened such an Inflammation. But when a Person recovers, there can be no anatomical Search for such Inflammations, or its Effects, the real or imaginary Cure of which may well amaze the Patient, and must greatly redound to the Honour of his Prescriber, so that there may be Policy sometimes in giving a moderate Disease a very bad Name. K

Consequences have I seen, from blundering Temerity, Imprudence and Ignorance. The Effect of such Medicines, in these Circumstances, are much the same with those we might reasonably expect, from the Application of Salt and Pepper to a dry, inflamed and foul Tongue, in Order to moisten and clean it.

§ 30. Every Person of sound plain Sense is capable of perceiving the Truth of whatever I have advanced in this Chapter: and there would be some Degree of Prudence, even in those who do not perceive the real good Tendency of my Advice, not to defy nor oppose it too hardily. The Question relates to a very important Object; and in a Matter quite foreign to themselves, they undoubtedly owe some Deference to the Judgment of Persons, who have made it the Study and Business of their whole Lives. It is not to myself that I hope for their Attention, but to the greatest Physicians, whose feeble Instrument and Eccho I am. What Interest have any of us in forbidding sick People to eat, to be stifled, or to drink such heating things as heighten their Fever? What Advantage can accrue to us from opposing the fatal Torrent, which sweeps them off? What Arguments can persuade People, that some thousand Men of Genius, of Knowledge, and of Experience, who pass their Lives among a Croud and Succession of Patients, who are entirely employed to take Care of them, and to observe all that passes, have been only amusing and deceiving themselves, on the Effects of Food, of

Regimen

Regimen and of Remedies? Can it enter into any sensible Head, that a Nurse, who advises Soup, an Egg, or a Biscuit, deserves a Patients Confidence, better than a Physician who forbids them? Nothing can be more disagreeable to the latter, than his being obliged to dispute continually in Behalf of the poor Patients; and to be in constant Terror, lest this mortally officious Attendance, by giving such Food as augments all the Causes of the Disease, should defeat the Efficacy of all the Remedies he administers to remove it; and should fester and aggravate the Wound, in Proportion to the Pains he takes to dress it. The more such absurd People love a Patient, the more they urge him to eat, which, in Effect, verifies the Proverb of *killing one with Kindness*.

CHAPTER III.

Of the Means that ought to be used, at the Beginning of Diseases, and of the Diet in acute Diseases.

SECT. 31.

I Have clearly shewn the great Dangers of the Regimen, or Diet, and of the principal Medicines too generally made Use of by the Bulk of the People, on these Occasions. I must now point out
the

the actual Method they may pursue, without any Risque, on the Invasion of some acute Diseases; and the general Diet which agrees with them all. As many as are desirous of reaping any Benefit from this Treatise, should attend particularly to this Chapter; since, throughout the other Parts of it, in Order to avoid Repetitions, I shall say nothing of the Diet, except the particular Distemper shall require a different one, from that of which I am now to give an exact Detail. And whenever I shall say in general, that a Patient is to be put upon a Regimen, it will signify, that he is to be treated according to the Method prescribed in this Chapter; and all such Directions are to be observed, with Regard to Air, Food, Drink and Glisters; except when I expresly order something else, as different Ptisans, Glysters, &c.

§ 32 The greater Part of Diseases (by which I always understand acute and feverish ones) often give some Notice of their Approach a few Weeks, and, very commonly, some Days before their actual Invasion, such as a light Lassitude, or Weariness, Stiffness or Numbness, less Activity than usual, less Appetite, a small Load or Heaviness at Stomach; some Complaint in the Head, a profounder Degree of Sleep, yet less composed, and less refreshing than usual; less Gayety and Liveliness, sometimes a light Oppression of the Breast, a less regular Pulse; a Propensity to be Cold, an Aptness to sweat; and sometimes a Suppression of a former Disposition

sition to sweat. At such a Term it may be practicable to prevent, or at least considerably to mitigate, the most perplexing Disorders, by carefully observing the four following Points.

1. To omit all violent Work or Labour, but yet not so, as to discontinue a gentle easy Degree of Exercise

2. To bring the Complainant to content himself without any, or with very little, solid Food; and especially to renounce all Flesh, Flesh-broth, Eggs and Wine.

3. To drink plentifully, that is to say, at least three Pints, or even four Pints daily, by small Glasses at a Time, from half hour to half hour, of the Ptisans Nº 1 and 2, or even of warm Water, to each Quart of which may be added half a Glass of Vinegar. No Person can be destitute of this very attainable Assistance. But should there be a Want even of Vinegar, a few Grains of common * Salt may be added to a Quart of warm Water for Drink. Those who have Honey will do well to add two or three Spoonfuls of it to the Water. A light Infusion of Elder Flowers, or of those of the Linden, the Lime-tree, may also be advantageously used, and even well settled and clear sweet Whey.

4. Let

* This Direction of our Author's, which may surprize some, probably arises from his preferring a small Quantity of the marine Acid to no Acid at all. For though a great Proportion of Salt, in saving and seasoning Flesh and other Food, generally excites Thirst, yet a little of it seems to have rather a different Effect, by gently stimulating the salivary Glands. And we find that Nature very seldom leaves the great diluting Element wholly void of this quickening, antiputrescent Principle.

4. Let the Person, affected with such previous Complaints, receive Glysters of warm Water, or the Glyster N°. 5. By pursuing these Precautions some grievous Disorders have often been happily rooted out: and although they should not prove so thoroughly efficacious, as to prevent their Appearance, they may at least be rendered more gentle, and much less dangerous.

§ 33. Very unhappily People have taken the directly contrary Method. From the Moment these previous, these forerunning Complaints are perceived, they allow themselves to eat nothing but gross Meat, Eggs, or strong Meat-Soups. They leave off Garden-Stuff and Fruits, which would be so proper for them; and they drink heartily (under a Notion of strengthening the Stomach and expelling Wind) of Wine and other Liquors, which strengthen nothing but the Fever, and expel what Degree of Health might still remain. Hence all the Evacuations are restrained, the Humours causing and nourishing the Diseases are not at all attempered, diluted, nor rendered proper for Evacuation. Nay, on the very contrary, they become more sharp, and more difficult to be discharged: while a sufficient Quantity of diluting refreshing Liquor, assuages and separates all Matters foreign to the Blood, which it purifies; and, at the Expiration of some Days, all that was noxious in it is carried off by Stool, by Urine, or by Sweat.

§ 34 When the Distemper is further advanced, and the Patient is already seized with that
Coldness

Coldness or Shuddering, in a greater or less Degree, which ushers in all Diseases; and which is commonly attended with an universal Oppression, and Pains over all the Surface of the Body; the Patient, thus circumstanced, should be put to Bed, if he cannot keep up; or should sit down as quietly as possible, with a little more Covering than usual: he should drink every Quarter of an Hour a small Glass of the Ptisan, N°. 1 or 2, warm, or, if that is not at Hand, of some one of those Liquids I have recommended § 32.

§ 35. These Patients earnestly covet a great Load of covering, during the Cold or Shivering; but we should be very careful to lighten them as soon as it abates, so that when the succeeding Heat begins, they may have no more than their usual Weight of Covering. It were to be wished *perhaps*, they had rather less. The Country People lie upon a Feather-bed, and under a downy Coverlet, or Quilt, that is commonly extremely heavy; and the Heat which is heightened and retained by Feathers, is particularly troublesome to Persons in a Fever. Nevertheless, as it is what they are accustomed to, this Custom may be complied with for one Season of the Year: but during our Heats, or whenever the Fever is very violent, they should lie on a Pallet (which will be infinitely better for them) and should throw away their Coverings of Down, so as to remain covered only with Sheets, or something else, less injurious than Feather-Coverings. A Person could scarcely believe, who had not been,

E   as

as I have, a Witness of it, how much Comfort a Patient is sensible of, in being eased of his former Coverings. The Distemper immediately puts on a different Appearance.

§ 36. As soon as the Heat after the *Rigor*, or Coldness and Shuddering, approaches, and the Fever is manifestly advanced, we should provide for the Patient's *Regimen*. And

1, Care should be taken that the Air, in the Room where he lies, should not be too hot, the mildest Degree of Warmth being very sufficient, that there be as little Noise as possible, and that no Person speak to the Sick, without a Necessity for it. No external Circumstance heightens the Fever more, nor inclines the Patient more to a *Delirium* or Raving, than the Persons in the Chamber, and especially about the Bed. They lessen the Spring, the elastic and refreshing Power, of the Air; they prevent a Succession of fresh Air, and the Variety of Objects occupies the Brain too much. Whenever the Patient has been at Stool, or has made Urine, these Excrements should be removed immediately. The Windows should certainly be opened Night and Morning, at least for a Quarter of an Hour each Time, when also a Door should be opened, to promote an entire Renovation or Change of the Air in the Room. Nevertheless, as the Patient should not be exposed at any Time to a Stream or Current of Air, the Curtains of his Bed should be drawn on such Occasions, and, if he lay without any, Chairs, with Blankets or Cloaths

hung

hung upon them, should be substituted in the Place of Curtains, and surround the Bed, while the Windows continued open, in Order to defend the Patient from the Force of the rushing Air. If the Season, however, be rigidly cold, it will be sufficient to keep the Windows open, but for a few Minutes, each Time. In Summer, at least one Window should be set open Day and Night. The pouring a little Vinegar upon a red-hot Shovel also greatly conduces to restore the Spring, and correct the Putridity, of the Air. In our greatest Heats, when that in the Room seems nearly scorching, and the sick Person is sensibly and greatly incommoded by it, the Floor may be sprinkled now and then; and Branches of Willow or Ash-trees dipt a little in Pails of Water

§ 37. 2. With Respect to the Patient's Nourishment, he must entirely abstain from all Food; but he may always be allowed, and have daily prepared, the following Sustenance, which is one of the wholesomest, and indisputably the simplest one Take half a Pound of bread, a Morsel of the freshest Butter about the Size only of a Hazel Nut (which may even be omitted too) three Pints and one quarter of a Pint of Water. Boil them 'till the Bread be entirely reduced to a thin Consistence. Then strain it, and give the Patient one eighth Part of it every three, or every four, Hours; but still more rarely, if the Fever be vehemently high. Those who have Groats, Barley, Oatmeal, or Rice, may boil and prepare them in the same Manner, with some Grains of Salt.

§ 38. The Sick may also be sometimes indulged, in lieu of these different Spoon-Meats, with raw Fruits in Summer, or in Winter with Apples baked or boiled, or Plumbs and Cherries dried and boiled. Persons of Knowledge and Experience will be very little, or rather not at all, surprized to see various Kinds of Fruit directed in acute Diseases, the Benefit of which they may here have frequently seen. Such Advice can only disgust those who remain still obstinately attached to old Prejudices. But could they prevail on themselves to reflect a little, they must perceive that these Fruits which allay Thirst, which cool and abate the Fever, which correct and attemper the putrid and heated Bile; which gently dispose the Belly to be rather open, and promote the Secretion and Discharge of the Urine, must prove the properest Nourishment for Persons in acute Fevers. Hence we see, as it were by a strong Admonition from Nature herself, they express an ardent Longing for them, and I have known several, who would not have recovered, but for their eating secretly large Quantities of these Fruits they so passionately desired, and were refused. As many however, as are not convinced by my Reasoning in this Respect, may at least make a Trial of my Advice, on my Affirmation and Experience, when I have no doubt but their own will speedily convince them of the real Benefit received from this Sort of Nourishment. It

will

will then be evident, that we may safely and boldly allow, in all continual Fevers, Cherries red and black, Strawberries, the best cured Raisins, Raspberries, and Mulberries, provided that all of them be perfectly ripe. Apples, Pears and Plumbs are less melting and diluting, less succulent, and rather less proper. Some kinds of Pears however are extremely juicy, and even watery almost, such as the Dean or Valentia Pear, different Kinds of the Buree Pear; the St. Germain, the Virgoleuse, the green sugary Pear, and the Summer Royal, which may all be allowed, as well as a little Juice of very ripe Plumbs, with the Addition of Water to it. This last I have known to assuage Thirst in a Fever, beyond any other Liquor. Care should be taken, at the same Time, that the Sick should never be indulged in a great Quantity of any of them at once, which would overload the Stomach, and be injurious to them; but if they are given a little at a Time and often, nothing can be more salutary. Those whose Circumstances will afford them China Oranges, or Lemons, may be regaled with the Pulp and Juice as successfully, but without eating any of their Peel, which is hot and inflaming.

§ 39. 3. Their Drink should be such as allays Thirst, and abates the Fever, such as dilutes, relaxes, and promotes the Evacuations by Stool, Urine and Perspiration. All these which I have recommended in the preceding Chapters, jointly and severally possess these Qualities. A Glass of a Glass and a half of the Juice of such Fruits as I have just mentioned, may also be added to three full Pints of Water.

§ 40. The Sick should drink at least twice or thrice that Quantity daily, often, and a little at once, between three or four Ounces, every Quarter of an Hour. The Coldness of the Drink should just be taken off.

§ 41. 4. If the Patient has not two Motions in the 24 Hours, if the Urine be in small Quantity and high coloured; if he rave, the Fever rage, the Pain of the Head and of the Loins be considerable, with a Pain in the Belly, and a Propensity to vomit, the Glyster N°. 5 should be given at least once a Day. The People have generally an Aversion to this kind of Remedy; notwithstanding there is not any more useful in feverish Disorders, especially in those I have just recounted; and one Glyster commonly gives more Relief, than if the Patient had drank four or five Times the Quantity of his Drinks. The Use of Glysters, in different Diseases, will be properly ascertained in the different Chapters, which treat of them. But it may be observed in this Place, that they are never to be given at the very Time the Patient is in a Sweat, which seems to relieve him

§ 42. 5 As long as the Patient has sufficient Strength for it, he should sit up out of Bed one Hour daily, and longer if he can bear it; but at least half an Hour It has a Tendency to lessen the Fever, the Head-ach, and a Light-headiness, or Raving. But he should not be raised, while he has a hopeful Sweating; though such Sweats hardly ever occur, but at the Conclusion of Diseases, and after the Sick has had several other Evacuations.

§ 43 6. His Bed should be made daily while he sits up, and the Sheets of the Bed, as well as the Patient's Linen, should be changed every two Days, if it can be done with Safety. An unhappy Prejudice has established a contrary, and a really dangerous, Practice. The People about the Patient dread the very Thought of his rising out of Bed, they let him continue there in nasty Linen loaded with putrid Steams and Humours, which contribute, not only to keep up the Distemper, but even to heighten it into some Degree of Malignity. I do again repeat it here, that nothing conduces more to continue the Fever and Raving, than confining the Sick constantly to Bed, and witholding him from changing his foul Linen: by relieving him from both of which Circumstances I have, without the Assistance of any other Remedy, put a Stop to a continual Delirium of twelve Days uninterrupted Duration. It is usually said, the Patient is too weak, but this is a very weak Reason. He must be in very nearly a dying Condition, not to be able to bear these small Commotions, which, in the very Moment when he permits them, increase his Strength, and immediately after abate his Complaints. One Advantage the Sick gain by sitting up a little out of Bed, is the increased

Quantity of their Urine, with greater Facility in passing it. Some have been observed to make none at all, if they did not rise out of Bed.

A very considerable Number of acute Diseases have been radically, effectually, cured by this Method, which mitigates them all. Where it is not used, as an Assistance at least, Medicines are very often of no Advantage. It were to be wished the Patient and his Friends were made to understand, that Distempers were not to be expelled at once with rough and precipitate Usage; that they must have their certain Career or Course; and that the Use of the violent Methods and Medicines they chuse to employ, might indeed abridge the Course of them, by killing the Patient, yet never otherwise shortened the Disease, but on the contrary, rendered it more perplexing, tedious and obstinate, and often entailed such unhappy Consequences on the Sufferer, as left him feeble and languid for the rest of his Life.

§ 44. But it is not sufficient to treat, and, as it were, to conduct the Distemper properly. The Term of Recovery from a Disease requires considerable Vigilance and Attention, as it is always a State of Feebleness, and, thence, of Depression and Faintness. The same Kind of Prejudice which destroys the Sick, by compelling them to eat, during the Violence of the Disease, is extended also into the Stage of Convalescence, or Recovery, and either renders it troublesome and tedious, or produces fatal Relapses, and often chronical Distempers. In Proportion to the Abatement and in the Decline, of the Fever, the
Quantity

in acute Diseases.

Quantity of Nourishment may be gradually increased: but as long as there are any Remains of it, their Qualities should be those I have already recommended. Whenever the Fever is compleatly terminated, some different Foods may be entered upon; so that the Patient may venture upon a little white Meat, provided it be tender; some * Fish, a little Flesh-Soup, a few Eggs at times, with Wine properly diluted. It must be observed at the same Time, that those very proper Aliments which restore the Strength, when taken moderately, delay the perfect Cure, if they exceed in Quantity, tho' but a little; because the Action of the Stomach being extremely weakened by the Disease and the Remedies, is capable only, as yet, of a small Degree of Digestion, and if the Quantity of its Extents exceed its Powers, they do not digest, but become putrid. Frequent Returns of the Fever supervene; a continual Faintishness, Head-achs; a heavy Drowsiness without a Power of Sleeping comfortably; flying Pains and Heats in the Arms and Legs, Inquietude, Peevishness, Propensity to Vomit, Looseness, Obstructions, and sometimes a slow Fever, with a Collection of Humours, that comes to Suppuration.

All these bad Consequences are prevented, by the recovering Sick contenting themselves, for some

---

* The most allowable of these are Whitings, Flounders, Plaice, Dabbs, or Gudgeons, especially such of the last as are taken out of clear current Streams with gravelly Bottoms. Salmon, Eels, Carp, all the Skate kind, Haddock, and the like, should not be permitted, before the Sick return to their usual Diet when in Health. *K.*

some Time, with a very moderate Share of proper Food. We are not nourished in Proportion to the Quantity we swallow, but to that we digest. A Person on the mending Hand, who eats moderately, digests it and grows strong from it. He who swallows abundantly does not digest it, and instead of being nourished and strengthened, he withers insensibly away.

§ 45. We may reduce, within the few following Rules, all that is most especially to be observed, in Order to procure a compleat, a perfect Termination of acute Diseases; and to prevent their leaving behind them any Impediments to Health.

1 Let these who are recovering, as well as those who are actually sick, take very little Nourishment at a time, and take it often.

2 Let them take but one sort of Food at each Meal, and not change their Food too often.

3 Let them chew whatever solid Victuals they eat, very carefully.

4 Let them diminish their Quantity of Drink. The best for them in general is Water, * with a fourth or third Part of white Wine. Too great a Quantity of Liquids at this time prevents the Stomach

---

* We have known many who had an Aversion to Water, and with whom, on that very Account, it might probably agree less, and Wine very grateful, in which a thoroughly baked and hot, or burnt, Slice of Bread had been infused, 'till it attained the Colour of a fine clear small Beer, or light Amber coloured Beer, and we never saw an Inconvenience result from it. Doubtless pure, untasted elemental Water may be preferable for those who use, and have been accustomed to it. K.

Stomach from recovering its Tone and Strength; impairs Digestion; keeps up Weakness; increases the Tendency to a Swelling of the Legs; sometimes even occasions a slow Fever; and throws back the Person recovering into a languid State.

5. Let them go abroad as often as they are able, whether on Foot, in a Carriage, or on Horseback. This last Exercise is the healthiest of all, and three fourths of the labouring People in this Country, who have it in their Power to procure it, without Expence, are in the wrong to neglect it. They, who would practice it, should mount before their principal Meal, which should be about Noon, and never ride after it. Exercise taken before a Meal strengthens the Organs of Digestion, which is promoted by it. If the Exercise is taken soon after the Meal, it impairs it.

6. As People in this State are seldom quite as well towards Night, in the Evening they should take very little Food. Then Sleep will be the less disturbed for this, and repair them the more, and sooner.

7 They should not remain in Bed above seven, or eight Hours.

8. The Swelling of the Legs and Ancles, which happens to most Persons at this time, is not dangerous, and generally disappears of itself; if they live soberly and regularly, and take moderate Exercise.

9. It

9. It is not necessary, in this State, that they should go constantly every Day to Stool, though they should not be without one above two or three. If their Costiveness exceeds this Term, they should receive a Glyster the third Day, and even sooner, if they are heated by it, if they feel puffed up, are restless, and have any Pains in the Head.

10. Should they, after some time, still continue very weak, if their Stomach is disordered, if they have, from time to time, a little irregular Fever, they should take three Doses daily of the Prescription N° 14. which fortifies the Digestors, recovers the strength, and drives away the Fever.

11. They must by no means return to their Labour too soon. This erroneous Habit daily prevents many Peasants from ever getting perfectly well, and recovering their former Strength. From not having been able to confine themselves to Repose and Indolence for some Days, they never become as hearty hardy Workmen as they had been, and this premature hasty Labour makes them lose in the Consequence, every following Week of their Lives, more time than they ever gained, by the over-early resuming of their Labour. I see every Day weakly Labourers, Vinegroers, and other Workmen, who date the Commencement of their Weakness from that of some acute Disease, which, for want of proper Management through the Term of their Recovery, was never perfectly cured. A Repose of
seven

seven or eight Days, more than they allowed themselves, would have prevented all these Infirmities, notwithstanding it is very difficult to make them sensible of this. The Bulk, the Body of the People, in this and in many other Cases, look no further than the present Day, and never extend their Views to the following one. They are for making no Sacrifice to Futurity, which nevertheless must be done, to render it favourable to us.

Chapter IV.

Of an Inflammation of the Breast

Sect. 46

THE Inflammation of the Breast, or Peripneumony, or a Fluxion upon the Breast, is an Inflammation of the Lungs, and most commonly of one only, and consequently on one Side. The Signs by which it is evident, are a Shivering, of more or less Duration, during which the Person affected is sometimes very restless and in great Anguish, an essential and inseparable Symptom, and which has helped me more than once to distinguish this Disease certainly, at the very Instant of its Invasion. Besides this, a considerable Degree of Heat succeeds the Shivering, which Heat, for a few

few enfuing Hours, is often blended as it were, with fome Returns of Chillinefs. The Pulfe is quick, pretty ftrong, moderately full, hard and regular, when the Diftemper is not very violent; but fmall, foft and irregular, when it is very dangerous. There is alfo a Senfation of Pain, but rather light and tolerable, in one Side of the Breaft, fometimes a kind of ftraitning or Preffure on the Heart, at other times Pains through the whole Body, efpecially along the Reins; and fome Degree of Oppreffion, at leaft very often, for fometimes it is but very inconfiderable. The Patient finds a Neceffity of lying almoft continually upon his Back, being able to lie but very rarely upon either of his Sides. Sometimes his Cough is dry, and then attended with the moft Pain; at other times it is accompanied with a Spitting or Hawking up, blended with more or lefs Blood, and fometimes with pure fheer Blood. There is alfo fome Pain, or at leaft a Senfation of Weight and Heavinefs in the Head: and frequently a Propenfity to rave. The Face is almoft continually flufhed and red: though fometimes there is a Degree of Palenefs and an Air of Aftonifhment, at the Beginning of the Difeafe, which portend no little Danger. The Lips, the Tongue, the Palate, the Skin are all dry; the Breath hot; the Urine little and high coloured in the firft Stage: but more plentiful, lefs flaming, and letting fall much Sediment afterwards. There is a frequent Thirft, and fometimes an Inclination

tion to vomit, which impofing on the ignorant Affiftants, have often inclined them to give the Patient a Vomit, which is mortal, efpecially at this Juncture. The Heat becomes univerfal. The Symptoms are heightened almoft every Night, during which the Cough is more exafperated, and the Spitting or Expectoration in lefs Quantity. The beft Expectoration is of a middling Confiftence, neither too thin, nor too hard and tough, like thofe which are brought up at the Termination of a Cold; but rather more yellow, and mixed with a little Blood, which gradually becomes ftill lefs, and commonly difappears entirely, before the feventh Day. Sometimes the Inflammation afcends along the Wind-pipe, and in fome Meafure fuffocates the Patient, paining him confiderably in Swallowing, which makes him think he has a fore Throat.

§ 47. Whenever the Difeafe is very violent at firft, or increafes to be fuch, the Patient cannot draw his Breath, but when he fits up. The Pulfe becomes very fmall and very quick, the Countenance livid, the Tongue black, the Eyes ftare wildly; and he fuffers inexpreffible Anguifh, attended with inceffant Reftlefsnefs and Agitation in his Bed. One of his Arms is fometimes affected with a fort of Palfy; he raves without Intermiffion, can neither thoroughly wake nor fleep. The Skin of his Breaft and of his Neck is covered (efpecially in clofe fultry Weather, and when the Diftemper is extremely violent) with livid Spots, more or lefs remarkable, which

which should be called *petechial* ones, but are improperly termed the *pourpre*, or purple. The natural Strength becomes exhausted; the Difficulty of breathing increases every Moment, he sinks into a Lethargy, and soon dies a terrible Death in Country Places, by the very Effects of the inflaming Medicines they employ on such Occasions. It has been known in Fact, that the Use of them has raised the Distemper to such a Height, that the very Heart has been rent open, which the Dissection of the Body has demonstrated.

§ 48. If the Disease rushes on at once, with a sudden and violent Attack, if the Horror, the Cold and Shivering last many Hours, and are followed with a nearly scorching Degree of Heat; if the Brain is affected from the very Onset; if the Patient has a small Purging, attended with a *Tnesmus*, or straining to Stool, often termed a *Needy*; if he abhors the Bed, if he either sweat excessively, or if his Skin be extremely dry; if his natural Manner and Look are considerably changed; and if he spits up with much Difficulty, the Disease is extremely dangerous.

§ 49. He must directly, from the first Seizure in this State, be put upon a Regimen, and his Drink must never be given cold. It should either be the Barley Water N°. 2, the Almond Emulsion N° 4, or that of N°. 7. The Juices of the Plants, which enter into the last of these Drinks, are excellent Remedies in this Case; as they

Of an Inflammation of the Breast.

they powerfully attenuate, or melt down, the viscid thick Blood, which causes the Inflammation.

As long as the Fever keeps up extremely violent, while the Patient does not expectorate sufficiently; continues raving; has a violent Headach, or raises up pure Blood, the Glyster N°. 5 must be given thrice, or at least twice, in twenty four Hours. However the principal Remedy is Bleeding. As soon as ever the preceding cold Assault is over, twelve Ounces of Blood must be taken away at once; and, if the Patient be young and strong, fourteen or even sixteen. This plentiful Bleeding gives him more Ease, than if twenty four Ounces had been drawn, at three different Times.

§ 50. When the Disease is circumstanced as described (§ 46) that first Bleeding makes the Patient easy for some Hours; but the Complaint returns; and to obviate its Violence, as much as possible, we must, except things promise extremely well, repeat the Bleeding four Hours after the first, taking again twelve Ounces of Blood, which pretty often proves sufficient. But if, about the Expiration of eight or ten Hours, it appears to kindle up again, it must be repeated a third, or even a fourth Time. Yet, with the Assistance of other proper Remedies, I have seldom been obliged to bleed a fourth Time, and have sometimes found the two first Bleedings sufficient.

If the Disease has been of several Days Duration, when I have first been called, if the Fever is still very high, if there be a Difficulty of Breathing, if the Patient does not expectorate at all, or brings up too much Blood, without being too scrupulous about the Day of the Disease, the Patient should be bled, though it were on the tenth. (a)

§ 51. In this, and in all other inflammatory Diseases, the Blood is in a very thick viscid State: and almost immediately on its being drawn, a white tough Skin, somewhat like Leather, is formed on its Top, which most People have seen, and which is called the *pleuritic Crust*. It is thought a promising Appearance, when at each Bleeding it seems less hard, and less thick, than it was at the preceding ones, and this is very generally true, if the Sick feels himself, at the same Time, sensibly better: but whoever shall attend *solely* to the Appearance of the Blood, will find himself often deceived. It will happen, even in the most violent Inflammation of the Breast, that this Crust is not formed, which is supposed to be a very unpromising Sign. There are also, in this Respect, many odd Appearances, which

arise

(a) We should however with the greater Circumspection (of which the ascertaining the Disease has been, and by how much more difficult the viscous Humours are to be melted and discharged) attend to the Coction of the Matter, the operation, which Nature does not often easily effect, and when she effects the more imperfectly and slowly, the more her Efforts have often been attended with certain Paroxysms have imposed even upon very competent Doctors, who have made them open a Vein a few Hours before the Patient's Death, from their Pulses being strong, hard ... But the Weakness is the Sign, by which we ... their languishing Efforts to be the last. *E. L.*

arise from the smallest Circumstances, so that we must not regulate the Repetitions of our bleeding, solely by this Crust: and in general we must not be over credulous in supposing, that the Appearances in the Blood, received into the Bason, can enable us to determine, with Certainty, of its real State in the Body.

§ 52 When the sick Person is in the Condition described (§ 47) the Bleeding is not only unattended with Ease, but sometimes it is also pernicious, by the sudden Weakness to which it reduces him. Generally in such a Case all Medicines and Means are insignificant: and it is a very bad Sign in this Disease, when this Discharge is not attended with Ease and Benefit to the Sick, or when there are some Circumstances, which oblige us to be sparing of it.

§ 53. The Patient's Legs should every Day, for one half Hour, be put into a Bath of warm Water, wrapping him up closely, that the Cold may not check that Perspiration, which the Bath promotes.

§ 54. Every two Hours he should take two Spoonfuls of the Mixture N°. 8, which promotes all the Discharges, and chiefly that of Expectoration.

§ 55. When the Oppression and Straitness are considerable, and the Cough dry, the Patient may receive the Vapour of boiling Water, to which a little Vinegar has been added. There are two ways of effecting this, either by placing below his Face, after setting him up, a Vessel filled with

such

such boiling hot Water, and covering the Patient's Head and the Vessel with a Linen Cloth, that may inclose the Steam; or else by holding before his Mouth a Spunge dipped in the same boiling Liquor. This last Method is the least effectual, but it fatigues the Patient considerably less. When this bad Symptom is extremely pressing, Vinegar alone should be used without Water; and the Vapour of it has often saved Patients, who seemed to have one Foot in the Grave: but it should be continued for several Hours.

§ 56. The outward Remedies directed in N°. 9. are also applied with Success to the Breast, and to the Throat.

§ 57. When the Fever is extremely high, the Sick should take every Hour, a Spoonful of the Mixture N°. 10. in a Cup of the Ptisan (a) but

* The Use of Acids, in Inflammations of the Breast, requires no little Consideration. Whenever the sick Person has an Aversion to them, when the Tongue is moist, the Stomach is heavy and disordered, and the Habit and Temperament of the Patient is mild and soft, when the Cough is very sharp without great Thirst, we ought to abstain from them. But when the Inflammation is joined to a dry Tongue, to great Thirst, Heat and Fever, they are of great Service. Slices of China Oranges sprinkled with Sugar may be given first, a light Limonade may be allowed afterwards; and at last small Doses of the Mixture N° 10 if it becomes necessary. E L—I have chosen to retain this Note of the Editor of Lyons, from having frequently seen the Inefficacy, and sometimes, I have even thought, the ill Effects of Acids in Peripneumonies and Pleurisies, in a Country far South of Switzerland, and where these Diseases are very frequent, acute and fatal. On the other hand I find the Substance of what Dr Tissot says on this Head in a Note

but without diminishing on this Account the usual Quantity of his other Drinks, which may be taken immediately after it.

§ 58. As long as the Patient shall grow worse, or only continue equally bad, the same Medicines are to be repeated. But if on the third Day (tho' it rarely happens so soon) or fourth, or fifth, the Disease takes a more favourable Turn; if the Exasperation returns with less Violence; the Cough be less severe; the Matter coughed up less bloody: if Respiration becomes easier, the Head be less affected, the Tongue not quite so dry; if the high Colour of the Urine abates, and its Quantity be increased, it may be sufficient

then

a Note to his Table of Remedies, wherein he affirms, that he has given in this Disease very large Doses of them, rising gradually from small ones, and always with great Success, intreating other Physicians to order this Acid (the Spirit of Sulphur) in the same large Doses which he directs in this Chapter, and assuring himself of their thanks, for its good Consequences—Now the only ill Effect I can surmize here, from shewing this Diversity of Opinion in these two learned Physicians, and my own Doubts, is, that the Subjects of this Disease in Country Places may prove somewhat confused and irresolute by it, in their Conduct in such Cases But as all of us certainly concur in the great Intention of doing all possible Good, by the extensive Publication of this Treatise, I shall take leave to observe that in this Disease, and in Pleurisies, more solid Benefit has been received in *Carolina*, *Virginia*, &c. from the Use of the *Seneka* Rattle-snake Root, than from any other Medicine whatever Bleeding indeed is necessarily premised to it, but it has often saved the Necessity of many repeated Bleedings This Medicine, which is termed in Latin, the *Polygala Virginiana*, is certainly rather of a saponaceous attenuating Quality, and betrays not any Marks of Acidity, being rather moderately acrid. There will be Occasion to mention it more particularly in the subsequent Chapter, as such a Liberty can need no Apology to any philosophical Physician K.

then to keep the Patient carefully to his Regimen, and to give him a Glyster every Evening. The Exasperation that occurs the fourth Day is often the highest.

§ 59. This Distemper is most commonly terminated and carried off by Expectoration, and often by Urine, which on the seventh, the ninth, or the eleventh Day, and sometimes on the Days between them, begins to let fall a plentiful Sediment, or Settling, of a pale red Colour, and sometimes real *Pus* or ripe Matter. These Discharges are succeeded by Sweats, which are as serviceable then, as they were injurious at the Beginning of the Disease.

§ 60 Some Hours before these Evacuations appear, there come on, and not seldom, some very alarming Symptoms, such as great Anguish, Palpitations, some Irregularity in the Pulse, an increased Oppression, convulsive Motions (this being what is called the *Crisis*, the Height, or Turn of the Distemper) but they are no ways dangerous, provided they do not occasion any improper Treatment. These Symptoms depend on the morbid and purulent Matter, which, being dislodged, circulates with the Humours, and irritates different Parts, until the Discharge of it has fairly begun, after which all such Symptoms disappear, and Sleep generally ensues. However I cannot too strongly insist on the Necessity of great Prudence in such Circumstances. Sometimes it is the Weakness of the Patient, and at other times Convulsions, or some other Symptoms

toms, that terrify the By-ſtanders. If, which is moſt generally the Caſe, the abſurd Practice of directing particular Remedies for ſuch Accidents takes place, ſuch as ſpirituous Cordials, Venice Treacle, Confections, Caſtor and Rue, the Conſequence is, that Nature being diſturbed in her Operations, the *Criſis* or Turn is not effected; the Matter which ſhould be diſcharged by Stool, by Urine, or by Sweat, is not diſcharged out of the Body; but is thrown upon ſome internal or external part of it. Should it be on ſome inward part, the Patient either dies at once; or another Diſtemper ſucceeds, more troubleſome and incurable than the firſt. Should it be expelled to ſome outward part, the Danger indeed is leſs, and as ſoon as ever ſuch a Tumour appears, ripening Pultices ſhould be apply'd to bring it to a Head, after which it ſhould immediately be opened.

§ 61. In order to prevent ſuch unhappy Conſequences, great Care muſt be taken, whenever ſuch terrifying Symptoms come on, [about the Time of the *Criſis*] to make no Change in the Diet, nor in the Treatment of the Patient; except in giving him the looſening Glyſter No. 5, and applying every two Hours a Flannel, ſqueezed out of warm Water, which may cover all the Belly, and in a Manner go round the Body behind the Reins. The Quantity of his Drink may alſo be increaſed a little, and that of his Nouriſhment leſſened, as long as this high and violent State continues

§ 62. I have not spoken of Vomits or Purges, as being directly contrary to the Nature of this Disease. Anodynes, or Opiates, to procure Sleep are also, in general, very improper. In a few Cases, however, they may possibly be useful; but these Cases are so very difficult to be sufficiently distinguished, that Opiates should never be admitted in this Disease, without the Presence and Advice of a Physician. I have seen many Patients, who have been thrown into an incurable Hectic, by taking them improperly. When the Disease is not received in a mortal Degree, nor has been injudiciously treated, and proceeds in a benign regular Manner, the Patient may be called very well and safe by the fourteenth Day; when he may, if he has an Appetite, be put upon the Diet of People who are recovering. But if he still retains an Aversion to Food, if his Mouth is foul and furred, and he is sensible of some Heaviness in his Head, he should take the purging Potion N° 11.

§ 63. Bleedings from the Nose occur sometimes naturally in this Disease, even after repeated Bleedings by Art, these are very benign and favourable, and are commonly attended with more Ease and Relief than artificial Bleedings. Such voluntary Discharges may sometimes be expected, when the Patient is sensibly mended in many Respects after the Use of the Lancet; and yet complains of a great Pain in his Head, accompanied with quick sparkling Eyes, and a Redness of the Nose. Nothing should be done to stop this

these voluntary Bleedings, since it would be very dangerous: For when Nature has fulfilled her Intention by them, they cease of themselves. At other times, but more rarely, the Distemper is carried off by a natural Purging, attended with moderate Pain, and the Discharge of bilious Matter.

§ 64. If the Expectoration, or hawking up of Matter, stops very suddenly, and is not speedily attended with some other Evacuation; the Oppression and Anguish of the Patient immediately return, and the Danger is great and pressing. If the Distemper, at this Juncture, is not of many Days standing; if the Patient is a strong Person; if he has not as yet been plentifully bled; if there be still some Blood mixed with the Humour he expectorates, or if the Pulse be strong and hard, he should be bled immediately in the Arm, and constantly receive the Steam of hot Water and Vinegar by the Mouth, and drink plentifully of the Ptisan N° 2, something hotter than ordinary. But if his Circumstances, after this Suppression, are different from these just mentioned, instead of bleeding him, two Blisters should be applied to the Legs; and he should drink plentifully of the Ptisan N° 12.

The Causes which oftenest produce this Suppression of his Expectoration are, 1, a sharp and sudden cold Air 2, too hot a one 3, over hot Medicines 4, excessive Sweating. 5, a Purge prematurely and injudiciously timed. and 6, some immoderate Passion of the Mind.

§ 65 When

§ 65. When the Sick has not been sufficiently bled, or not soon enough; and even sometimes, which I have seen, when he has been greatly weakened by excessive Bleeding; so that the Discharges by Stool, Urine, Expectoration and Perspiration, have not been sufficiently made, when these Discharges have been confused by some other Causes; or the Disease has been injudiciously treated; then the Vessels that have been inflamed, do not unload themselves of the Humours, which stuff up and oppress them: but there happens in the Substance of the affected Lung, the same Circumstance we see daily occur on the Surface of the Body. If an inflammatory Tumour or Swelling does not disperse itself, and disappears insensibly, it forms an Imposthume or Abscess. Thus exactly also in the inflamed Lung, if the Inflammation is not dissipated, it forms an Abscess, which, in that part, is called a *Vomica:* and the Matter of that Abscess, like the external ones, remains often long inclosed in its Sac or Bag, without bursting open its Membrane or Case, and discharging the Matter it contains.

§ 66. If the Inflammation was not very deeply seated in the inward Substance of the diseased Lung, but was extended to its Surface, that is, very near the Ribs, the Sac will burst on the Surface of the Lung, and the Matter contained in it must be discharged into the Cavity, or Hollowness of the Breast, between the Lung, the Ribs, and the Diaphragm or Midriff, which is

the

the Membrane that divides the Breast and the Belly. But when the Inflammation is considerably deeper, the Imposthume bursts withinside of the Lung itself. If its Orifice, or Opening is so small, that but little can get out at once; if the Quantity of all the Matter be inconsiderable, and the Patient is at the same Time pretty strong, he coughs up the Matter, and is very sensibly relieved. But if this *Vomica* be large, or if its Orifice is wide, and it throws out a great Quantity of Matter at once; or if the Patient is very weak, he dies the Moment it bursts, and that sometimes when it is least expected. I have seen one Patient so circumstanced expire, as he was conveying a Spoonful of Soup to his Mouth; and another, while he was wiping his Nose. There was no present Symptom in either of these Cases, whence a Physician might suppose them likelier to die at that Instant, than for some Hours before. The *Pus*, or Matter, is commonly discharged through the Mouth after Death, and the Bodies very soon become putrified.

§ 67. We call that *Vomica* which is not burst, an *occult* or hidden, and that which is, an evident or open one. It is of considerable Importance to treat exactly and clearly of this Topic, as a great Number of Country People die of these Imposthumes, even without a Suspicion of the Cause of their Death. I had an Instance of it some Days since, in the School-master of a Village. He had an occult and very considerable *Vomica* in the left Lung, which was the Consequence

quence of an Inflammation of the Breast, that had been treated improperly at the Beginning. He seemed to me not likely to live twenty four Hours, and really died in the Night, after inexpressible Anguish.

§ 68. Whatever Distemper is included within the Breast of a living Patient, is neither an Object of the Sight or Touch; whence these *Vomicas*, these inward Tumours, are so often unknown, and indeed unsuspected. The Evacuations that were necessary for the Cure, or sometimes for the Prevention, of them, have not taken place, during the first fourteen Days. At the End of this Term, the Patient, far from being cured, is not very considerably relieved, but, on the contrary, the Fever continues to be pretty high, with a Pulse continually quick; in general soft and weak, though sometimes pretty hard, and often fluctuating, or, as it were, waving. His Breathing is still difficult and oppressed, with small cold Shudderings from Time to Time, an Exasperation of the Fever, flushed Cheeks, dry Lips, and Thirst.

The Increase of these Symptoms declare, that *Pus* or Matter is thoroughly formed: the Cough then becomes more continual; being exasperated with the least Motion, or as soon as ever the Patient has taken any Nourishment. He can repose only on the Side affected. It often happens indeed, that he cannot lie down at all; but is obliged to be set up all Day, sometimes even without daring to lean a little upon his

Loins,

Loins, for fear of increasing the Cough and Oppression. He is unable to sleep; has a continual Fever, and his Pulse frequently intermits.

The Fever is not only heightened every Evening; but the smallest Quantity of Food, the gentlest Motion, a little Coughing, the lightest Agitation of the Mind, a little more than usual Heat in the Chamber, Soup either a little too strong, or a little too salt, increase the Quickness of his Pulse the Moment they occur, or are given. He is quite restless, has some short Attacks of the most terrible Anguish, accompanied and succeeded by Sweatings on his Breast, and from his whole Countenance. He sweats sometimes the whole Night; his Urine is reddish, now frothy, and at other times oily, as it were. Sudden Flushings, hot as Flames, rise into his whole Visage. The greater Number of the Sick are commonly sensible of a most disagreeable Taste in their Mouth, some of old strong Cheese; others of rotten Eggs, and others again of stinking Meat, and fall greatly away. The Thirst of some is unquenchable, their Mouths and Lips are parched; their Voice weak and hoarse; their Eyes hollow, with a kind of Wildness in their Looks. They have a general Disgust to all Food; and if they should ask for some particular Nourishment without seeing it, they reject it the Moment it is brought them; and their Strength at length seems wholly exhausted.

Besides these Symptoms, a little Inflation, or *Bloatedness,* as it were, is sometimes observed on the

the Breaſt, towards the Side affected; with an almoſt inſenſible Change of Colour. If the *Vomica* be ſituated at the Bottom of the affected Lobe of the Lungs, and in its internal Part, that is, nearly in the Middle of the Breaſt, ſome *Puffineſs* or light Swelling may be perceived in ſome Bodies, by gently preſſing the Pit of the Stomach; eſpecially when the Patient coughs. In ſhort, according to the Obſervations of a German Phyſician, if one ſtrike the open Hand on the Breaſt, covered only with a Shirt, it retains in the Spot, which is directly oppoſite to the *Vomica*, a flat heavy Sound, as if one ſtruck a Piece of Fleſh; while in ſtriking on the other Side it gives a clear loud Sound, as from a Drum. I ſtill doubt however, whether this Obſervation will generally hold true; and it would be hazardous to affirm there is no Abſceſs in a Breaſt, which does not return this heavy Sound.

§ 69. When a *Vomica* is formed, as long as it is not emptied, all the Symptoms I have already enumerated increaſe, and the *Vomica* grows in Size: the whole Side of the Lung affected ſometimes becomes a Bag or Sac of Matter. The ſound Side is compreſſed; and the Patient dies after dreadful Anguiſh, with the Lung full of *Pus*, and without having ever brought up any.

To avoid ſuch fatal Conſequences, it is neceſſary to procure the Rupture and Diſcharge of this inward Abſceſs, as ſoon as we are certain of its Exiſtence: And as it is ſafer it ſhould break within the Lobe affected, from whence it may be be discharged by hawking up; than that it should burst and void itself into the Cavity of the Breast, for Reasons I shall give hereafter, we must endeavour, that this Rupture may be effected within the internal Substance of the Lungs.

§ 70. The most effectual Methods to procure this are, 1. To make the Patient continually receive, by his Mouth, the Vapour of warm Water. 2. When by this Means that part of the Sac or Abscess is softened, where we could wish the Rupture of it to happen, the Patient is to swallow a large Quantity of the most emollient Liquid, such as Barley Water, Almond Milk, light Veal Broth, or Milk and Water. By this Means the Stomach is kept always full: so that the Resistance to the Lungs being considerable on that Side, the Abscess and its Contents will naturally be pressed towards the Side of the Wind-pipe, as it will meet with less Resistance there. This Fulness of the Stomach will also incline the Patient to cough, which may concur to produce a good Event. Hence, 3, we should endeavour to make the Patient cough, by making him smell to some Vinegar, or even snuff up a little; or by injecting into his Throat, by the Means of a small Syringe or Pipe, such as Children make out of short Pieces of Elder-Boughs, a little Water or Vinegar. 4. He should be advised to bawl out aloud, to read loud, or to laugh heartily, all which Means contribute to burst open the Abscess, as well as those two following ones. 5. Let him take every two Hours a Soup-

Ladle of the Potion N°. 8. 6. He should be put into a Cart, or some other Carriage; but not before he has drank plentifully of such Liquors as I have just mentioned: after which the Shaking and Jolting in the Carriage have sometimes immediately procured that Rupture, or breaking of the Bag or Abscess, we wished for.

§ 71. Some Years since I saw a Country Maid Servant, who was left in a languishing Condition after an Inflammation of the Breast; without any Person's suspecting her Ailment. This Woman being put into a Cart, that was sent for a Load of Hay; one of the Wheels run violently against a Tree: she swooned away, and at the same Time brought up a great Quantity of digested Matter. She continued to bring up more; during which I was informed of her Case, and of the Accident, which effectually cured her.

A *Swiss* Officer, who served in *Piedmont*, had been in a languid State of Health for some Months; and returned home to set himself down as easily as he could, without conceiving any considerable Hopes of Recovery. Upon entering into his own Country, by the Way of *Mount Bernard*, and being obliged to go some Paces on Foot, he fell down; and remained in a Swoon above a Quarter of an Hour: during which Time he threw up a large Quantity of Matter, and found himself that very Moment very greatly relieved. I ordered him a proper Diet, and suitable Medicines: his Health became
perfectly

perfectly established; and the Preservation of his Life was principally owing to this lucky Fall.

Many Persons afflicted with a *Vomica*, faint away the very Instant it breaks. Some sharp Vinegar should be directly held to their Nose. This small Assistance is generally sufficient, where the bursting of it is not attended with such Appearances as shew it to be mortal, in which Case every Application is insignificant.

§ 72. If the sick Person was not extremely weak before the Bursting of the Abscess; if the Matter was white, and well conditioned; if the Fever abates after it; if the Anguish, Oppression and Sweats terminate, if the Cough is less violent; if the Patient is sensibly easier in his Situation or Posture; if he recovers his Sleep and Appetite; if his usual Strength returns; if the Quantity he expectorates, or brings up, becomes daily and gradually less, and if his Urine is apparently better, we may have Room to hope, that by the Assistance of these Remedies I shall immediately direct, he may be radically, compleatly cured.

§ 73 But if on the contrary; when his Strength is exhausted before the bursting of the Abscess, when the Matter is too thin and transparent, brown, green, yellow, bloody and of an offensive Smell; if the Pulse continues quick and weak, if the Patient's Appetite, Strength and Sleep do not improve, there remains no hope of a Cure, and the best Medicines are ineffectual: Nevertheless we ought to make some Tryal of them.

§ 74. They confist of the following Medicines and Regulations. 1 Give every four Hours a little Barley or Rice Cream. 2. If the Matter brought up is thick and glewy, so that it is very difficult to be loosened and discharged, give every two Hours a Soup-ladle of the Potion N°. 8, and between the giving these two, let the Patient take every half Hour a Cup of the Drink N°. 13. 3. When the Consistence of the Matter is such, that there is no Occasion for these Medicines to promote the Discharge of it, they must be omitted, tho' the same Sort and Quantity of Food are to be continued, but with the Addition of an equal Quantity of Milk; or, which would be still more beneficial, instead of this Mixture, we should give an equal Quantity of sweet Milk, taken from a good Cow, which, in such a Case, may compose the whole Nourishment of the Patient 4 He should take four Times a Day, beginning early in the Morning, and at the Distance of two Hours, a Dose of the Powder N°. 14, diluted in a little Water, or made into a *Bolus*, or Morsel, with a little Syrup or Honey. His common Drink should be Almond Emulsion, commonly called Almond Milk, or Barley Water, or fresh Water with a fourth part Milk 5. He should air and exercise every Day on Horseback, or in a Carriage, according as his Strength and his Circumstances will allow him. But of all Sorts of Exercise, that upon a trotting Horse is, beyond all Comparison, the very best, and the easiest to be procured by every Body;

provided

provided the Disease be not too far advanced, since in such a Situation, any Exercise, that was only a little violent, might prove pernicious.

§ 75. The Multitude, who are generally illiterate, seldom consider any thing as a Remedy, except they swallow it. They have but little Confidence in *Regimen*, or any Assistance in the Way of Diet, and consider Riding on Horseback as wholly useless to them. This is a dangerous Mistake, of which I should be glad to undeceive them: since this Assistance, which appears so insignificant to them, is probably the most effectual of any: it is that in Fact, without which they can scarcely expect a Cure, in the highest Degrees of this Disease: it is that, which perhaps alone may recover them, provided they take no improper Food. In brief it is considered, and with Reason, as the real Specific for this Disease

§ 76 The Influence of the Air is of more Importance in this Disorder, than in any others; for which Reason great Care should be taken to procure the best, in the Patient's Chamber. For this Purpose it should often be ventilated, or have an Admission of fresh Air, and be sweetened from Time to Time, tho' very lightly, with a little good Vinegar; and in the Season it should be plentifully supplied with agreeable Herbs, Flowers and Fruits. Should the Sick be unfortunately situated, and confined in an unwholsome Air, there can be but little Prospect of curing him, without altering it.

§ 77. Out of many Persons affected with these Disorders, some have been cured by taking nothing whatsoever but Butter-milk; others by Melons and Cucumbers only; and others again by Summer Fruits of every Sort. Nevertheless, as such Cases are singular, and have been but few, I advise the Patient to observe the Method I have directed here, as the surest.

§ 78. It is sufficient if he have a Stool once in two, or even in three, Days. Hence, there is no Reason for him, in this Case, to accustom himself to Glysters; they might excite a Looseness, which may be very dangerous.

§ 79. When the Discharge of the Matter from the Breast diminishes, and the Patient is perceivably mended in every Respect, it is a Proof that the Wound in the Abscess is deterged, or clean, and that it is disposed to heal up gradually. If the Suppuration, or Discharge, continues in great Quantity, if it seems but of an indifferent Consistence, if the Fever returns every Evening, it may be apprehended, that the Wound, instead of healing, may degenerate into an Ulcer, which must prove a most embarrassing Consequence. Under such a Circumstance, the Patient would fall into a confirmed Hectic, and die after some Months Sickness.

§ 80. I am not acquainted with any better Remedy, in such a dangerous Case, than a Perseverance in those already directed, and especially in moderate Exercise on Horseback. In some of them indeed Recourse may be had to the sweet

Vapours

Of an Inflammation of the Breast.

Vapours of some vulnerary Herbs in hot Water, with a little Oil of Turpentine, as directed N°. 15. I have seen them succeed; but the safest Way is to consult a Physician, who may examine and consider, if there is not some particular Circumstance combined with the Disease, that proves an Obstacle to the Cure of it. If the Cough prevents the Patient from Sleeping, he may take in the Evening two or three Table Spoonfuls of the Prescription N°. 16, in a Glass of Almond Milk or Barley Water.

§ 81. The very same Causes which suddenly suppress the Expectoration, in an Inflammation of the Breast, may also check the Expectoration from a *Vomica* already begun: in which Circumstance the Patient is speedily afflicted with an Oppression and Anguish, a Fever and evident Feebleness. We should immediately endeavour to remove this Stoppage, by the Vapour of hot Water, by giving a Spoonful of the Mixture N°. 3 every Hour; by a large Quantity of the Ptisan N°. 12, and by a proper Degree of Motion or Exercise. As soon as ever the Expectoration returns, the Fever and the other Symptoms disappear. I have seen this Suppression in strong Habits quickly followed with an Inflammation about the Seat of the *Vomica*, which has obliged me to bleed, after which the Expectoration immediately returned.

§ 82 It happens sometimes, that the *Vomica* is entirely cleansed; the Expectoration is entirely finished,

finished, or drained off, the Patient seems well, and thinks himself compleatly cured: but soon after, the Uneasiness, Oppression, Cough and Fever are renewed, because the Membrane or Bag of the *Vomica* fills again: again it empties itself, the Patient expectorates for some Days, and seems to recover. After some Time however, the same Scene is repeated; and this Vicissitude, or Succession, of moderate and of bad Health, often continues for some Months and even some Years. This happens when the *Vomica* is emptied, and is gradually deterged; so that its Membranes, or Sides touch or approach each other, but without cicatrizing or healing firmly, and then there drops or leaks in very gradually fresh Matter. For a few Days this seems no ways to incommode the Patient; but as soon as a certain Quantity is accumulated, he is visited again with some of the former Symptoms, 'till another Evacuation ensues. People thus circumstanced, in this Disease, sometimes appear to enjoy a tolerable Share of Health. It may be considered as a kind of internal Issue, which empties and cleanses itself from Time to Time, pretty frequently in some Constitutions, more slowly in others; and under which some may attain a good middling Age. When it arrives however at a very considerable Duration, it proves incurable. In its earliest State, it gives way sometimes to a Milk-diet, to riding on Horseback, and to the Medicine N°. 14.

§ 83

§ 83. Some may be surprized, that in treating of an Abscess of the Lungs, and of the Hectic, which is a Consequence of it, I say nothing of those Remedies, commonly termed *Balsamics*, and so frequently employed in them, for Instance, Turpentines, Balsam of Peru, of Mecca, Frankincense, Mastich, Myrrh, Storax and Balsam of Sulphur. I shall however say briefly here (because it is equally my Design to destroy the Prejudice of the People, in favour of improper Medicines, and to establish the Reputation of good ones) that I never in such Cases made use of these Medicines; because I am convinced, that their Operation is generally hurtful in such Cases, because I see them daily productive of real Mischief; that they protract the Cure, and often change a slight Disorder into an incurable Disease. They are incapable of perfect Digestion, they obstruct the finest Vessels of the Lungs, whose Obstructions we should endeavour to remove; and evidently occasion, except their Dose be extremely small, Heat and Oppression. I have very often seen to a Demonstration, that Pills compounded of Myrrh, Turpentine and Balsam of Peru, have, an Hour after they were swallowed, occasioned a Tumult and Agitation in the Pulse, high Flushings, Thirst and Oppression. In short it is demonstrable to every unprejudiced Person, that these Remedies, as they have been called, are truly prejudicial in this Case, and I heartily wish People may be disabused with Respect to them, and that they may lose that Reputation so unhappily ascribed to them.

I know that many Persons, very capable in other Respects, daily make use of them in these Distempers: such however cannot fail of disusing them, as soon as they shall have observed their Effects, abstracted from the Virtues of the other Medicines to which they add them, and which mitigate the Danger of them. I saw a Patient, whom a foreign Surgeon, who lived at *Orbe*, attempted to cure of a Hectic with melted Bacon, which aggravated the Disease. This Advice seemed, and certainly was, absurd; nevertheless the Balsamics ordered in such Cases are probably not more digestible than fat Bacon. The Powder N°. 14 possesses whatever these Balsamics pretend to; it is attended with none of the Inconveniencies they produce; and has all the good Qualites ascribed to them. Notwithstanding which, it must not be given while the Inflammation exists, nor when it may revive again, and no other Aliment should be mixed with the Milk.

The famous Medicine called the *Antihectic*, (*Aut Hecticum Poterii*) has not, any more than these Balsamics, the Virtues ascribed to it in such Cases. I very often give it in some obstinate Coughs to Infants with their Milk, and then it is very useful: but I have seldom seen it attended with considerable Effects in grown Persons, and in the present Cases I should be fearful of its doing Mischief.

§ 82. If the *Vomica*, instead of breaking within

in the Substance of the Lungs affected, should break without it, the Pus must be received into the Cavity of the Breast. We know when that has happened, by the Sensation or Feeling of the Patient, who perceives an uncommon, a singular kind of Movement, pretty generally accompanied with a Fainting. The Oppression and Anguish cease at once; the Fever abates, the Cough however commonly continues, tho' with less Violence, and without any Expectoration. But this seeming Amendment is of a short Duration, since from the daily Augmentation of the Matter, and its becoming more acrid or sharp, the Lungs become oppressed, irritated and eroded. The Difficulty of Breathing, Heat, Thirst, Wakefulness, Distaste, and Deafness, return, with many other Symptoms unnecessary to be enumerated, and especially with frequent Sinkings and Weakness. The Patient should be confined to his *Regimen*, to retard the Increase of the Disease as much as possible, notwithstanding no other effectual Remedy remains, except that of opening the Breast between two of the Ribs, to discharge the Matter, and to stop the Disorder it occasions. This is called the Operation for the *Empyema* I shall not describe it here, as it should not be undertaken but by Persons of Capacity and Experience, for whom this Treatise was not intended. I would only observe, it is less painful than terrifying, and that if it is delayed too long, it proves useless, and the Patient dies miserably

§ 85. We may daily see external Inflammations

mations turn gangrenous, or mortify. The same Thing occurs in the Lungs, when the Fever is excessive, the Inflammation either in its own Nature, extremely violent, or raised to such a Height by hot Medicines. Intolerable Anguish, extreme Weakness, frequent Faintings, Coldness of the Extremities, a livid and fœtid thin Humour brought up instead of concocted Spitting, and sometimes blackish Stripes on the Breast, sufficiently distinguish this miserable State. I have smelt in one Case of this Kind, where the Patient had been attacked with this Disease (after a forced March on Foot, having taken some Wine with Spices to force a Sweat) his Breath so horribly stinking, that his Wife had many Sinkings from attending him. When I saw him, I could discern neither Pulse nor Intellect, and ordered him nothing. He died an Hour afterwards, about the Beginning of the third Hour.

§ 86 An Inflammation may also become hard, when it forms what we call a *Scirrhus*, which is a very hard Tumour, indolent, or unpainful. This is known to occur, when the Disease is not terminated in any of those Manners I have represented; and where, tho' the Fever and the other Symptoms disappear, the Respiration, or Breathing, remains always a little oppressed; the Patient still retains a troublesome Sensation in one Side of his Breast, and has from Time to Time a dry Cough, which increases after Exercise, and after eating. This Malady is but seldom cured, though some Persons attacked with it last many Years,

Years, without any other confiderable Complaint. They fhould avoid all Occafions of over-heating themfelves; which might readily produce a new Inflammation about this Tumour, the Confequences of which would be highly dangerous.

§ 87. The beft Remedies againft this Diforder, and from which I have feen fome good Effects, are the medicated Whey N°. 17, and the Pills N°. 18. The Patient may take twenty Pills, and a Pint and a half of the Whey every Morning for a long Continuance; and receive inwardly, now and then, the Vapour of hot Water.

§ 88. Each Lung, in a perfect State of Health, touches the *Pleura*, the Membrane, that lines the Infide of the Breaft; though it is not connected to it. But it often happens, after an Inflammation of the Breaft, after the Pleurify, and in fome other Cafes, that thefe two Parts adhere clofely to each other, and are never afterwards feparated. However this is fcarcely to be confidered as a Difeafe; and remains commonly unknown, as the Health is not impaired by it, and nothing is ever prefcribed to remove it. Neverthelefs I have feen a few Cafes, in which this Adhefion was manifeftly prejudicial.

Chapter V.

Of the Pleurisy.

Sect. 89

THE Pleurisy, which is chiefly known by these four Symptoms, a strong Fever, a Difficulty of Breathing, a Cough, and an acute Pain about the Breast, the Pleurisy, I say, is not a different Malady from the Peripneumony, or Inflammation of the Breast, the Subject of the preceding Chapter; so that I have very little to say of it, particularly, or apart.

§ 90. The Cause of this Disease then is exactly the same with that of the former, that is, an Inflammation of the Lungs, but an Inflammation, that seems rather a little more external. The only considerable Difference in the Symptoms is, that the Pleurisy is accompanied with a most acute Pain under the Ribs, and which is commonly termed a *Stitch*. This Pain is felt indifferently over every Part of the Breast; though more commonly about the Sides, under the more fleshy Parts of the Breast, and oftenest on the right Side. The Pain is greatly increased whenever the Patient coughs or draws in the Air in breathing, and hence a Fear of increasing it,

by

by making some Patients forbear to cough or respire, as much as they possibly can, and that aggravates the Disease, by stopping the Course of the Blood in the Lungs, which are soon overcharged with it. Hence the Inflammation of this Bowel becomes general, the Blood mounts up to the Head, the Countenance looks deeply red, or as it were livid, the Patient becomes nearly suffocated, and falls into the State described § 47

Sometimes the Pain is so extremely violent, that if the Cough is very urgent at the same Time, and the Sick cannot suppress or restrain it, they are seized with Convulsions, of which I have seen many Instances, but these occur almost always to Women, though they are much less subject than Men to this Disease, and indeed to all inflammatory ones. It may be proper however to observe here, that if Women should be attacked with it, during their monthly Discharges, that Circumstance should not prevent the repeated and necessary Bleedings, nor occasion any Alteration in the Treatment of the Disease. And hence it appears, that the Pleurisy is really an Inflammation of the Lungs, accompanied with acute Pain

§ 91 I am sensible that sometimes an Inflammation of the Lungs is communicated also to that Membrane, which lines the Inside of the Breast; and which is called the *Pleura*, and from thence to the Muscles, the fleshy Parts, over and between the

the Ribs. This however is not very frequently the Case.

§ 92. Spring is commonly the Season most productive of Pleurisies: in general there are few in Summer: notwithstanding that in the Year 1762, there were a great many during the hottest Season, which then was excessively so. The Disease usually begins with a violent Shivering, succeeded by considerable Heat, with a Cough, an Oppression, and sometimes with a sensible Straitning, or Contraction, as it were, all over the Breast, and also with a Head-ach, a Redness of the Cheeks, and with Reachings to vomit. The Stitch does not always happen at the very first Onset, often not 'till after several Hours from the first Complaint, sometimes not before the second, or even the third Day. Sometimes the Patient feels two Stitches, in different Parts of the Side; though it seldom happens that they are equally sharp, and the lightest soon ceases. Sometimes also the Stitch shifts its Place, which promises well, if the Part first attacked by it continues perfectly free from Pain: but it has a bad Appearance, if, while the first is present, another also supervenes, and both continue. The Pulse is usually very hard in this Distemper; but in the dreadful Cases described § 47 and 90, it becomes soft and small. There often occur at, or very quickly after, the Invasion, such an Expectoration, or hawking up, as happens in an Inflammation of the Breast, at other Times there is not the least

least Appearance of it, whence such are named dry Pleurisies, which happen pretty often. Sometimes the Sick cough but little, or not at all. They often lie more at Ease upon the Side affected, than on the sound one. The Progress of this Disease advances exactly like that described in the preceding Chapter: for how can they differ considerably? and the Treatment of both is the same. Large Hæmorrhages, or Bleedings from the Nose, frequently happen, to the great Relief of the Patient, but sometimes such Discharges consist of a kind of corrupted Blood, when the Patient is very ill, and these portend Death.

§ 93. This Distemper is often produced by drinking cold Water, while a Person is hot; from which Cause it is sometimes so violent, as to kill the Patient in three Hours. A young Man was found dead at the Side of the Spring, from which he had quenched his Thirst: neither indeed is it uncommon for Pleurisies to prove mortal within three Days.

Sometimes the Stitch disappears, whence the Patient complains less, but at the same Time his Countenance changes; he grows pale and sad; his Eyes look dull and heavy, and his Pulse grows feeble. This signifies a Translation of the Disease to the Brain, a Case which is almost constantly fatal.

There is no Disease in which the critical Symptoms are more violent, and more strongly marked, than in this. It is proper this should be be known, as it may prevent or lessen our excessive Terror. A perfect Cure supervenes sometimes, at the very Moment when Death was expected.

§ 94. This Malady is one of the most common and the most destroying kind, as well from its own violent Nature, as through the pernicious Treatment of it in Country Places. That Prejudice, which insists on curing all Diseases by Sweating, entirely regulates their Conduct in treating a Pleurisy; and as soon as a Person is afflicted with a Stitch, all the hot Medicines are immediately set to Work. This mortal Error destroys more People than Gunpowder; and it is by so much the more hurtful, as the Distemper is of the most violent kind; and because, as there is commonly not a Moment to be lost, the whole depends on the Method immediately recurred to.

§ 95. The proper Manner of treating this Disease, is exactly the same in all Respects, with that of the Peripneumony, because, I again affirm, it is the very same Disease. Hence the Bleedings, the softening and diluting Drinks, the Steams, the Glysters, the Potion N°. 8, and the emollient Poultices are the real Remedies. These last perhaps are still more effectual in the Pleurisy, and therefore they should be continually applied over the very Stitch.

The first Bleeding, especially if there has been a considerable Discharge, almost constantly abates the Stitch, and often entirely removes it: though it more commonly returns, after an Intermission of some Hours, either in the same Spot, or sometimes in another. This shifting of it is rather favourable, especially if the Pain, that was first felt under the Breast, shifts into the Shoulders, to the Back, the Shoulder-blade, or the Nape of the Neck.

When the Stitch is not at all abated, or only a little; or if, after having abated, it returns as violently as at first, and especially if it returns in the same Spot, and the Height of the other Symptoms continue, Bleeding must be repeated. But if a sensible Abatement of the Stitch continues; and if, though it returns, it should be in a smaller Degree, and by Intervals, or in these Places I have mentioned above; if the Quickness, or the Hardness of the Pulse, and all the other Symptoms are sensibly diminished, this repeated Bleeding may sometimes be omitted. Nevertheless, in a very strong Subject, it seems rather prudent not to omit it, since in such Circumstances it can do no Mischief; and a considerable Hazard may sometimes be incurred by the Omission. In very high and dangerous Pleurisies a frequent Repetition of bleeding is necessary; except some Impediment to it should arise from the particular Constitution of the Patient, or from his Age, or some other Circumstances.

If, from the Beginning of the Disease, the Pulse is but a little quicker and harder than in a healthy State; if it is not manifestly strong; if the Head-ach and the Stitch are so moderate as to prove supportable; if the Cough is not too violent; if there is no sensible Oppression or Straitness, and the Patient expectorate, or cough up, Bleeding may be omitted.

With Respect to the administering of other Remedies, the same Directions are to be exactly followed, which have been already given in the preceding Chapter, to which the Reader is referred from § 53 to 66.

§ 96. When the Disease is not very acute and pressing, I have often cured it in a very few Days by a single Bleeding, and a large Quantity of a Tea or Infusion of Elder-flowers, sweetened with Honey. It is in some Cases of this kind, that we often find the Water *Faltranc* succeed, with the Addition of some Honey, and even of Oil: though the Drink I have just directed is considerably preferable. That Drink which is compounded of equal Quantities of Wine and Water, with the Addition of much Venice Treacle, annually destroys a great Number of People in the Country.

§ 97. In those dry Pleurisies, in which the Stitch, the Fever, and the Head-ach are strong and violent, and where the Pulse is very hard and very full, with an excessive Dryness of the Skin and of the Tongue, Bleeding should be frequently repeated, and at small Intervals from each other. This Method frequently cures the Disease effectually, without using any other Evacuation.

§ 98. The Pleurisy terminates, like any other inward Inflammation, either by some Evacuation; by an Abscess; in a Mortification; or in a Scirrhosity or hard Tumour; and it often leaves Adhesions in the Breast.

The Gangrene or Mortification sometimes appears on the third Day, without having been preceded by very vehement Pains. In such Cases the dead Body often looks very black, especially in the Parts near the Seat of the Disease; and in such the more superstitious ascribe it to some supernatural Cause; or draw some unhappy Presage from it, with Respect to those who are yet unattacked by it. This Appearance however is purely a natural Consequence, quite simple, and cannot be otherwise; and the hot Regimen and Medicines are the most prevailing Causes of it. I have seen it thus circumstanced in a Man in the Flower of his Age, who had taken Venice Treacle in Cherry Water, and the Ingredients of *Faltranc* infused in Wine.

§ 99 *Vomicas* are sometimes the Consequences of Pleurisies; but their particular Situation disposes them more to break * outwardly, which is the most frequent Cause of an *Empyema* § 84.
" To prevent this, it is highly proper to apply,
" at the first Invasion of the Disease, to the Spot
" where the Pain chiefly rages, a small Plaister,
" which may exactly fit it, since if the Pleurisy
" should terminate in an Abscess or Imposthume,

---

* That is, into the Cavity of the Breast, rather than within the Substance of the Lungs.

"the purulent Matter will be determined to that
"Side

"As soon then as it is foreseen that an Abscess
"is forming (see § 68) we should erode, by a
"light Caustic, the Place where it is expected;
"and as soon as it is removed, Care should be
"taken to promote Suppuration there. By this
"Means we may entertain a reasonable Hope,
"that the Mass of Matter will incline its Course
"to that Spot, where it will meet with the least
"Resistance, and be discharged from thence.
"For this Heap of Matter is often accumulated
"between the *Pleura*, and the Parts which ad-
"here to it."

This is the Advice of a very * great Physician;
but I must inform the Reader, there are many
Cases, in which it can be of no Service; neither
ought it to be attempted, but by Persons of un-
doubted Abilities.

With Regard to the Scirrhosity, or Hardness,
and to the Circumstances of Adhesions, I can add
nothing to what I have said in § 86 and 87.

§ 100. It has been observed that some Persons, who have been once attacked by this Disease, are often liable to Relapses of it, especially
such as drink hard. I knew one Man, who
reckoned up his Pleurisies by Dozens. A few
Bleedings, at certain proper Intervals, might prevent these frequent Returns of it; which, joined

to

---

* This is, undoubtedly, Baron *Van Swieten*, with whom he
has permised, re agreed considerably, in all the Diseases they
have took treated of   K

to their excessive Drinking, make them languid and stupid, in the very Flower of their Age. They generally fall into some Species of an Asthma, and from that into a Dropsy, which proves the melancholy, though not an improper, Conclusion of their Lives. Such as can confine themselves to some proper Precautions, may also prevent these frequent Returns of this Disease, even without bleeding; by a temperate Regimen; by abstaining from Time to Time, from eating Flesh and drinking Wine; at which Times they should drink Whey, or some of those Diet-Drinks N°. 1. 2. 4; and by bathing their Legs sometimes in warm Water; especially in those Seasons, when this Disease is the most likely to return.

§. 101. Two Medicines greatly esteemed in this Disease among the Peasantry, and even extolled by some Physicians, are the Blood of a wild He Goat, and the * Soot in an Egg. I do not contest the Cure or Recovery of many Persons, who have taken these Remedies; notwithstanding it is not less true, that both of them, as well as the Egg in which the Soot is taken, are dangerous. For which Reason it is prudent, at least, never to make use of them; as there is great Probability, they may do a little Mischief; and a Certainty that they can do no Good. The

Gempi,

---

* This, with great Probability, means that small black Substance often visible in a rotten Egg, which is undoubtedly of a violent, or even poisonous Quality. Dr *Tissot* terms it expressly —*la suie dans un Oeuf.*

Genipi, or † Wormwood of the Alps, has also acquired great Reputation in this Disease, and occasioned many Disputes between some very zealous Ecclesiastics, and a justly celebrated Physician. It seems not difficult however to ascertain the proper Use of it. This Plant is a powerful Bitter, it heats and excites Sweat: it seems clear, that, from such Consequences, it should never be employed in a Pleurisy, while the Vessels are full, the Pulse hard, the Fever high, and the Blood inflamed. In all such Circumstances it must aggravate the Disease; but towards the Conclusion of it, when the Vessels are considerably emptied, the Blood is diluted, and the Fever abated, it may then be recurred to; but with a constant Recollection that it is hot, and not to be employed without Reflection and Prudence (a)

† Dr *Lewis*, who has not taken Notice of this Species of Wormwood in his Improvement of *Quincy*'s Dispensatory, has mentioned it in his late *Materia Medica* K.

(a) This being a proper Place for directing the Seneka Rattle Snake Root, I shall observe, that the best Way of exhibiting it is in Decoction, by gradually simmering and boiling two Ounces of it in gross Powder, in two Pints and a half of Water, to a Pint and a quarter; and then giving three Spoonfuls of it to a grown Person, every six Hours. If the Stitch should continue, or return, after taking it, Bleeding, which should be premised to it, must be occasionally repeated, though it seldom proves necessary, after a few Doses of it. It greatly promotes Expectoration, keeps the Body gently open, and sometimes operates by Urine and by Sweat, very seldom proving at all emetic in Decoction. The Regimen of Drinks directed here in Pleurisies are to be given as usual. Dr *Tennent*, the Introducer of this valuable Medicine, confided solely in it, in Bastard Peripneumonies, without Bleeding, Blistering, or any other Medicines K.

CHAP-

CHAPTER VI.

Of the Diseases of the Throat.

SECT. 102.

THE Throat is subject to many Diseases: One of the most frequent and the most dangerous, is that Inflammation of it, commonly termed a Quinsey. This in Effect is a Distemper of the same Nature with an Inflammation of the Breast; but as it occurs in a different Part, the Symptoms, of Course, are very different. They also vary, not a very little, according to the different Parts of the Throat which are inflamed.

§ 103. The general Symptoms of an Inflammation of the Throat are, the Shivering, the subsequent Heat, the Fever, the Head-ach, red high-coloured Urine, a considerable Difficulty, and sometimes even an Impossibility, of swallowing any thing whatever. But if the nearest Parts to the *Glottis*, that is, of the Entrance into the Windpipe, or Conduit through which we breathe, are attacked, Breathing becomes excessively difficult; the Patient is sensible of extreme Anguish, and great Approaches to Suffocation, the Disease is then extended to the *Glottis*, to the Body of the Wind-pipe, and even to the Substance of the Lungs, whence it becomes speedily fatal.

The Inflammation of the other Parts is attended with less Danger; and this Danger becomes still less, as the Disease is more extended to the outward and superficial Parts. When the Inflammation is general, and seizes all the internal Parts of the Throat, and particularly the Tonsils or Almonds, as they are called, the *Uvula*, or Process of the Palate, and the *Basis*, or remotest deepest Part of the Tongue, it is one of the most dangerous and dreadful Maladies. The Face is then swelled up and inflamed; the whole Inside of the Throat is in the same Condition; the Patient can get nothing down; he breathes with a Pain and Anguish, which concur, with a Stuffing or Obstruction in his Brains, to throw him into a kind of furious *Delirium*, or Rave. His Tongue is bloated up, and is extended out of his Mouth; his Nostrils are dilated, as tho' it were to assist him in his Breathing; the whole Neck, even to the Beginning of the Breast, is excessively tumified or swelled up; the Pulse is very quick, very weak, and often intermits; the miserable Patient is deprived of all his Strength, and commonly dies the second or third Day. Very fortunately this Kind, or Degree of it, which I have often seen in *Languedoc*, happens very rarely in *Switzerland*, where the Disease is less violent; and where I have only seen People die of it, in Consequence of its being

ing perniciously treated; or by Reason of some accidental Circumstances, which were foreign to the Disease itself. Of the Multitude of Patients I have attended in this Disorder, I have known but one to fail under it, whose Case I shall mention towards the Close of this Chapter.

§ 104. Sometimes the Disease shifts from the internal to the external Parts: the Skin of the Neck and Breast grows very red, and becomes painful, but the Patient finds himself better.

At other Times the Disorder quits the Throat; but is transferred to the Brain, or upon the Lungs. Both these Translations of it are mortal, when the best Advice and Assistance cannot be immediately procured; and it must be acknowledged, that even the best are often ineffectual.

§ 105. The most usual kind of this Disease is that which affects only the Tonsils (the Almonds) and the Palate, or rather its Process, *commonly called* the Palate. It generally first invades one of the Tonsils, which becomes enlarged, red and painful, and does not allow the afflicted to swallow, but with great Pain. Sometimes the Disorder is confined to one Side, but most commonly it is extended to the *Uvula*, (the Palate) from whence it is extended to the other Tonsil. If it be of a mild kind, the Tonsil first affected is generally better, when the second is attacked. Whenever they are both affected at once, the Pain and the Anguish of the Patient are very considerable, he cannot swallow, but with great Difficulty and Complaint, and the Torment of

this

this is so vehement, that I have seen Women affected with Convulsions, as often as they endeavoured to swallow their Spittle, or any other Liquid. They continue, even for several Hours sometimes, unable to take any thing whatever, all the upper inward Part of the Mouth, the Bottom of the Palate, and the descending Part of the Tongue become lightly red, or inflamed.

A considerable Proportion of Persons under this Disease swallow Liquids more difficultly than Solids, by Reason that Liquids require a greater Action of some Part of the Muscles, in order to their being properly directed into their Conduit or Chanel. The Deglutition (the Swallowing) of the Spittle is attended with still more Uneasiness than that of other Liquids, because it is a little more thick and viscid, and flows down with less Ease. This Difficulty of swallowing, joined to the Quantity thence accumulated, produces that almost continual hawking up, which oppresses some Patients so much the more, as the Inside of their Cheeks, their whole Tongue, and their Lips are often galled, and even flead as it were. This also prevents their Sleeping, which however seems no considerable Evil, Sleep being *sometimes* but of little Service in Diseases attended with a Fever, and I have often seen those, who thought their Throats almost entirely well in the Evening, and yet found them very bad after some Hours Sleep.

The Fever, in this Species of the Disease, is sometimes very high, and the Shivering often endures

endures for many Hours. It is succeeded by considerable Heat, and a violent Head-ach, which yet is sometimes attended with a Drowsiness. The Fever is commonly pretty high in the Evening, though sometimes but inconsiderable, and by the Morning perhaps there is none at all.

A light Invasion of this Disease of the Throat often precedes the Shivering; though most commonly it does not become manifest 'till after it, and at the same Time when the Heat comes on.

The Neck is sometimes a little inflated, or puffed up; and many of the Sick complain of a pretty smart Pain in the Ear of that Side, which is most affected. I have but very seldom observed that they had it in both.

§ 106. The Inflammation either disappears by Degrees, or an Abscess is formed in the Part which was chiefly affected. It has never happened, at least within my Knowledge, that this Sort of the Disease, prudently treated, has ever terminated either in a Mortification, or a Scirrhus: but I have been a Witness to either of these supervening, when Sweating was extorted in the Beginning of it, by hot Medicines.

It is also very rare to meet with those highly dangerous Translations of this Disease upon the Lungs, such as are described in that Species of it from § 103, 104. It is true indeed it does not occur more frequently, even in that Species, whenever the Disease is thrown out upon the more external Parts.

§ 107.

§ 107. The Treatment of the Quinfey, as well as of all other inflammatory Difeafes, is the fame with that of an Inflammation of the Breaft.

The Sick is immediately to be put upon a Regimen; and in that Sort defcribed § 103, Bleeding muft be repeated four or five Times within a few Hours; and fometimes there is a Neceffity to recur ftill oftner to it. When it affaults the Patient in the moft vehement Degree, all Medicines, all Means, are very generally ineffectual; they fhould be tried however. We fhould give as much as can be taken of the Drinks N°. 2 and 4. But as the Quantity they are able to fwallow is often very inconfiderable; the Glyfter N°. 5 fhould be repeated every three Hours; and then Legs fhould be put into a Bath of warm Water, thrice a Day.

§ 108. Cupping Glaffes, with Scarification, applied about the Neck, after bleeding twice or thrice, have often been experienced to be highly ufeful. In the moft defperate Cafes, when the Neck is exceffively fwelled, one or two deep Incifions made with a Razor, on this external Tumour, have fometimes faved a Patient's Life.

§ 109 In that kind, and thofe Circumftances, of this Difeafe defcribed § 105 we muft have very frequent Recourfe to Bleeding, and it fhould never be omitted, when the Pulfe is very perceivably hard and full. It is of the utmoft Confequence to do it inftantaneoufly, fince it is the only Means to prevent the Abfcefs, which forms very readily, if Bleeding has been neglected, only for a few Hours. Sometimes it is neceſſary to repeat it a ſecond Time, but very rarely a third.

This Diſeaſe is frequently ſo gentle and mild, as to be cured without Bleeding, by the Means of much good Management. But as many as are not Maſters of their own Time, nor in ſuch an eaſy Situation, as to be properly attended, ought, without the leaſt Heſitation, to be bled directly, which is ſometimes ſufficient to remove the Complaint; eſpecially if, after Bleeding, the Patient drinks plentifully of the Ptiſan Nº. 2

In this light Degree of the Diſeaſe, it may ſuffice to bathe the Legs, and to receive a Glyſter, once a Day each; the firſt to be uſed in the Morning, and the laſt in the Evening. Beſides the general Remedies againſt Inflammations, a few particular ones, calculated preciſely for this Diſeaſe, may be applied in each kind or Degree of it. The beſt are, firſt the emollient Poultices, Nº. 9, laid over the whole Neck. (1) Some have highly extolled the Application of Swallows Neſts in this Diſeaſe; and though I make no Objection to it, I think it certainly leſs efficacious than any of thoſe which I direct.

2 Of the Gargariſms (Nº 19) a great Variety may be prepared, of pretty much the ſame Properties, and of equal Efficacy. Thoſe I direct

---

(1) The *Engliſh* avail themſelves conſiderably, in this Diſeaſe, of a Mixture of equal Parts of Sallad Oil, and Spirit of Sal Ammoniac, or of Oil and Spirit of Hartſhorn, as a Liniment and Application round the Neck. This Remedy correſponds with many Indications, and deſerves perhaps, the firſt Place amongſt local Applications againſt the inflammatory Quinſey

rect here are what have succeeded best with me; and they are very simple. (2)

3. The Steam of hot Water, as directed § 55, should be repeated five or six Times a Day; a Poultice should be constantly kept on, and often renewed; and the Patient should often gargle.

There are some Persons, besides Children, who cannot gargle themselves. and in fact the Pain occasioned by it makes it the more difficult. In such a Case, instead of gargling, the same Gargarism (N°. 19) may be injected with a small Syringe. The Injection reaches further than Gargling, and often causes the Patient to hawk up a considerable Quantity of glarey Matter (which has grown still thicker towards the Bottom of the Throat) to his sensible Relief. This Injection should be often repeated. The little hollowed Pipes of Elder Wood, which all the Children in the Country can make, may be conveniently employed for this Purpose. The Patient should breath out, rather than inspire, during the Injection.

§ 110. Whenever the Disease terminates without Suppuration, the Fever, the Head-ach, the Heat in the Throat, and the Pain in swallowing, begin to abate from the fourth Day, sometimes from the third, often only from the fifth; and from such Period that Abatement increases at a great

---

(2) Dr *Pringle* is apprehensive of some ill Effects from Acids in Gargarisms [which is probably from their supposed repelling Properties] and prefers a Decoction of Figs in Milk and Water, to which he adds a small Quantity of Spirit of Sal Ammoniac

a great Rate; so that at the End of two, three, or four Days, on the sixth, seventh, or eighth, the Patient is entirely well. Some few however continue to feel a light Degree of Pain, and that only on one Side, four or five Days longer, but without a Fever, or any considerable Uneasiness.

§ 111. Sometimes the Fever and the other Symptoms abate, after the Bleeding and other Remedies, without any subsequent Amendment in the Throat, or any Signs of Suppuration. In such Cases we must chiefly persist in the Gargarisms and the Steams; and where an experienced and dexterous Surgeon can be procured, it were proper he should scarify the inflamed Tonsils. These discharge, in such Cases, a moderate Quantity of Blood; and this Evacuation relieves, very readily, as many as make use of it.

§ 112. If the Inflammation is no ways disposed to disperse, so that an Abscess is forming, which almost ever happens, if it has not been obviated at the Invasion of the Disease; then the Symptoms attending the Fever continue, though raging a little less after the fourth Day: the Throat continues red, but of a less florid and lively Redness: a Pain also continues, though less acute, accompanied sometimes with Pulsations, and at other Times intirely without any; of which it is proper to take Notice: the Pulse commonly grows a little softer; and on the fifth or sixth Day, and sometimes sooner, the Abscess is ready to break. This may be discovered by the Appearance of a

small

small white and soft Tumour, when the Mouth is open, which commonly appears about the Centre or Middle of the Inflammation. It bursts of itself; or, should it not, it must be opened. This is effected by strongly securing a Lancet to one End of a small Stick or Handle, and enveloping, or wrapping up the whole Blade of it, except the Point and the Length of one fourth or a third of an Inch, in some Folds of soft Linnen; after which the Abscess is pierced with the Point of this Lancet. The Instant it is opened, the Mouth is filled with the Discharge of a Quantity of *Pus*, of the most intolerable Savour and Smell. The Patient should gargle himself after the Discharge of it with the detersive, or cleansing Gargarism N°. 19. It is surprising sometimes to see the Quantity of Matter discharged from this Imposthumation. In general there is but one; though sometimes I have seen two of them.

§ 113. It happens, and not seldom, that the Matter is not collected exactly in the Place, where the Inflammation appeared, but in some less exposed and less visible Place: whence a Facility of swallowing is almost entirely restored, the Fever abates; the Patient sleeps, he imagines he is cured, and that no Inconvenience remains, but such as ordinarily occurs in the earliest Stage of Recovery. A Person who is neither a Physician, nor a Surgeon, may easily deceive himself, when in this State. But the following Signs may enable him to discover that there is an Abscess, viz. A certain Inquietude and general Uneasiness, a

Pain

Pain throughout the Mouth, some Shiverings from Time to Time, frequently sharp, but short and transient, Heat: a Pulse moderately soft, but not in a natural State; a Sensation of Thickness and Heaviness in the Tongue, small white Eruptions on the Gums, on the Inside of the Cheek, on the Inside and Outside of the Lips, and a disagreeable Taste and Odour.

§ 114. In such Cases Milk or warm Water should frequently be retained in the Mouth; the Vapour of hot Water should be conveyed into it; and emollient Cataplasms may be applied about the Neck. All these Means concur to the softening and breaking of the Abscess. The Finger may also be introduced to feel for its Situation; and when discovered, the Surgeon may easily open it. I happened once to break one under my Finger, without having made the least Effort to do it. Warm Water may be injected pretty forcibly, either by the Mouth or the Nostrils: this sometimes occasions a kind of Cough, or certain Efforts which tend to break it. I have seen this happen even from laughing. As to the rest, the Patient should not be too anxious or uneasy about the Event. I never saw a single Instance of a Person's dying of a Quinsey of this kind, after the Suppuration is truly effected, neither has it happened perhaps after the Time it is forming for Suppuration

§ 115. The glairy Matter with which the Throat is over-charged, and the very Inflammation of that Part, which, from its Irritation, produces the same Effect, as the Introduction of a Finger into it, occasions some Patients to complain of incessant Propensities to vomit. We must be upon our Guard here, and not suppose that this Heart-Sickness, as some have called it, results from a Disorder of, or a Load within, the Stomach, and that it requires a Vomit for its Removal. The giving one here would often prove a very unfortunate Mistake. It might, in a high Inflammation, further aggravate it, or we might be obliged (even during the Operation of the Vomit) to bleed, in order to lessen the Violence of the Inflammation. Such Imprudence with its bad Consequences, often leaves the Patient, even after the Disease is cured, in a State of Languor and Weakness for a considerable Time. Nevertheless, there are some particular Disorders of the Throat, attended with a Fever, in which a Vomit may be prudently given. But this can only be, when there is no Inflammation, or after it is dispersed, and there still remains some putrid Matter in the first Passages. Of such Cases I shall speak hereafter. (a)

§ 116. We often see in *Swisserland* a Disorder different from these of the Throat, of which we have

---

In Diseases of the Throat, which have been preceded by such Excesses in Food or strong Drink as occur too often in many Countries, when the Patient has very strong Reachings to vomit, and the Tongue is moist at the same Time, we should not hesitate, after decreasing the first Symptoms of the Inflammation [by a little Bleeding, &c.] to assist the Efforts of Nature, and give a small Dose of Tartar emetic, dissolved in some Spoonfuls of Water. This Remedy in this Case promotes the Dispersion of the Inflammation, beyond any other. *E. L.*

have just treated, though, like these, attended with a Difficulty of swallowing. It is termed in French the *Oreillons*, and often the *Ourles*, or swelled Ears. It is an Overfulness and Obstruction of those Glands and their Tubes, which are to furnish the *Saliva* or Spittle; and particularly of the two large Glands which lie between the Ear and the Jaw; which are called the *Parotides*, and of two under the Jaw, called the *Maxillares*. All these being considerably swelled in this Disease, do not only produce a great Difficulty of swallowing; but also prevent the Mouth from opening; as an Attempt to do it is attended with violent Pain. Young Children are much more liable to this Disease than grown Persons. Being seldom attended with a Fever, there is no Occasion for Medicines: It is sufficient to defend the Parts affected from the external Air; to apply some proper Poultice over them; to lessen the Quantity of their Food considerably, denying them Flesh and Wine; but indulging them plentifully in some light warm Liquid, to dilute their Humours and restore Perspiration. I cured myself of this Disorder in 1754, by drinking nothing, for four Days, but Balm Tea, to which I added one fourth part Milk, and a little Bread. The same *Regimen* has often cured me of other light Complaints of the Throat

§ 117 In the Spring of 1761, there were an astonishing Number of Persons attacked with Disorders of the Throat, of two different Kinds. Some of them were seized with that common

Sort which I have already described. Without adding any thing more particularly, in Respect to this Species, it happened frequently to grown Persons, who were perfectly cured by the Method already recited. The other Species, on which I shall be more particular in this Place (because I know they have abounded in some Villages, and were very fatal) invaded Adults, or grown Persons also, but especially Children, from the Age of one Year, and even under that, to the Age of twelve or thirteen.

The first Symptoms were the same with those of the common Quinsey, such as the Shivering, the ensuing Heat or Fever, Dejection, and a Complaint of the Throat: but the following Symptoms distinguished these from the common inflammatory Quinseys.

1. The Sick had often something of a Cough, and a little Oppression.

2. The Pulse was quicker, but less hard, and less strong, than generally happens in Diseases of the Throat.

3. The Patients were afflicted with a sharp, stinging and dry Heat, and with great Restlessness.

4. They spat less than is usual in a common Quinsey, and their Tongues were extremely dry.

5. Though they had some Pain in swallowing, this was not their principal Complaint, and they could drink sufficiently.

6. The

Of the Diseases of the Throat.

6 The Swelling and Redness of the Tonsils, of the Palate, and of its Process were not considerable, but the parotid and maxillary Glands, and especially the former, being extremely swelled and inflamed, the Pain they chiefly complained of, was this outward one.

7 When the Disease proved considerably dangerous, the whole Neck swelled; and some times even the Veins, which return the Blood from the Brain, being overladen, as it were, the Sick had some Degree of Drowsiness, and of a *Delirium,* or Raving.

8 The Paroxysms, or Returns, of the Fever were considerably irregular.

9 The Urine appeared to be less inflamed, than in other Diseases of the Throat.

10. Bleeding and other Medicines did not relieve them, as soon as in the other kind; and the Disease itself continued a longer Time.

11. It did not terminate in a Suppuration like other Quinsies, but sometimes the Tonsils were ulcerated.

12. * Almost every Child, and indeed a great many of the grown Persons assaulted with this Disease, threw out, either on the first Day, or on some succeeding one, within the first six Days, a certain Efflorescence, or Eruptions, resembling the Measles considerably in some, but of a less lively Colour, and without any Elevation, or ri-

---

* This seems to have been the same kind of Quinsey, of which Drs *Huxham, Fothergil, Cotton* and others wrote, though under different Appellations.

sing above the Skin. It appeared first in the Face, next in the Arms, and descended to the Legs, Thighs and Trunk; disappearing gradually at the End of two or three Days, in the same Order it had observed in breaking out. A few others (I have seen but five Instances of it) suffered the most grievous Symptoms before the Eruption, and threw out the genuine *purpura*, or white miliary Eruption.

13. As soon as these Efflorescences or Eruptions appeared, the sick generally found themselves better. That, last mentioned, continued four, five, or six Days, and frequently went off by Sweats. Such as had not these Ebullitions, which was the Case of many Adults, were not cured without very plentiful Sweats towards the Termination of the Disease; those which occurred at the Invasion of it being certainly unprofitable, and always hurtful.

14. I have seen some Patients, in whom the Complaint of the Throat disappeared entirely, without either Eruptions or Sweats: but such still remained in very great Inquietude and Anguish, with a quick and small Pulse. I ordered them a sudorific Drink, which being succeeded by the Eruption, or by Sweating, they found themselves sensibly relieved.

15. But whether the Sick had, or had not, these external Redneffes or Eruptions, every one of them parted with their Cuticle or Scarf Skin, which fell off, in large Scales, from the whole Surface of the Body. So great was the Acrimony

or

or Sharpness of that Matter, which was to be discharged through the Skin.

16. A great Number suffered a singular Alteration in their Voice, different from that which occurs in common Quinsies, the Inside of their Nostrils being extremely dry.

17. The Sick recovered with more Difficulty after this, than after the common Quinsies: and if they were negligent or irregular, during their Recovery, particularly, if they exposed themselves too soon to the Cold, a Relapse ensued, or some different Symptoms, such as a Stuffing with Oppression, a Swelling of the Belly, windy Swellings in different Parts, Weakness, Loathings, Ulcerations behind the Ears, and something of a Cough and Hoarseness.

18. I have been sent for to Children, and also to some young Folks, who, at the End of several Weeks, had been taken with a general Inflammation of the whole Body, attended with great Oppression, and a considerable Abatement of their Urine, which was also high-coloured and turbid, or without Separation. They seemed also in a very singular State of Indifference, or Disregard, with Respect to any Object, or Circumstance. I recovered every one of them entirely by Blisters, and the Powder N°. 25. The first Operation of this Medicine was to vomit them: to this succeeded a Discharge by Urine, and at last very plentiful Sweating, which compleated the Cure. Two Patients only, of a bad Constitution, who were a little ricketty, and disposed to

glandular

glandular Scirrhofity or Knottineſs, relapſed and died, after being recovered of the Diſeaſe itſelf for ſome Days.

§ 118 I have bled ſome adult Perſons, and made Uſe of the cooling Regimen, as long as there was an evident Inflammation: it was neceſſary after this to unload the firſt Paſſages, and at laſt to excite moderate Sweats. The ſame Powders N°. 25 have often effected both theſe Diſcharges, and with entire Succeſs. In other Caſes I have made Uſe of Ipecacuanha, as directed N°. 35.

In ſome Subjects there did not appear any inflammatory Symptom, and the Diſtemper reſulted ſolely from a Load of putrid Matter in the firſt Paſſages. Some Patients alſo diſcharged Worms. In ſuch Caſes I never bled, but the Vomit had an excellent Effect, at the very Onſet of the Diſeaſe; it produced a perceivable Abatement of all the Symptoms, Sweating enſued very kindly and naturally, and the Patient recovered entirely a few Hours after.

§ 119 There were ſome Places, in which no Symptom or Character of Inflammation appeared, and in which it was neceſſary to omit Bleeding, which was attended with bad Conſequences.

I never directed Infants to be bled. After opening the firſt Paſſages, Bliſters and diluting Drinks proved their only Remedies. A ſimple Infuſion of Elder Flower, and thoſe of the Lime Tree,

Tree, has done great Service to those who drank plentifully of it.

§ 120. I am sensible that in many Villages a great Number of Persons have died, with a prodigious Inflation or Swelling of the Neck. Some have also died in the City, and among others a young Woman of twenty Years of Age, who had taken nothing but hot sweating Medicines and red Wine, and died the fourth Day, with violent Suffocations, and a large Discharge of Blood from the Nose. Of the great Number I have seen in Person, only two died. One was a little Girl of ten Months old. She had an Efflorescene which very suddenly disappeared at this Time I was called in, but the Humour had retreated to the Breast, and rendered her Death inevitable. The other was a strong Youth from sixteen to seventeen Years old, whose sudden Attack from the Disease manifested, from the very Beginning, a violent Degree of it. Nevertheless, the Symptoms subsiding, and the Fever nearly terminating, the Sweats which approached would probably have saved him. But he would not suffer them to have their Course, continually stripping himself quite naked. The Inflammation was immediately repelled upon the Lungs, and destroyed him within the Space of thirty Hours. I never saw a Person die with so very dry a Skin. The Vomit affected him very little upwards, and brought on a purging. His own bad Conduct seems to have been the Occasion of his Death; and may this serve as one Example of it.

§ 121. I chose to expatiate on this Disease, as it may happen to reach other Places, where it may be useful to have been apprized of its Marks, and of its Treatment, which agrees as much with that of putrid Fevers, of which I shall speak hereafter, as with that of the inflammatory Diseases I have already considered: since in some Subjects the Complaint of the Throat has evidently been a Symptom of a putrid Fever, rather than of the chiefly apparent Disease, a Quinsey. (a)

§ 122. Disorders of the Throat are, with Respect to particular Persons, an habitual Disease returning every Year, and sometimes oftner than once a Year. They may be prevented by the same Means, which I have directed for the Preservation from habitual Pleurisies § 100; and by defending the Head and the Neck from the Cold; especially after being heated by Hunting, or any violent Exercise, or even by singing long and loud, which may be considered as an extraordinary Exercise of some of the Parts affected in this Disease.

(a) I reserve some other interesting Reflections on this Disease, for the second Edition of my Treatise on Fevers, and the Editor at *Paris* has very well observed, that it has some Relation to the gangrenous sore Throat, which has been epidemical these twenty Years past, in many Parts of *Europe*——This Note is from Dr. Tissot himself.

CHAPTER

Chapter VII.

Of Colds.

Sect. 123.

THERE are many erroneous Prejudices, with Regard to Colds, all of which may be attended with pernicious Consequences. The first is, that a Cold is never dangerous; an Error which daily destroys the Lives of many. I have already complained of it for many Years past; and I have since beheld a Multitude of such Examples of it, as have but too sufficiently warranted my Complaints.

No Person however, it is certain, dies merely of a Cold, as long as it is nothing but a Cold simply, but when, from Inattention and Neglect, it is thrown upon, and occasions Distempers of the Breast, it may, and often does, prove mortal. *Colds destroy more than Plagues*, was the Answer of a very sagacious and experienced Physician to one of his Friends, who, being asked, how he was in Health, replied, Very well, I have nothing but a Cold.

A second erroneous Prejudice is, that Colds require no Means, no Medicines, and that they last the longer for being nursed, or tampered with. The last Article may be true indeed, with
Respect

Respect to the Method, in which the Person affected with them treats them; but the Principle itself is false. Colds, like other Disorders, have their proper Remedies, and are removed with more or less Facility, as they are conducted better or worse.

§ 124. A third Mistake is, that they are not only considered as not dangerous, but are even supposed wholesome too. Doubtless a Man had better have a Cold than a more grievous Disease; though it must be still better to have neither of them. The most that can reasonably be said and admitted on this Point, is, that when a checked, or an obstructed Perspiration becomes the Cause of a Distemper, it is fortunate that it produces rather a Cold, than any very dreadful Disease, which it frequently does; though it were to be wished, that neither the Cause, nor its Effect existed. A Cold constantly produces some Disorder or Defect in the Functions of some Part or Parts of the Body, and thus becomes the Cause of a Disease. It is indeed a real Disorder itself, and which, when in a violent Degree, makes a very perceivable Effect upon our whole Machine. Colds, with their Defluxions, considerably weaken the Breast, and sooner or later considerably impair the Health. Persons subject to frequent Colds are never robust or strong; they often sink into languid Disorders; and a frequent Aptitude to take Cold is a Proof, that their Perspiration may be easily checked and retained, whence the Lungs become oppressed and obstructed; which

must

muſt always be attended with conſiderable Danger.

§ 125. We may be convinced of the Weakneſs and Fallacy of theſe Prejudices, by conſidering attentively the Nature of Colds, which are nothing elſe than the very Diſeaſes already deſcribed in the three preceding Chapters, though in their greateſt Degree only.

A Cold in Truth is almoſt conſtantly an inflammatory Diſeaſe, a light Inflammation of the Lungs, or of the Throat, of the Membrane or very thin Skin, which lines the Noſtrills, and the Inſide of certain Cavities in the Bones of the Cheeks and Forehead. Theſe Cavities communicate with the Noſe, in ſuch a Manner, that when one Part of this Membrane is affected with an Inflammation, it is eaſily communicated to the other Parts.

§ 126 It is ſcarcely neceſſary to deſcribe the Symptoms of a Cold, and it may be ſufficient to remark, 1 That their chief Cauſe is the ſame with that, which moſt commonly produces the Diſeaſes already treated of, that is, an obſtructed Perſpiration, and a Blood ſomewhat inflamed. 2. That whenever theſe Diſeaſes affect great Numbers, many Colds prevail at the ſame Time. 3. That the Symptoms which manifeſt a violent Cold, greatly reſemble thoſe which precede or uſher in theſe Diſeaſes. People are rarely attacked by great Colds, without a ſhivering and Fever, which laſt ſometimes continues for many Days. There is a Cough, a dry Cough, for ſome Time,

Time; after which some Expectoration ensues; which allays the Cough, and lightens the Oppression; at which Time the Cold may be said to be maturated, or ripe. There are pretty often slight Stitches, but unfixed or flying about, with a little Complaint of the Throat. When the Nostrills happen to be the Seat of the Disorder, which is then very improperly termed a Cold of the Brain, it is often attended with a vehement Head-ach; which sometimes depends on an Irritation of the Membrane, that lines the Cavities in the Bone of the Forehead, or the maxillary Sinusses, that is, the Cavities in the Jaws. At first the Running from the Nose is very clear, thin and sharp; afterwards, in Proportion to the Abatement of the Inflammation, it becomes thicker; and the Consistence and Colour of it resemble those of what others cough up. The Smell, the Taste and the Appetite are commonly impaired by it.

§ 127. Colds seem to be of no certain Duration or Continuance. Those of the Head or Brain generally last but a few Days; of the Breast longer. Some Colds nevertheless terminate in four or five Days. If they extend beyond this Term they prove really hurtful. 1. Because the Violence of the Cough disorders the whole Machine, and particularly, by forcing up the Blood to the Head. 2. By depriving the Person afflicted of his usual Sleep, which is almost constantly diminished by it. 3. By impairing the Appetite, and confusing the Digestion,

which

which is unavoidably leſſened by it. 4. By weakening the very Lungs, by the continual Agitations from Coughing; whence all the Humours being gradually determined towards them, as the weakeſt Part, a continual Cough ſubſiſts. Hence alſo they become overcharged with Humours, which grow viſcid there; the Reſpiration is overloaded and oppreſſed, a ſlow Fever appears; Nutrition almoſt ceaſes, the Patient becomes very weak; ſinks into a Waſting; an obſtinate Wakefulneſs and Anguiſh, and often dies in a ſhort Time. 5. By Reaſon that the Fever, which almoſt conſtantly accompanies great Cold, concurs to wear the body down.

§ 128. Wherefore, ſince a Cold is a Diſeaſe of the ſame kind with Quinſies, Peripneumonies and Inflammations of the Breaſt, it ought to be treated in the ſame Manner. If it is a violent one, Blood ſhould be taken from the Arm, which may conſiderably ſhorten its Duration: and this becomes moſt eſſentially neceſſary, whenever the Patient is of a ſanguineous ruddy Complexion, abounds with Blood, and has a ſtrong Cough, and great Head-ach The Drinks N°. 1, 2, 3, 4, ſhould be very plentifully uſed It is advantagious to bathe the Feet in warm Water every Night at going to Bed (a) In a Word, if the Patient

---

(a) It frequently happens, that the Bathings alone remove the Head ach, and the Cough too, by relaxing the lower Parts, and the entire Surface of the Body If the Patient is coſtive, he ſhould receive Glyſters of warm Water, in which ſome Bran has been boiled, with the addition of a little common Soap or Butter. *L*

is put into a Regimen, the Cure is very speedily effected.

§ 129. The Disorder indeed, however, is often so very slight, that it may be thought to require very little, if any, medical Treatment, and may be easily cured without Physick, by abstaining from Flesh, Eggs, Broth, and Wine, from all Food that is sharp, fat and heavy; and by dieting upon Bread, Pulse, Fruit, and Water; particularly by eating little or no Supper, and drinking, if thirsty, a simple Ptisan of Barley, or an Infusion of Elder Flowers, with the Addition of a third or fourth Part of Milk. Bathing the Feet, and the Powder N°. 20 contribute to dispose the Patient to sleep. Five Tea-Cups of an Infusion of the Red, or wild Poppy Leaves may also be ventured on safely.

§ 130. When the Fever, Heat and Inflammation wholly disappear, when the Patient has kept to his Regimen for some Days, and his Blood is well diluted, if the Cough and Want of Sleep still continues, he may take in the Evening a Dose of Storax * Pill, or of Venice Treacle with Elder

---

* Under these Circumstances of a tickling Cough from a Cold, without a Fever, and with very little Inflammation, I have known great and very frequent Success from a Dose of *Elixir paregoric*, taken at Bed time, after a very light thin Supper. If the Patient be sanguine, strong and costive, bleeding in a suitable Quantity, and a gentle opening Potion or purging Glyster, may be prudently premised to it. Grown Persons may take from 30 to 80, or even 100 Drops of it, in Barley Water, or any other pectoral Drink, and Children in the Cure of it from five to twenty Drops, in an Ounce of any Medicine containing about one
Grain

Elder Flower Water, after bathing his Feet. These Remedies by stilling the Cough, and restoring Perspiration, frequently cure the Cold in the Space of one Night. I confess at the same Time, I have seen bad Consequences from such Opiates, when given too early in the Complaint. It is also necessary, when they are given, that the Patient should have supt but very moderately, and that his Supper should be digested.

§ 131. An immense Number of Remedies are cried up for the Cure of Colds; such as Ptisans of Apples or Pippins, of Liquorice, of dry Raisins, of Figs, of Borage, of Ground-Ivy, of *Veronica* or Speedwell, of Hysop, of Nettles, &c &c I have no Design to depreciate them; as all of them may possibly be useful: But unfortunately, those who have seen any particular one of them succeed in one Case, readily conclude it to be the most excellent of them all; which is a dangerous Error, because no one Case is a sufficient Foundation to decide upon: which besides none are qualified to do, who have not often seen a great Number of such Cases; and who do not so attentively observe the Effects of different Medicines, as to determine on those which most frequently agree with the Disorder;

K and

Grain of Opium, which is the Quantity contained in less than quite six Grains of the Storax Pill, this last being a very available pectoral Opiate too in Coughs from a Distillation, in more adult Bodies, who may also prefer a Medicine in that small Size, and Form *K*.

and which, in my Judgment, are those I have just enumerated. I have known a Tea or Infusion of Cherry Stalks, which is not a disagreeable Drink, to cure a very inveterate Cold.

§ 132 In Colds of the Head or Brain, the Steam of warm Water alone, or that in which Elder Flowers, or some other mild aromatic Herbs, have been boiled, commonly afford a pretty speedy Relief. These are also serviceable in Colds fallen on the Breast. See § 55.

It has been a Practice, though of no very long standing, to give the Fat of a Whale in these Cases, but this is a very crude indigestible kind of Fat, and greasy oily Medicines seldom agree with Colds. Besides, this Whales' Fat is very disagreeable and rancid, that is rank, so that it were better to forbear using it: I have sometimes seen ill Effects from it, and rarely any good ones. *

§ 133. Such Persons as abate nothing of the usual Quantity of their Food, when seized with a Cold, and who swallow down large Quantities of hot Water, ruin their Health. Their Digestion ceases, the Cough begins to affect the Stomach, without ceasing to afflict the Breast; and they incur a Chance of sinking into the Condition described § 127, N°. 4.

Burnt Brandy and spiced Wine are very pernicious

* This seems but too applicable to the very popular Use of *Spermaceti*, &c. in such Cases, which can only grease the Passage to the Stomach, must impair its digestive Faculty, and cannot operate against the Cause of a Cold, though that Cure of it, which is effected by the Oeconomy of Nature in due Time, is often ascribed to such Medicines, as may rather have retarded it *K*

nicious in the Beginning of Colds, and the Omiſſion of them muſt be a very prudent Omiſſion. If any good Effects have ever been known to attend the Uſe of them, it has been towards the going off of the Cold; when the Diſorder maintained its Ground, ſolely from the Weakneſs of the Patient. Whenever this is the Caſe, there is not the leaſt Room for farther Relaxation, but the Powders N°. 14, ſhould be taken every Day in a little Wine; and ſhould the Humours ſeem likely to be thrown upon the Lungs, Bliſters ought to be applied to the fleſhy Part of the Legs.

§ 134. Drams, or *Liqueurs*, as they are called in *French*, agree ſo very little in this laſt State, that frequently a very ſmall Quantity of them revives a Cold that was juſt expiring. There really are ſome Perſons who never drink them without taking Cold, which is not to be wondered at, as they occaſion a light Inflammation in the Breaſt, which is equivalent to a Cold or Diſtillation.

Nevertheleſs, People in this Diſorder ſhould not expoſe themſelves to violent cold Weather, if there is a Poſſibility of avoiding it: though they ſhould equally guard too againſt exceſſive Heat. Thoſe, who incloſe themſelves in very hot Rooms, never get quite cured; and how is it poſſible they ſhould be cured in ſuch a Situation? Such Rooms, abſtracted from the Danger of coming out of them, produce Colds in the ſame Manner that Drams do, by producing a light Inflammation in the Breaſt.

§ 135 Persons subject to frequent Colds, which Habits are sometimes termed *fluxionary*, or liable to Distillations, imagine, they ought to keep themselves very hot. This is an Error which thoroughly destroys their Health. Such a Disposition to take Cold arises from two Causes, either because their Perspiration is easily impaired, or sometimes from the Weakness of the Stomach or the Lungs, which require particular Remedies. When the Complaint arises from the Perspiration's being easily disturbed and lessened, the hotter they keep themselves, the more they sweat, and increase their Complaint the more. This incessantly warm Air lets down and weakens the whole Machine, and more particularly the Lungs; where the Humours finding less Resistance, are continually derived, and are accumulated there. The Skin, being constantly bathed in a small Sweat, becomes relaxed, soft, and incapable of compleating its Functions. from which Failure the slightest Cause produces a total Obstruction of Perspiration, and a Multitude of languid Disorders ensue.

These Patients thus circumstanced, redouble their Precautions against the Cold, or even the Coolness of the Air, while their utmost Cautions are but so many effectual Means to lower their Health, and this the more certainly, as their Dread of the free Air necessarily subjects them to a sedentary Life, which increases all their Symptoms, while the hot Drinks they indulge in, compleat their Severity. There is but one Method

thod to cure People thus situated; that is, by accustoming them gradually to the Air; to keep them out of hot Chambers; to lessen their Cloathing by Degrees; to make them sleep cool; and to let them eat or drink nothing but what is cold, Ice itself being wholesome in their Drink: to make them use much Exercise, and finally, if the Disorder be inveterate, to give them for a considerable Time the Powder N°. 14, and make them use the cold Bath. This Method succeeds equally too with those, in whom the Disease originally depended on a Weakness of the Stomach, or of the Lungs; and in fact, at the End of a certain Period, these three Causes are always combined. Some Persons who have been subject, for many Years, to catch Colds throughout the Winter, and who, during that Season, never went out, and drank every thing warm, have been evidently the better, during the Winter of 1761, and 1762, for the Directions I have given here. They now walk out every Day, drink their Liquids cold, and by this Means entirely escape Colds, and enjoy perfect Health.

§ 136 It is more customary indeed in Town, than in the Country, to have different Troches, and Compositions in the Mouth. I am not for excluding this Habit; though I think nothing is so efficacious as Juice of Liquorice, and provided a sufficient Dose be taken, it affords certain Relief. I have taken an Ounce and a half in one Day, and have felt the good Consequences of it very remarkably.

CHAPTER

Chapter VIII.

Of Diseases of the Teeth.

Sect. 137.

THE Diseases of the Teeth, which are sometimes so tedious and so violent, as to cause obstinate Wakefulness, a considerable Degree of Fever, Raving, Inflammations, Abscesses, Rottenness of the Bones, Convulsions and Faintings, depend on three principal Causes. 1. On a *Caries* or Rottenness of the Teeth. 2. On an Inflammation of the Nerves of the Teeth, or of the Membrane which invests and covers them; and which affects the Membrane of the Gums. 3. A cold Humour or Defluxion that is determined to the Teeth, and to their Nerves and Membrane.

§ 138. In the first of these Cases, the *Caries* having eat down to, and exposed the naked Nerve, the Air, Food and Drink irritate, or, as it were sting it, and this Irritation is attended with Pain more or less violent. Every thing that increases the Motion or Action of the affected Part, as Exercise, Heat or Food, will be attended with the same Consequence.

When the Tooth is greatly decayed, there is no other Cure besides that by extracting it, without

out which the Pain continues, the Breath becomes very offensive; the Gum is eat down; the other Teeth, and sometimes even the Jawbone, are infected with the Rottenness: besides, that it prevents the Use of the other Teeth, which are infested with a kind of tartarous Matter, and decay.

But when the Disorder is less considerable, the Progress of it may sometimes be restrained, by burning the Tooth with a hot Iron, or by filling it with Lead, if it is fitted to receive and to retain it. Different corroding Liquids are sometimes used on these Occasions, *Aqua fortis* itself, and Spirit of Vitriol: but such Applications are highly dangerous, and ought to be excluded. When the Patients, from Dread, reject the Operations just mentioned, a little Oyl of Cloves may be applied, by introducing a small Pellet of Cotton, dipt in it, to the rotten hollow Tooth; which often affords considerable Ease, and Respite. Some make use of a Tincture of Opium, or Laudanum, after the same Manner, and indeed these two Medicines may be used together in equal Quantities. I have often succeeded with *Hoffman*'s mineral anodyne Liquor; which seemed indeed, for a few Moments, to increase the Pain; but Ease generally ensues after spitting a little Time. A Gargarism made of the Herb *Argentina*, that is Silver-weed or wild Tansey, in Water, frequently appeases the Pain that results from a *Caries* of the Teeth: and in such Cases many People have found themselves at Ease, under

der a constant Use of it. It certainly is an Application that cannot hurt, and is even beneficial to the Gums. Others have been relieved by rubbing their Faces over with Honey.

§ 139 The second Cause is the Inflammation of the Nerve within the Substance, or of the Membrane on the Outside, of the Tooth. This is discovered by the Patient's Temperament, Age and Manner of living. They who are young, sanguine, who heat themselves much, whether by Labour, by their Food, their Drink, by sitting up late, or by any other Excess: they who have been accustomed to any Discharges or Eruptions of Blood, whether natural or artificial, and who cease to have them as usual, are much exposed to the Tooth-ach, from this Cause.

This Pain, or rather Torment, if in an acute Degree, commonly happens very suddenly, and often after some heating Cause. The Pulse is strong and full; the Countenance considerably red, the Mouth extremely hot: there is often a pretty high Fever, and a violent Head-ach. The Gums, or some Part of them, become inflamed, swelled, and sometimes an Abscess appears. At other times the Humours throw themselves upon the more external Parts, the Cheek swells, and the Pain abates. When the Cheek swells, but without any Diminution of the Pain, it then becomes an Augmentation, but no essential Change, of the Disorder.

§ 140 In this Species of the Disease, we must have Recourse to the general Method of treating inflammatory Disorders, and direct Bleeding, which often produces immediate Ease, if performed early. After Bleeding, the Patient should gargle with Barley Water, or Milk and Water; and apply an emollient Cataplasm to the Cheek. If an Abscess or little Imposthume appears, the Suppuration or ripening of it is to be promoted, by holding continually in the Mouth some hot Milk, or Figs boiled in some Milk: and as soon as ever it seems ripe, it should be opened, which may be done easily, and without any Pain. The Disorder, when depending on this Cause, is sometimes not so violent, but of a longer Duration, and returns whenever the Patient heats himself; when he goes to Bed; when he eats any heating Food, or Drink, Wine or Coffee. In this Case he should be bled, without which his other Medicines will have little Effect, and he should bathe his Feet in warm Water for some Evenings successively, taking one Dose of the Powder N°. 20 Entire Abstinence from Wine and Meat, especially at Night, has cured several Persons of inveterate and obstinate Maladies of the Teeth.

In this Species of Tooth-ach, all hot Remedies are pernicious, and it often happens that Opium, Venice Treacle, and Storax Pills, are so far from producing the Relief expected from them, that they have aggravated the Pain.

§ 141 When the Disease arises from a cold Distillation, or Humour, tending to these Parts, it is commonly (though equally painful) attended with less violent Symptoms. The Pulse is
neither

neither strong, full nor quick; the Mouth is less heated, and less swelled. In such Cases, the afflicted should be purged with the Powder N°. 21, which has sometimes perfectly cured very obstinate Complaints of this Sort. After purging they should make Use of the Diet Drink of the Woods N°. 22. This has cured Tooth-achs, which have baffled other Attempts for many Years, but it must be added, this Drink would be hurtful in the Disease from a different Cause. Blisters to the Nape of the Neck, or * elsewhere, it matters not greatly where, have often extraordinary good Effects, by diverting the Humour, and restoring a compleat Perspiration. In short in this Species, we may employ, not only with Safety, but with Success (especially after due purging) Pills of Storax, Opium and Venice Treacle. Acrid sharp Remedies, such as hard-spun * Tobacco, Root of Pellitory of *Spain*, &c. by exciting much Spitting, discharge part of the Humour

---

* * A small Blister behind the Ear of the affected Side, or both Ears, has very often removed the Pain, when from a Defluxion. It is pretty common for the Subjects of this Disease to be very costive during the Exacerbations of it, which I have sometimes experienced to be pretty regularly and severely quotidian, for a Week or two. The Custom of smoking Tobacco very often, which the Violence of this Pain has sometimes introduced, often disposes to a Blackness, and premature Decay of the Teeth, to which the Chewers of it seem less obnoxious; and this Difference may result from some Particles of its chemical Oil rising by Fumigation, and being retained in the Teeth, which Particles are not extracted by Mastication. But with Regard to the habitual Use of this very acrid and in small violent Herb, for our chief after, this Disease, it should be considered well, whether in some Constitutions it may not prove the Way to more dangerous ones, than it was introduced to remove.

Humour which causes the Disease, and hence diminish the Pain. The Smoke of Tobacco also succeeds now and then in this Disorder, whether this happens from the Discharge of the Rheum or Spittle it occasions; or whether it is owing to any anodyne Efficacy of this Plant, in which it resembles Opium.

§ 142. As this last Cause is often the Consequence of a Weakness in the Stomach, it daily happens that we see some People, whose Disorder from this Cause is augmented, in Proportion as they indulge in a cooling, refreshing Way of living. The Increase of the Disorder disposes them to increase the Dose of what they mistake for its Remedy, in Proportion to which their Pain only increases. There is a Necessity that such Persons should alter this Method; and make use of such Medicines as are proper to strengthen the Stomach, and to restore Perspiration. The Powder N°. 14 has often produced the best Consequences, when I have ordered it in these Cases, and it never fails to dissipate the Tooth-ach very speedily, which returns periodically at stated Days and Hours. I have also cured some Persons who never drank Wine, by advising them to the Use of it.

§ 143. But besides the Diseases of the Teeth, that are owing to these three principal Causes, which are the most common ones, there are some very tedious and most tormenting Disorders of them, that are occasioned by a general Acrimony, or great Sharpness, of the Mass of Blood, and

and which are never cured by any other Medicines but such, as are proper to correct that Acrimony. When it is of a scorbutic Nature, the wild Horse-radish (Pepperwort) Water Cresses, Brooklime, Sorrel, and Wood-sorrell correct and cure it. If it is of a different Nature, it requires different Remedies. But very particular Details do not come within the Plan of this Work. As the Malady is of the chronical or tedious kind, it allows Time to consider and consult more particularly about it.

The Gout and the Rheumatism are sometimes transferred to the Teeth, and give Rise to the most excruciating Pains; which must be treated like the Diseases from which they arise

§ 144 From what has been said on this Disorder, the Reader will discern, in what that imaginary Oddness may consist, which has been ascribed to it, from the same Application's relieving one Person in it, and not affording the least Relief to another. Now the plain Reason of this is, that these Applications are always directed, without an exact Knowledge of the particular Cause of the Disease, in different Subjects and Circumstances, whence the Pain from a rotten Tooth, is treated like that from an Inflammation; that from an Inflammation, like the Pain from a cold Humour or Fluxion, and this last like a Pain caused by a scorbutic Acrimony. so that the Disappointment is not in the least surprizing. Perhaps Physicians themselves do not always attend distinctly enough to the Nature of each

particular

Of Diseases of the Teeth.

particular Disorder: and even when they do, they content themselves with directing some of the less potent Medicines, which may be inadequate to accomplish the necessary Effect. If the Distemper truly be of an inflammatory Disposition, Bleeding is indispensible to the Cure.

It happens in Fact, with Regard to the Diseases of the Teeth, as well as to all other Diseases, that they arise from different Causes, and if these Causes are not opposed by Medicines suited to them, the Disease, far from being cured, is aggravated.

I have cured violent Tooth-achs, of the lower Jaw, by applying a Plaister of Meal, the White of an Egg, Brandy and Mastich, at the Corner of that Jaw, over the Spot where the Pulsation of the Artery may be perceived. and I have also mitigated the most excruciating Pains of the Head, by applying the same Plaister upon the temporal Artery.

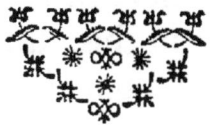

CHAPTER

Chapter IX.

Of the Apoplexy.

Sect. 145.

EVERY Person has some Idea of the Disease termed an Apoplexy, which is a sudden Privation or Loss of all Sense, and of all voluntary Motion; the Pulse at the same Time being kept up, but Respiration or Breathing, being oppressed. I shall treat of this Disease only in a brief Manner, as it is not common in our Country Villages; and as I have expatiated on it in a different Manner in a Letter to Dr. HALLER, published in 1761.

§ 146. This Disease is generally distinguished into two Kinds, the sanguineous and serous Apoplexy. Each of them results from an Overfulness of the Blood Vessels of the Brain, which presses upon, and prevents or impairs the Functions of the Nerves. The whole Difference between these two Species consists in this, that the sanguineous Apoplexy prevails among strong robust Persons, who have a rich, heavy, thick and inflammable Blood, and that in a large Quantity, in which Circumstance it becomes a genuine inflammatory Distemper. The serous, or humoral Apoplexy invades

Of the Apoplexy.

invades Perſons of a leſs robuſt Conſtitution; whoſe Blood is more dilute or watery; and rather viſcid, or lightly gelatinous, than heavy or rich; whoſe Veſſels are in a more relaxed State, and who abound more in other Humours than in red Blood.

§ 147 When the firſt Kind of this Diſeaſe exiſts in its moſt violent Degree, it is then ſometimes termed, an apoplectic Stroke, or thundering Apoplexy, which kills in a Moment or inſtantaneouſly, and admits of no Remedies. When the Aſſault is leſs violent, and we find the Patient with a ſtrong, full and raiſed Pulſe, his Viſage red and bloated, and his Neck ſwelled up, with an oppreſſed and loud hoarſe Reſpiration; being ſenſible of nothing, and capable of no other Motions, except ſome Efforts to vomit, the Caſe is not always equally deſperate We muſt therefore immediately,

1. Entirely uncover the Patient's Head, covering the reſt of his Body but very lightly; procure him inſtantly very freſh free Air, and leave his Neck quite unbound and open.

2. His Head ſhould be placed as high as may be, with his Feet hanging down.

3 He muſt loſe from twelve to ſixteen Ounces of Blood, from a free open Orifice in the Arm: the Strength or Violence with which the Blood ſallies out, ſhould determine the Surgeon to take a few Ounces more or leſs. It ſhould be repeated to the third or fourth Time, within the Space of

of three or four Hours, if the Symptoms seem to require it, either in the Arm, or in the Foot.

4. A Glyster should be given of a Decoction of the first emollient opening Herbs that can be got, with four Spoonfuls of Oil, one Spoonful of Salt: and this should be repeated every three Hours.

5. If it is possible, he should be made to swallow Water plentifully, in each Pot of which three Drams of Nitre are to be dissolved

6. As soon as the Height and Violence of the Pulse abates; when his Breathing becomes less oppressed and difficult, and his Countenance less inflamed, he should take the Decoction N°. 23; or, if it cannot be got ready in Time, he should take three Quarters of an Ounce of Cream of Tartar, and drink Whey plentifully after it. This Medicine succeeded extremely well with me in a Case, where I could not readily procure any other.

7. He should avoid all strong Liquor, Wine, distilled Spirit, whether inwardly or by outward Application, and should even be prevented from * smelling them.

8. The Patient should be stirred, moved, or even touched, as little as it is possible: in a Word every Thing must be avoided that can give him
the

---

* I have been very authentically assured of the Death of a pale Man, which happened in the very Act of pouring out a large Quantity of distilled Spirit, by Gallons or Bucketfulls, from one Vessel into another.

the least Agitation. This Advice, I am sensible, is directly contrary to the common Practice; notwithstanding which it is founded in Reason, approved by Experience, and absolutely necessary. In Fact, the whole Evil results from the Blood being forced up with too much Force, and in too great a Quantity, to the Brain; which being thence in a State of Compression, prevents every Movement and every Influence of the Nerves. In Order, therefore, to re-establish these Movements, the Brain must be unloaded, by diminishing the Force of the Blood. But strong Liquors, Wines, Spirits, volatile Salts, all Agitation and Frictions augment it, and by that very Means increase the Load, the Embarrassment of the Brain, and thus heighten the Disease itself. On the contrary, every Thing that calms the Circulation, contributes to recall Sensation and voluntary Motion the sooner.

9 Strong Ligatures should be made about the Thighs under the Ham: By this Means the Blood is prevented in its Ascent from the Legs, and less is carried up to the Head.

If the Patient seems gradually, and in Proportion as he takes proper Medicines, to advance into a less violent State, there may be some Hopes. But if he rather grows worse after his earliest Evacuations, the Case is desperate.

§ 148. When Nature and Art effect his Recovery, his Senses return: though there frequently remains a little *Delirium* or Wandering for some Time; and almost always a paralytic Defect, more or less, of the Tongue, the Arm, the Leg, and the Muscles of the same Side of the Face. This Palsy sometimes goes off gradually, by the Help of cooling Purges from Time to Time, and a Diet that is but very moderately and lightly nourishing. All hot Medicines are extremely hurtful in this Case, and may pave the Way to a repeated Attack. A Vomit might be even fatal, and has been more than once so. It should be absolutely forbidden; nor should we even promote, by Draughts of warm Water, the Efforts of the Patient to vomit. They do not any ways depend on any Humour or Mass in the Stomach, but on the Oppression and Embarrassment of the Brain, and the more considerable such Efforts are, the more such Oppression is increased: by Reason that as long as they continue, the Blood cannot return from the Head, by which Means the Brain remains overcharged.

§ 149 The other Species of Apoplexy is attended with the like Symptoms, excepting the Pulse not being so high nor strong, the Countenance being also less red, sometimes even pale, the Breathing seems less oppressed, and sometimes the Sick have a greater Facility to vomit, and discharge more upwards.

As this Kind of the Disease attacks Persons who abound less in Blood, who are less strong, and less heated or inflamed, Bleeding is not often at all necessary; at least the Repetition of it is scarcely ever so: and should the Pulse have but a small Fulness, and not the least unnatural Hardness, Bleeding might even be pernicious.

1. The Patient however should be placed as was directed in the former Mode of this Disease; though it seems not equally necessary here.

2. He should receive a Glyster, but without Oil, with double the Quantity of Salt, and a Bit of Soap of the Size of a small Egg; or with four or five Sprigs of Hedge Hyssop. It may be repeated twice a Day.

3. He should be purged with the Powder N°. 4. (a)

4. His common Drink may be a strong Infusion of Leaves of Balm.

5. The

(a) Vomits which are so pernicious in the sanguineous Apoplexy, where the Patient's Countenance and Eyes are inflamed, and which are also dangerous or useless, when a Person has been very moderate in his Meals, or is weakened by Age or other Circumstances, and whose Stomach is far from being overloaded with Aliment, are nevertheless very proper for gross Feeders, who are accustomed to exceed at Table, who have Indigestions, and have a Mass of viscid glairy Humours in their Stomachs, more especially, if such a one has a little while before indulged himself excessively, whence he has vomited without any other evident Cause, or at least had very strong *Nauseas*, or Loathings. In brief, Vomits are the true Specific for Apoplexies, occasioned by any narcotic or stupifying Poisons, the pernicious Effects of which cease, the Moment the Persons so poisoned vomit them up. An attentive Consideration of what has occured to the Patient before his Seizure, his small natural Propensity to this Disease and great and incessant Loathings, render it manifest whether it has been caused by such Poisons, or such poisonous Excesses. In these two last Cases a double Dose of Tartar emetic should be dissolved in a Goblet or Cup of Water, of which the Patient should immediately take a large Spoonful, which should be repeated every Quarter of an Hour, till it operates *E L*

5. The Purge should be repeated the third Day.

6. Blisters should immediately be applied to the fleshy Part of the Legs, or between the Shoulder Blades. (a)

7. Should Nature seem disposed to relieve herself by Sweatings, it should be encouraged; and I have often known an Infusion of the *Carduus benedictus*, or blessed Thistle, produce this Effect very successfully. If this Method be entered upon, the Sweat ought to be kept up (without stirring if possible) for many Days. It has then sometimes happened, that at the End of nine Days, the Patient has been totally freed from the Palsy, which commonly succeeds this Species of the Apoplexy, just as it does the other

§ 150. Persons who have been attacked with either kinds of this Disease are liable to subsequent ones; each of which is more dangerous than that preceding. whence an Endeavour to obviate or prevent such Relapses becomes of the utmost Importance. This is to be effected in each Sort by a very exact, and rather severe Diet, even to diminishing the usual Quantity of the Patient's Food, the most essential Precaution, to be observed by any who have been once assaulted with it, being entirely to leave off Suppers Indeed

---

These Blisters may be preceded by Cupping with Scarification on the Nape of the Neck. This Remedy, often used by the ancient Physicians, but too little practiced in France, is one of the most speedy, and not the least efficacious, Applications in both general and particular Apoplexies. E. L.

deed those, who have been once attacked with the *first*, the *sanguineous Apoplexies*, should be still more exact, more upon their Guard, than the others. They should deny themselves whatever is rich and juicy, hot or aromatic, sharp, Wine, distilled Liquors and Coffee. They should chiefly confine themselves to Garden-Stuff, Fruits and Acids; such should eat but little Flesh, and only those called white; taking every Week two or three Doses of the Powder N° 24, in a Morning fasting, in a Glass of Water. They should be purged twice or thrice a Year with the Draught N°. 23; use daily Exercise; avoid very hot Rooms, and the violent Heat of the Sun. They should go to Bed betimes, rise early, never lie in Bed above eight Hours: and if it is observed that their Blood increases considerably, and has a Tendency towards the Head, they should be bled without Hesitation: and for some Days restrain themselves entirely to a thin and low Regimen, without taking any solid Food. In these Circumstances warm Bathings are hurtful. In the other, the serous, Apoplexy, instead of purging with N°. 23, the Patient should take the Purge N°. 21

§ 151. The same Means, that are proper to prevent a Relapse, might also obviate or keep off a primary or first Assault, if employed in Time: for notwithstanding it may happen very suddenly, yet this Disease foreshews itself many Weeks, sometimes many Months, nay even Years beforehand, by Vertigos, Heaviness of the Head, small

Defects of the Tongue or Speech; short and momentary Palsies, sometimes of one, sometimes of another, Part: sometimes by Loathings and Reachings to vomit; without supposing any Obstruction or Load in the first Passages, or any other Cause in the Stomach, or the adjoining Parts. There happens also some particular Change in the Looks and Visage not easy to be described: sharp and short Pains about the Region of the Heart, an Abatement of the Strength, without any discernible Cause of it. Besides there are still some other Signs, which signify the Ascent of the Humours too much to the Head, and shew, that the Functions of the Brain are embarrassed.

Some Persons are liable to certain Symptoms and Appearances, which arise from the same Cause as an Apoplexy; and which indeed may be considered as very light benign Apoplexies, of which they sustain many Attacks, and yet without any considerable Annoyance of their Health. The Blood all at once as it were, flushes up to their Heads: they appear heedless or blundering; and have sometimes Disgusts and *Nauseas*, and yet without any Abatement of their Understanding, their Senses, or Motion of any Sort. Tranquillity of Mind and Body, once Bleeding, and a few Glisters usually carry it off soon after its Invasion. The Returns of it may be prevented by the Regimen directed § 150, and especially by a frequent Use of the Powder N°. 24. At the long Run however, one of these Attacks commonly degene-

degenerates into a mortal Apoplexy: though this may be retarded for a very long Time by an exact Regimen, and by avoiding all strong Commotions of the Mind, but especially that of Anger or violent Rage.

CHAPTER X.

Of the violent Influence, or Strokes, of the Sun.

SECT. 152.

THIS Appellation is applied to those Disorders, which arise from too violent an Influence of the Heat of the Sun, immediately upon the Head, and which in one Word may be termed *Insolation*.

If we consider that Wood, Stone and Metals, when long exposed to the Sun, become very hot, and that even in temperate Climates, to such a Degree, that they can scarcely be touched without some Sensation of burning, we may easily conceive the Risk a Person undergoes, in having his Head exposed to the same Degree of Heat. The Blood-Vessels grow dry, the Blood itself becomes condensed or thickened, and a real Inflammation is formed, which has proved mortal in a very little Time. It was this Distemper, a Stroke of the Sun, which killed *Manasses* the Husband of *Judith* ' For as he was among the

' Labourers

'Labourers who bound up the Sheafs in the
'Fields, the Heat struck upon his Head, and
'he was taken ill; he went to Bed and he died.'
The Signs which precede and attend this Disease are, being exposed in a Place where the Sun shines forth with great Force and Ardour; a violent Head-ach, attended with a very hot and extremely dry Skin: the Eyes are also dry and red, being neither able to remain open, nor yet to bear the Light, and sometimes there is a kind of continual and involuntary Motion in the Eyelid, while some Degree of Relief is perceivable from the Application of any cooling Liquor. It often happens that some cannot possibly sleep, and at other times they have a great Drowsiness, but attended with outrageous Wakenings: there is a very strong Fever, a great Faintness, and a total Disrelish and Loathing. Sometimes the Patient is very thirsty, and at other times not at all. And the Skin of his Face often looks as though it were burnt.

§ 153 People may be affected with the Disease from this Cause at two different Seasons of the Year; that is, either in the Spring, or during the very raging Heats, but their Events are very different. Country People and Labourers are but little liable to the former. They chiefly affect the Inhabitants of Cities, and delicate Persons, who have used very little Exercise in the Winter, and abound with superfluous Humours. If thus circumstanced they expose themselves to the Sun, as even in the Spring he attains a considerable

Of Strokes of the Sun

fiderable Force; and, by the Course of Life they have led, their Humours are already much disposed to mount to the Head, while the Coolness of the Soil, especially when it has rained, prevents their Feet from being so easily warmed; the Power of the Sun acts upon their Head like a Blister, attracting a great Quantity of Humours to it. This produces excruciating Pains of the Head, frequently accompanied with quick and violent Shootings, and with Pain in the Eyes; notwithstanding this Degree of the Malady is seldom dangerous. Country People, and even such Inhabitants of Cities and Towns, as have not forbore to exercise themselves in Winter, have no Sort of Dread of these Strokes of the Sun, in the Spring of the Year. Its Summer Strokes are much more vehement and troublesome, and assault Labourers and Travellers, who are for a long Time exposed to the Fervour of it. Then it is that the Disease is aggravated to its highest Pitch, those who are thus struck often dying upon the Spot. In the hot Climates this Cause destroys many in the very Streets, and makes dreadful Havock among Armies on the March, and at Sieges. Some tragical Effects of it, on such Occasions, are seen even in the temperate Countries. After having marched a whole Day in the Sun, a Man shall fall into a Lethargy, and die within some Hours, with the Symptoms of raving Madness. I have seen a Tyler in a very hot Day, complaining to his Comrade of a violent Pain in his Head, which increased every Moment almost;

almost, and at the very Instant when he purposed to retire out of the Sun, he sunk down dead, and fell down from the House he was slating. This same Cause produces very often in the Country some most dangerous Phrenzies, which are called there hot or burning Fevers. Every Year furnishes but too many of them.

§ 154. The Vehemence of the Sun is still more dangerous to those, who venture to sleep exposed to it. Two Mowers who fell asleep on a Haycock, being wakened by some others, immediately on waking, staggered, and pronouncing a few incoherent unmeaning Words, died. When the Violence of Wine and that of the Sun are combined, they kill very suddenly: nor is there a single Year in which Peasants are not found dead on the Highroads; who being drunk endeavoured to lie down in some Corner, where they perished by an Apoplexy, from the Heat of the Sun and of strong Drink. Those of them who escape so speedy and premature a Death, are subject for the Remainder of their Lives, to chronical, or tedious Head-achs; and to suffer some little Disorder and Confusion in their Ideas. I have seen some Cases, when after violent Head-achs of some Days Continuance, the Disease has been transferred to the Eyelids, which continued a long Time red and distended, so that they could not be kept asunder or open. It has also been known, that some Persons have been struck by the Sun into a *Delirium* or Raving, without a Fever, and without complaining of a Headach.

ach. Sometimes a *Gutta Serena* has been its Consequence; and it is very common to see People, whose long Continuance under the strong Light and Influence of the Sun, has made such an Impression upon the Eyes, as presents them with different Bodies flying about in the Air, which distract and confuse their Sight.

A Man of forty two Years of Age, having been exposed for several Hours to the violent Heat of the Sun, with a very small Cap or Bonnet, and having past the following Night in the open Air, was attacked the next Day with a most severe Head-ach, a burning Fever, Reachings to vomit, great Anguish, and red and sparkling Eyes. Notwithstanding the best Assistance of several Physicians, he became phrenitic on the fifth Day, and died on the ninth. Suppurated Matter was discharged from his Mouth, one of his Nostrils, and his right Ear, a few Hours before his Death; and upon Dissection a small Abscess was found within the Skull, and the whole Brain, as well as all the Membranes inclosing it, were entirely corrupted.

§ 155. In very young Children, who are not, or never should be, exposed for any long Time to such excessive Heat (and whom a slight Cause will often affect) this Malady discovers itself by a heavy deep Drowsiness, which lasts for several Days; also by incessant Ravings mingled with Rage and Terror, much the same as when they are affected with violent Fear, and sometimes by convulsive Twitchings, by Head-achs which returned

returned at certain Periods, and continual Vomitings. I have seen Children, who, after a Stroke of the Sun, have been harrassed a long Time with a little Cough.

§ 156. Old Men who often expose themselves imprudently to the Sun, are little apprized of all the Danger they incur by it. A certain Person, who purposely sunned himself for a considerable Time, in the clear Day of an intermitting tertian Fever, underwent the Assault of an Apoplexy, which carried him off the following Day. And even when the Disease may not be so speedy and violent, yet this Custom (of sunning in hot Weather) certainly disposes to an Apoplexy, and to Disorders of the Head. One of the slightest Effects of much solar Heat upon the Head is, to cause a Defluxion from the Brain, a Swelling of the Glands of the Neck, and a Dryness of the Eyes, which sometimes continues for a considerable Term after it.

§ 157. The Effect of too much culinary, or common Fire, is of the same Quality with that of the Sun. A Man who fell asleep with his Head directly opposite, and probably, very near to the Fire, went off in an Apoplexy, during his Nap.

§ 158. The Action of too violent a Sun is not only pernicious, when it falls upon the Head; but it is also hurtful to other Parts, and those who continue long exposed to it, though their Heads should not be affected, experience violent Pains, a disagreeable Sensation of Heat, and a considerable Stiffness in the Parts that have been, in some Manner, parched by it; as in the Legs, the Knees, the Thighs, Reins and Arms; and sometimes they prove feverish.

§ 159. In contemplating the Case of a Patient, *Sun-struck*, as we may term it, we must endeavour to distinguish, whether there may not be also some other joint Causes concurring to the Effect. A Traveller, a labouring Man, is often as much affected by the Fatigue of his Journey, or of his Labour, as he is by the Influence of solar Heat.

§ 160. It is necessary to set about the Cure of this Disease, as soon as ever we are satisfied of its Existence: for such as might have been easily preserved by an early Application, are considerably endangered by a Neglect of it. The Method of treating this is very much the same, with that of the inflammatory Diseases already mentioned; that is, by Bleeding, and cooling Medicines of various Kinds in their Drinks, by Bathings, and by Glysters. And 1 If the Disease be very high and urgent, a large Quantity of Blood should be taken away, and occasionally repeated. Lewis the XIV. was bled nine Times to prevent the Fatality of a Stroke of the Sun, which he received in Hunting in 1658.

2 After Bleeding, the Patient's Legs should be plunged into warm Water. This is one of the Applications that affords the most speedy Relief, and I have seen the Head-ach go off and return again, in Proportion to the Repetition, and the Duration, of these Bathings of the Legs. When the Disorder is highly dangerous, it will be necessary

cessary to treat the Patient with *Semicupia*, or warm Baths, in which he may sit up to his Hips; and in the most dangerous Degrees of it, even to bathe the whole Body: but the Water in this Case, as well as in Bathings of the Feet, should be only sensibly warm: the Use of hot would be highly pernicious.

3. Glysters made from a Decoction of any of the emollient Herbs are also very effectual.

4. The Patient should drink plentifully of Almond Emulsion N°. 4; of Limonade, which is a Mixture of the Juice of Lemons and Water, (and is the best Drink in this Disease) of Water and Vinegar, which is a very good Substitute for Limonade, and of, what is still more efficacious, very clear Whey, with the Addition of a little Vinegar. These various Drinks may all be taken cold; Linen Cloths dipt in cold Water and Vinegar of Roses may be applied to the Forehead, the Temples, or all over the Head, which is equivalent to every other Application used upon such Occasions. Those which are the most cried up, are the Juice of Purslain, of Lettuce, of Houseleek, and of Vervain. The Drink N°. 32 is also serviceable, taken every Morning fasting.

§ 161. Cold Baths have sometimes recovered Persons out of such violent Symptoms, from this Cause, as have been almost quite despaired of

A Man twenty Years of Age, having been a very long Time exposed to the scorching Sun, became violently delirious, without a Fever, and proved really mad After repeated Bleedings, he he was thrown into a cold Bath, which was also frequently repeated; pouring cold Water, at the same Time, upon his Head. With such Assistance he recovered, though very gradually.

An Officer who had rode Post for several Days successively, in very hot Weather, swooned away, immediately on dismounting; from which he could not be recovered by the ordinary Assistance in such Cases. He was saved however, in Consequence of being plunged into a Bath of freezing Water. It should be observed however, that in these Cases the cold Bath should never be recurred to, without previous Bleeding.

§ 162. It is past Doubt, that if a Person stands still in the violent Heat of the Sun, he is more liable to be struck with it, than if he walks about, and the Use of white Hats, or of some Folds of clean white Paper under a black one, may sensibly contribute to prevent any Injury from the considerable Heat of the Sun; though it is a very incompetent Defence against a violent Degree of it.

The natural Constitution, or even that Constitution, which has been formed from long Custom and Habit, make a very great Difference between the Effects of solar Heat on different Persons. People insensibly accustom themselves to the Impressions of it, as they do to those of all the other Bodies and Elements, which are continually acting upon us, and by Degrees we arrive at a Power of sustaining his violent Heat with Impunity: just as others arrive at the Hardiness of

bearing

bearing the most rigid Colds, with very little Complaint or Inconvenience. The human Body is capable of supporting many more Violences and Extremes, than it commonly does. Its natural Force is scarcely ever ascertained among civilized Nations, because their Education generally tends to impair and lessen it, and always succeeds in this Respect. If we were inclined to consider a purely natural, a simply physical Man, we must look for him among savage Nations; where only we can discover what we are able to be, and to bear. We certainly could not fail of being Gainers, by adopting their corporal Education, neither does it seem as yet to have been infallibly demonstrated, that we should be great Losers in commuting our moral Education for theirs. *

CHAPTER.

---

* As some may think an Apology necessary for a Translation of this Chapter on a Disease, which never, or very seldom, exists in this or the adjacent Island, I shall observe here, that, abstracted from the Immorality of a narrow and local Solicitude only for ourselves, we are politically interested as a Nation always in Trade, and often at War (and whose Subjects are extended into very distant and different Climates) to provide against a sudden and acute Distemper, to which our Armies, our Sailors and Colonies are certainly often exposed. A Fatality from this Cause is not restrained to our Islands within the Tropic, where several Instances of it have occurred during the late War but it has also been known to prevail as far Northward as *Pensylvania*, in their Summers, and even in their Harvests. I once received a sensible Scald on the Back of my Thumb, from the Sun suddenly darting out through a clear Hole, as it were, in a Cloud, after a short and impetuous Shower in Summer, which Scald manifestly blistered within some Minutes after. Had this concentered Ray been darted on my bare Head, the Consequence might have been more dangerous, or perhaps as fatal as some of the Cases recorded by Dr. Tissot, in this Chapter. K

Chapter XI.

Of the Rheumatism.

Sect. 163.

THE Rheumatism may exist either with or without a Fever. The first of these may be classed among the Diseases, of which I have already treated; being an Inflammation which is manifested by a violent Fever, preceded by Shivering, a subsequent Heat, hard Pulse, and a Head-ach. Sometimes indeed an extraordinary Coldness, with general Uneasiness and Inquietude, exists several Days before the Fever is perceived. On the second or third Day, and sometimes even on the first, the Patient is seized with a violent Pain in some Part of his Body, but especially about the Joints, which entirely prevents their Motion, and which is often accompanied with Heat, Redness and a Swelling of the Part. The Knee is often the first Part attacked, and sometimes both the Knees at once. When the Pain is fixed, an Abatement of the Fever frequently happens; though in some other Persons it continues for several Days, and increases every Evening. The Pain diminishes in one Part after a Duration of some Days, and then invades some other. From the Knee it descends to the Foot, or mounts to the Hip, to the Loins, the Shoulder-blades, Elbow, Wrist, the Nape of the Neck, and frequently is felt in the intermediate Parts. Sometimes one Part is quite free from Pain, when another is attacked; at other Times many Parts are seized nearly at the same Instant, and I have sometimes seen every Joint afflicted at once. In this Case the Patient is in a very terrible Situation, being incapable of any Motion, and even dreading the Assistance of his Attendants, as he can scarcely admit of touching, without a sensible Aggravation of his Pains. He is unable to bear even the Weight of the Bed-cloths, which must be, as it were, arched over his Limbs by a proper Contrivance, to prevent their Pressure, and the very walking across the Chamber increases his Torments. The Parts in which they are the most excruciating, and obstinate, are the Region of the Loins, the Hips, and the Nape or hinder Part of the Neck.

§ 164. This Disease is also often extended over the Scalp and the Surface of the Head; and there the Pains are excessive. I have seen them affect the Eyelids and the Teeth with inexpressible Torment. As long as the Distemper is situated in the more external Parts, the Patient, however painful his Situation may prove, is in no great Danger, if he be properly treated: but if by some Accident, some Error, or by any latent Cause, the Disease be repelled upon an internal Part or Organ, his Case is extremely dangerous. If the Brain is attacked, a frantic raging *Delirium* is the Consequence; if it falls upon the Lungs, the Patient is suffocated: and if it attacks the Stomach or the Bowels, it is attended with the most astonishing Pains, which are caused by the Inflammation of those Parts, and which Inflammation, if violent, is * speedily fatal. About two Years since I was called to a robust Man, whose Guts were already in a gangrenous State, which was the Consequence of a Rheumatism, that first attacked one Arm and one Knee; the Cure of which had been attempted by sweating the Patient with some hot Remedies. These indeed brought on a plentiful Sweat; but the inflammatory Humour seized the Intestines, whose Inflammation degenerated into a Gangrene, after a Duration of the most acute Pain for thirty-six Hours; his Torments terminating in Death two Hours after I saw him.

§ 165. This Malady however is often in a less violent Degree; the Fever is but moderate, and ceases entirely when the Pain begins; which is also confined to one, or not more than two Parts.

§ 166 If the Disease continues fixed, for a considerable Time, in one Joint, the Motion of it is impaired for Life. I have seen a Person, who has now a wry Neck, of twenty Years standing, in Consequence of a Rheumatism in the Nape of the Neck; and I also saw a poor young Man from *Jurat*, who was Bed-ridden, and who had lost the Motion of one Hip and both Knees.

* See Note * to Page 59.

He could neither stand nor sit, and there were but a few Postures in which he could even lie in Bed.

§ 167. An obstructed Perspiration, an inflammatory Thickness of the Blood, constitute the most general Cause of the Rheumatism. This last concurring Cause is that we must immediately encounter, since, as long as that subsists, Perspiration cannot be perfectly re-established, which follows of Course, when the Inflammation is cured. For which Reason this Distemper must be conducted like the other inflammatory ones, of which I have already treated.

§ 168. As soon as it is sufficiently manifest, the Glyster N° 5, should be injected, and twelve Ounces of Blood be taken from the Arm an Hour after. The Patient is to enter upon a Regimen, and drink plentifully of the Ptisan N°. 2, and of Almond Milk or Emulsion N° 4. As this last Medicine may be too costly in Country Places for the poor Peasantry, they may drink, in Lieu of it, very clear Whey, sweetened with a little Honey. I have known a very severe Rheumatism cured, after twice bleeding, without any other Food or Medicine, for the Space of thirteen Days. The Whey also may be happily used by Way of Glyster.

§ 169. If the Distemper is not considerably assuaged by the first Bleeding, it should be repeated some Hours after. I have ordered it four times within the first two Days; and some time after I have even directed a fifth Bleeding. But

But in general the Hardness of the Pulse becomes less after the second; and notwithstanding the Pains may continue as severe as before, yet the Patient is sensible of less Inquietude. The Glyster must be repeated every Day, and even twice a Day, if each of them is attended only with a small Discharge; and particularly if there be a violent Head-ach. In such Cases as are excessively painful, the Patient can scarcely dispose himself into a proper Attitude or Posture to receive Glysters: and in such Circumstances his Drinks should be made as opening as possible, and a Dose of the Cream of Tartar N°. 24 should be given Night and Morning. This very Medicine, with the Assistance of Whey, cured two Persons I advised it to, of rheumatic Pains, of which they had been infested with frequent Returns for many Years, and which were attended with a small Fever.

Apples coddled, Prunes stewed, and well ripened Summer Fruits are the properest Nourishment in this Disease.

We may save the Sick a good deal of Pain, by putting one strong Towel always under their Back, and another under their Thighs, in order to move them the more easily. When their Hands are without Pain, a third Towel hung upon a Cord, which is fastened across the Bed, must considerably assist them in moving themselves.

§ 170. When the Fever entirely disappears, and the Hardness of the Pulse is removed, I have ordered

ordered the Purge N°. 23 with a very good Effect; and if it is attended with five or six Motions, the Patient is very sensibly relieved. The Day but one after it may be repeated successfully, and a third Time, after an Interval of a greater Number of Days.

§ 171. When the Pains are extremely violent, they admit of no Application: Vapour-Baths however may be employed, and provided they are often used, and for a considerable Time, they prove very efficacious. The Purpose of these Baths is only to convey the Steam of boiling Water to the Parts affected; which may always easily be effected, by a Variety of simple and easy Contrivances; the Choice of which must depend on the different Circumstances and Situation of the Sick.

Whenever it is possible, some of the emollient Applications N°. 9, should be continually employed. A half Bath, or an entire Bath of warm Water, in which the Patient should remain an Hour, after sufficient Bleedings and many Glysters, affords the greatest Relief. I have seen a Patient, under the most acute Pains of the Loins, of the Hips, and of one Knee, put into one. He continued still under extreme Torment in the Bath, and on being taken out of it. but an Hour after he had been put to Bed, he sweated, to an incredible Quantity, for thirty six Hours, and was cured. The Bath should never be made use of, until after repeated Bleedings, or at least other

equi-

equivalent Evacuations: for otherwise timed, it would aggravate the Disease.

§ 172. The Pains are generally most severe in the Night; whence it has been usual to give composing soporific Medicines. This however has been very erroneous, as Opiates really augment the Cause of the Disease, and destroy the Efficacy of the proper Remedies; and, even not seldom, far from assuaging the Pains, they increase them. Indeed they agree so little in this Disease, that even the Patient's natural Sleep at the Invasion of this Complaint, is rather to his Detriment. They feel, the very Moment they are dropping asleep, such violent Jirks as awaken them with great Pain: or if they do sleep a few Minutes, the Pains are stronger when they awake.

§ 173. The Rheumatism goes off either by Stool, by turbid thick Urine which drops a great Proportion of a yellowish Sediment, or by Sweats: and it generally happens that this last Discharge prevails towards the Conclusion of the Disease. It may be kept up by drinking an Infusion of Elder Flowers. At the Beginning however Sweating is pernicious.

§ 174 It happens also, though but very seldom, that Rheumatisms determine by depositing a sharp Humour upon the Legs; where it forms Vesications, or a kind of Blisterings; which burst open and form Ulcers, that ought not to be healed and dried up too hastily; as this would occasion a speedy Return of the rheumatic Pains.

They

They are disposed to heal naturally of themselves, by the Assistance of a temperate regular Diet, and a few gentle Purges.

§ 175. Sometimes again, an Abscess is formed either in the affected Part, or in some neighbouring one. I have seen a Vineyard Dresser, who after violent Pains of the Loins, had an Abscess in the upper Part of the Thigh, which he neglected for a long Time. When I saw him, it was of a monstrous Size. I ordered it to be opened, when at once above three Pots of * Matter rushed out of it: but the Patient, being exhausted, died some Time after it.

Another Crisis of the Rheumatism has happened by a kind of Itch, which breaks out upon all the Parts adjacent to the Seat of this Disease. Immediately after this Eruption the Pains vanish: but the Pustules sometimes continue for several Weeks.

§ 176. I have never observed the Pains to last, with considerable Violence, above fourteen Days, in this Species of the Rheumatism; though there remains a Weakness, Numbness, and some Inflation, or Puffing, of the adjoining Parts: and it will also be many Weeks, and sometimes even Months,

---

* This according to our Author's Estimation of the Pot-Measure a *Derne* which is that he always means, and which he says contains exactly of Water we suppose, fifty one Ounces and a Quarter (though without a material Error it may be computed at three Pound and a Quarter) will amount at least to nine Pounds and three Quarters of Matter, supposing this no heavier than Water. By Measure it will want but little of five of our Quarts; a very extraordinary Discharge indeed of *Pus* at once, and not unlikely to be attended by the Event which soon followed. *K*

Months; especially if the Distemper attacked them in the Fall, before the Sick recover their usual Strength. I have known some Persons, who, after a very painful Rheumatism, have been troubled with a very disagreeable Sensation of Lassitude; which did not go off till after a great Eruption, all over the Body, of little Vesications or Blisterings, full of a watery Humour, many of them burst open, and others withered and dried up without bursting.

§ 177. The Return of Strength into the Parts affected may be promoted by Frictions Night and Morning, with Flannel or any other woollen Stuff; by using Exercise; and by conforming exactly to the Directions given in the Chapter on Convalescence, or Recovery from acute Diseases. The Rheumatism may also be prevented by the Means I have pointed out, in treating of Pleurisies and Quinsies.

§ 178. Sometimes the Rheumatism, with a Fever, invades Persons who are not so sanguine, or abounding in Blood; or whose Blood is not so much disposed to Inflammation, those whose Flesh and Fibres are softer; and in whose Humours there is more Thinness and Sharpness, than Viscidity and Thickness. Bleeding proves less necessary for Persons so constituted, notwithstanding the Fever should be very strong. Some Constitutions require more Discharges by Stool; and after they are properly evacuated, some Blisters should be applied, which often afford them a sensible Relief as soon as ever they begin to operate.

operate. Nevertheless they should never be used where the Pulse is hard. The Powder Nº. 25 answers very well in these Cases.

§ 179. There is another Kind of Rheumatism, called chronical, or lasting. It is known by the following Characters or Marks. 1. It is commonly unattended with a Fever. 2. It continues a very long Time. 3. It seldom attacks so many Parts at once as the former. 4. Frequently no visible Alteration apppears in the affected Part, which is neither more hot, red, or swelled than in its healthy State, though sometimes one or other of these Symptoms is evident. 5. The former, the inflammatory, Rheumatism assaults strong, vigorous, robust Persons: but this rather invades People arrived at a certain Period of Life, or such as are weak and languishing.

§ 180. The Pain of the chronical Rheumatism, when left to itself, or injudiciously treated, lasts sometimes many Months, and even Years. It is particularly and extremely obstinate, when it is exerted on the Head, the Loins, or on the Hip, and along the Thighs, when it is called the *Sciatica* There is no Part indeed which this Pain may not invade; sometimes it fixes itself in a small Spot, as in one Corner of the Head; the Angle of the Jaw, the Extremity of a Finger; in one Knee; on one Rib, or on the Breast, where it often excites Pains, which make the Patient apprehensive of a Cancer. It penetrates also to the internal Parts When it affects the Lungs, a most obstinate Cough is the Consequence;

quence; which degenerates at length into very dangerous Disorders of the Breast. In the Stomach and Bowels it excites most violent Pains like a Cholic; and in the Bladder, Symptoms so greatly resembling those of the Stone, that Persons, who are neither deficient in Knowlege nor Experience, have been more than once deceived by them.

§ 181. The Treatment of this chronical Rheumatism does not vary considerably from that of the former. Nevertheless, in the first Place, if the Pain is very acute, and the Patient robust, a single Bleeding at the Onset is very proper and efficacious. 2. The Humours ought to be diluted, and their Acrimony or Sharpness should be diminished, by a very plentiful Use of a Ptisan of (a) Burdock Roots N°. 26. 3. Four or five Days after drinking abundantly of this, the purging (b) Powder

(a) Half a Pint of a pretty strong Infusion of the Leaves of Buckbean, which grows wild here, taken once a Day rather before Noon, has also been found very serviceable in that Species of a chronical Rheumatism, which considerably results from a scorbutic State of the Constitution *K.*

(b) Another very good Purge, in this Kind of Rheumatism, may also be compounded of the best Gum Guiacum in Powder from 30 to 40 Grains, dissolved in a little Yolk of a fresh Egg, adding from 6 to 10 Grains of Jallap powdered, and from 3 to 5 Grains of powdered Ginger, with as much plain or surfeit Water, as will make a purging Draught for a stronger or weaker grown Patient. Should the Pains frequently infest the Stomach, while the Patient continues costive, and there is no other Fever than such a small symptomatic one, as may arise solely from Pain, he may safely take, if grown up, from 30 to 45 Drops of the volatile Tincture of Gum Guiacum, in any diluting Infusion, that may not coagulate or separate the Gum. It generally disposes at first to a gentle *Diaphoresis* or Sweat, and several Hours after to one, and sometimes to a second Stool, with little or no Griping *K*

Powder N°. 21 may be taken with Success. In this Species of the Rheumatism, a certain Medicine is sometimes found serviceable. This has acquired some Reputation, particularly in the Country, where they bring it from, *Geneva*, under the Title of the Opiate for the Rheumatism, tho' I cannot say for what Reason; as it is indeed neither more nor less than the Electuary *Caryocostinum*, which may be procured at our Apothecaries. I shall observe however, that this Medicine has done Mischief in the inflammatory Rheumatism, and even in this, as often as the Persons afflicted with it are feeble, thin and of a hot Temperament, and either when they have not previously taken diluting Drinks, or when it has been used too long. For, in such a Circumstance, it is apt to throw the Patient into an irrecoverable Weakness. The Composition consists of the hottest Spices, and of very sharp Purgatives.

§ 182 When general Remedies have been used, and the Disorder still continues, Recourse should be had to such Medicines, as are available to restore Perspiration, and these should be persisted in for a considerable Time. The Pills N°. 18, with a strong Infusion of Elder Flowers, have often succeeded in this Respect. and then after a long Continuance of diluting Drinks, if the Fever is entirely subdued, if the Stomach exerts its Functions well, the Patient is no ways costive, if he is not of a dry Habit of Body, and the Part affected remains without Inflammation, the

the Patient may safely take the Powder No. 29, at Night going to Bed, with a Cup or two of an Infusion of *Carduus benedictus*, or the blessed Thistle, and a Morsel of Venice Treacle of the Size of a Hazel Nut, or a Filberd. This Remedy brings on a very copious Sweating, which often expells the (a) Disease. These Sweats may be rendered still more effectual, by wrapping up the affected Part in a Flanel dipt in the Decoction N°. 27.

§ 183 But of all these Pains, the Sciatica is one of the most tedious and obstinate. Nevertheless I have seen the greatest Success, from the Application of seven or eight Cupping-Glasses on the tormented Part; by which, without the Assistance of any other Remedy, I have cured, in a few Hours, Sciaticas of many Years standing, which had baffled other Remedies. Blisters, or any such stimulating Plaisters, as bring on a Suppuration and Discharge from the afflicted Part, contribute also frequently to the Cure, tho' less effectually than Cupping, which should be repeated several Times. Green Cere-cloth, commonly called Oil-cloth, (whether the Ingredients be spread on Taffety or on Linen) being applied to the diseased Part, disposes it to sweat abundantly, and thus to discharge the sharp Humour which occasions the Pain. Sometimes both of these Appli-

---

(a) Gum Guaiacum, given from six to ten Grains Morning and Night, is often very successful in these Cases. It may be made into Pills or Bolusses with the Rob of Elder, or with the Extract of Juniper. *E L*

Applications, but especially that spread on Silk (which may be applied more exactly and closely to the Part, and which is also spread with a different Composition) raise a little Vesication on the Part as Blisters do. A Plaister of Quicklime and Honey blended together has cured inveterate Sciaticas. Oil of Eggs has sometimes succeeded in such Cases. A Seton has also been successfully made in the lower Part of the Thigh. Finally some Pains, which have not yielded to any of these Applications, have been cured by actual burning, inflicted on the very Spot, where the most violent Pain has been felt; except some particular Reason, drawn from an anatomical Knowlege of the Part, should determine the Surgeon not to apply it there. The Scull or Head should never be cauterized with a burning Iron.

§ 184. The hot Baths of *Bourbon*, *Plombiers*, *Aix-la-Chapelle* and many others are often very efficacious in these chronical Pains: notwithstanding I really think, there is no rheumatic Pain that may not be cured without them. The common People substitute to these a Bath made of the Husk of Grapes, after their Juice is expressed, which cures some by making them sweat abundantly. Cold Baths however are the best to keep off this Disease; but then they cannot always be safely ventured on. Many Circumstances render the Use of them impracticable to particular Persons. Such as are subject to this chronical Rheumatism, would do very well to rub their whole Bodies every Morning, if they could,

could, but especially the afflicted Parts, with Flanel. This Habit keeps up Perspiration beyond any other Assistance; and indeed sometimes even increases it too much. It would be serviceable too, if such Subjects of this cruel Disease wore Flanel all over their Skin, during the Winter.

After a violent Rheumatism, People should long be careful to avoid that cold and moist Air, which disposes them to relapse.

§ 185. Rheumatic People have too frequent a Recourse to very improper and hurtful Medicines, in this Distemper, which daily produce very bad Consequences. Such are spirituous Medicines, Brandy, and Arquebusade Water. They either render the Pain more obstinate and fixed, by hardening the Skin, or they repell the Humour to some inward Part. And Instances are not wanting of Persons who have died suddenly, from the Application of Spirit of Wine upon the Parts, that were violently afflicted with the Rheumatism. It also happens sometimes that the Humour, having no Outlet through the Skin, is thrown internally on the Bone and affects it. A very singular Fact occured in this Respect, an Account of which may be serviceable to some Persons afflicted with the Disease. A Woman at Night was chaffing the Arm of her Husband, who had the Rheumatism there, with Spirit of Wine; when a very lucky Accident prevented the Mischief she might have occasioned by it. The Spirit of Wine took Fire from the Flame of the Candle she made use of, and burned the diseased Part. It was

dress

dreſt of Courſe, and the Suppuration that attended it, entirely cured the Rheumatiſm.

Sharp and greaſy Unctions or Ointments produce very bad Effects, and are equally dangerous. A *Caries*, a Rottenneſs of the Bones, has enſued upon the Uſe of a Medicine called, The Balſam of Sulphur with Turpentine. I was conſulted in 1750, three Days before her Deceaſe, about a Woman, who had long endured acute rheumatic Pains. She had taken various Medicines, and, among the reſt, a conſiderable Quantity of a Ptiſan, in which Antimony was blended with ſome purging Medicines, and a greaſy ſpirituous Balſam had been rubbed into the Part. The Fever, the Pains, and the Dryneſs of the Skin ſoon increaſed, the Bones of the Thighs and Arms became carious: and in moving the Patient no more than was neceſſary for her Relief and Convenience, without taking her out of her Bed, both Thighs and one Arm broke So dreadful an Example ſhould make People cautious of giving or applying Medicines inconſiderately, even in ſuch Diſeaſes, as appear but trifling in themſelves. I muſt alſo inform the Readers, there are ſome rheumatic Pains, which admit of no Application, and that almoſt every Medicine aggravates them. In ſuch Caſes the afflicted muſt content themſelves with keeping the Parts affected from the Impreſſions of the Air, by a Flanel, or the Skin of ſome Animal with the Fur on

It

It is also more adviseable sometimes to leave a sufferable and inveterate Pain to itself, especially in old or weakly People, than to employ too many Medicines, or such violent ones, as should affect them more importantly than the Pains did.

§ 186. If the Duration of the Pains fixed in the same Place, should cause some Degree of Stiffness in the Joint affected, it should be exposed twice a Day to the Vapour of warm Water, and dried well afterwards with hot Linen: then it should be well chaffed, and lastly touched over with Ointment of Marsh-mallows. Pumping, if superadded to this Vapour, considerably increases its Efficacy. I directed, for a Case of this Sort, a very simple Machine of white Tin, or Lattin, which combined the Application of the Steam and the Pump.

§ 187. Very young Children are sometimes subject to such violent and extended Pains, that they cannot bear touching in any Part, without excessive Crying. We must be careful to avoid mistaking these Cases, and not to treat them like Rheumatisms. They sometimes are owing to Worms, and go off when these have been discharged.

Chapter XII.

Of the Bite of a mad Dog.

Sect. 188.

MEN may contract the particular and raging Symptom, which is very generally peculiar to this Disease from this Cause, and even without any Bite, but this happens very rarely indeed. It is properly a Distemper belonging to the canine *Genus*, consisting of the three Species of Dogs, Wolves, and Foxes, to whom only it seems inherent and natural, scarcely ever arising in other Animals, without its being inflicted by them. Whenever there occurs one of them who breeds it, he bites others, and thus the Poison, the Cause of this terrible Disease, is diffused. Other Animals besides the canine Species, and Men themselves being exposed to this Accident, do sometimes contract the Disease in all its Rage and Horror: though it is not to be supposed, that this is always an unfailing Consequence.

§ 189 If a Dog who used to be lively and active becomes all at once moapish and morose; if he has an Aversion to eat, a particular and unusual Look about his Eyes, a Restlessness, which appears from his continually running to and fro, we may

may be apprehensive he is likely to prove mad; at which very Instant he ought to be tied up securely, that it may be in our Power to destroy him as soon as the Distemper is evident. Perhaps it might be even still safer to kill him at once.

Whenever the Malady is certain, the Symptoms heighten pretty soon. His Aversion to Food, but especially to Drink, grows stronger. He no longer seems to know his Master, the Sound of his Voice changes, he suffers no Person to handle or approach him; and bites those who attempt it. He quits his ordinary Habitation, marching on with his Head and his Tail hanging downwards, his Tongue lolling half out, and covered with Foam or Slaver, which indeed not seldom happens indifferently to all Dogs. Other Dogs scent him, not seldom at a considerable Distance, and fly him with an Air of Horror, which is a certain Indication of his Disease. Sometimes he contents himself with biting only those who happen to be near him: while at other Times becoming more enraged, he springs to the right and left on all Men and Animals about him. He hurries away with manifest Dread from whatever Waters occur to him: at length he falls down as spent and exhausted; sometimes he rises up again, and drags himself on for a little Time, commonly dying the third, or, at the latest, on the fourth Day after the manifest Appearance of the Disease, and sometimes even sooner.

§ 190. When a Person is bit by such a Dog, the Wound commonly heals up as readily, as if it was not in the least poisonous: but after the Expiration of a longer or shorter Term, from three Weeks to three Months, but most commonly in about six Weeks, the Person bitten begins to perceive, in the Spot that was bit, a certain dull obtuse Pain. The Scar of it swells, inflames, bursts open, and weeps out a sharp, fœtid, and serous, or somewhat bloody Humour. At the same Time the Patient becomes sad and melancholy; he feels a kind of Indifference, Insensibility, and general Numbness, an almost incessant Coldness, a Difficulty of breathing, a continual Anguish, and Pains in his Bowels. His Pulse is weak and irregular, his Sleep restless, turbid, and confused with Ravings; with starting up in Surprize, and with terrible Frights. His Discharges by Stool are often much altered and irregular, and small cold Sweats appear at very short Intervals. Sometimes there is also a slight Pain or Uneasiness in the Throat. Such is the first Degree of this Disease, and it is called by some Physicians the dumb Rage, or Madness.

§ 191. Its second Degree, the confirmed or downright Madness, is attended with the following Symptoms. The Patient is afflicted with a violent Thirst, and a Pain in drinking. Soon after this he avoids all Drink, but particularly Water, and within some Hours after, he even abhors it. This Horror becomes so violent, that the

the bringing Water near his Lips, or into his Sight, the very Name of it, or of any other Drink; the Sight of Objects, which, from their Transparence, have any Resemblance of Water, as a Looking Glass, &c. afflicts him with extreme Anguish, and sometimes even with Convulsions. They continue however still to swallow (though not without violent Difficulty) a little Meat or Bread, and sometimes a little Soup. Some even get down the liquid Medicines that are prescribed them, provided there be no Appearance of Water in them, or that Water is not mentioned to them, at the same Time. Their Urine becomes thick and high-coloured, and sometimes there is a Suppression or Stoppage of it. The Voice either grows hoarse, or is almost entirely abolished: but the Reports of the bitten barking like Dogs are ridiculous and superstitious Fictions, void of any Foundation, as well as many other Fables, that have been blended with the History of this Distemper. The Barking of Dogs however is very disagreeable to them. They are troubled with short *Deliriums* or Ravings, which are sometimes mixed with Fury. It is at such times that they spit around them, that they attempt also to bite, and sometimes unhappily effect it. Their Looks are fixed, as it were, and somewhat furious, and their Visage frequently red. It is pretty common for these miserable Patients to be sensible of the Approach of their raging Fit, and to conjure the Bystanders to be upon their Guard. Many of them never have an Inclination to bite. The increasing Anguish and Pain they feel become inexpressible: they earnestly wish for Death; and some of them have even destroyed themselves, when they had the Means of effecting it.

§ 192. It is with the Spittle, and the Spittle only, that this dreadful Poison unites itself. And here it may be observed, 1, That if the Wounds have been made through any of the Patient's Cloaths, they are less dangerous than those inflicted immediately on the naked Skin. 2, That Animals who abound in Wool, or have very thick Hair, are often preserved from the mortal Impression of the Poison; because in these various Circumstances, the Cloaths, the Hair, or the Wool have wiped, or even dried up, the Slaver of their Teeth. 3. The Bites inflicted by an infected Animal, very soon after he has bitten many others, are less dangerous than the former Bites, because their Slaver is lessened or exhausted. 4, If the Bite happens in the Face, or in the Neck, the Danger is greater, and the Operation of the Venom is quicker too; by Reason the Spittle of the Person so bit is sooner infected. 5, The higher the Degree of the Disease is advanced, the Bites become proportionably more dangerous. From what I have just mentioned here it may be discerned, why, of many who have been bitten by the same Sufferer, some have been infected with this dreadful Disease, and others not.

§ 193. A great Number of Remedies have been highly cried up, as famous in the Cure of this

this Disease, and, in *Swisserland* particularly, the Root of the Eglantine or wild Rose, gathered at some particular times, under the favorable Aspects of the Moon, and dried with some extraordinary Precautions. There is also the Powder of *Paulmier*, of calcined Egg Shells, that of the *Lichen terrestris*, or Ground Liverwort, with one third Part of Pepper, a Remedy long celebrated in *England*, Powder of Oyster-Shells, of Vervain; bathing in Salt Water, St. Hubert's Key, &c. &c. But the Death of a Multitude of those who have been bitten, notwithstanding their taking the greatest Part of all these boasted Antidotes, and the Certainty of no one's escaping, who had been attacked with the high raging Symptom, the *Hydrophobia*, have demonstrated the Inefficacy of them all, to all *Europe*. It is incontestable that to the Year 1730, not a single Patient escaped, in whom the Disease was indisputably manifest, and that every Medicine then employed against it was useless. When Medicines had been given before the great Symptom appeared, in some of those who took them, it afterwards appeared, in others not. The same different Events occurred also to others who were bitten, and who took not the least Medicine, so that upon the whole, before that Date, no Medicine seemed to be of any Consequence. Since that Time, we have had the Happiness to be informed of a certain Remedy, which is Mercury, joined to a few others.

§ 194. In short there is a Necessity for destroying or expelling the Poison itself, which Mercury effects, and is consequently the Counter-poison of it. That Poison produces a general Irritation of the Nerves; this is to be removed or asswaged by Antispasmodics: so that in Mercury, or Quicksilver, joined to Antispasmodics, consists the whole that is indicated in the Cure of this Disease. There really have been many Instances of Persons cured by these Medicines, in whom the Distemper had been manifest in its Rage and Violence, and as many as have unfortunately received the Cause of it in a Bite, should be firmly persuaded, that in taking these Medicines, and using all other proper Precautions, they shall be entirely secured from all its ill Consequences Those also in whom the Rage and Fury of this Distemper is manifest, ought to use the same Medicines, with entire * Hope and Confidence, which may justly be founded on the many Cures effected by them. It is acknowledged however, that they have proved ineffectual in a few Cases; but what Disease is there, which does not sometimes prove incurable?

§ 195.

---

* This Advice is truly prudent and judicious, Hope, as I have observed on a different Occasion, being a powerful, though impalpable, Cordial and in such perilous Situations, we should excite the most agreeable Expectations we possibly can in the Patient, that Nature, being undepressed by any desponding melancholy ones, may exert her Functions the more firmly, and co-operate effectually with the Medicines, against her internal Enemy.
A

§ 195. The very Moment after receiving the Bite, if it happens to be in the Flesh, and if it can safely be effected, all the Part affected should be cut † away. The Ancients directed it to be cauterized, or burnt with a red hot Iron (meer Scarification being of very little Effect) and this Method would very probably prove effectual. It requires more Resolution, however, than every Patient is endued with. The Wound should be washed and cleansed a considerable Time with warm Water, with a little Sea-Salt dissolved in it. After this into the Lips and Edges of the Wound, and into the Surface of the Part all about it, should

---

† I knew a brave worthy Gentleman abroad, who above forty Years past thus preserved his Life, after receiving the Bite of a large Rattle Snake, by resolutely cutting it and the Flesh surrounding it out, with a sharp pointed Penknife. ——Perhaps those who would not suffer the Application of the actual Cautery, that is, of a red hot Iron (which certainly promises well for a Cure) might be persuaded to admit of a potential Cautery, where the Bite was inflicted on a fleshy Part. Though even this is far from being unpainful, yet the Pain coming on more gradually, is less terrifying and horrid. And when it had been applied quickly after, and upon the Bite, and kept on for 3 or 4 Hours, the Discharge, after cutting the *Eschar*, would sooner ensue, and in more Abundance, than that from the actual Cautery, the only Preference of which seems to consist in its being capable perhaps of absorbing, or otherwise consuming, all the poisonous *Saliva* at once. This Issue should be dressed afterwards according to our Author's Direction, and in the gradual healing of the Ulcer, it may be properly deterged by adding a little Præcipitate to the Digestive. Neither would this interfere with the Exhibition of the *Tonquin* Powder N° 30, nor the antispasmodic *Bolus* N° 31, if they should be judged necessary. And these perhaps might prove the most certain Means of preventing the mortal Effects of this singular animal Poison, which it is so impossible to analyze, and so extremely difficult to form any material Idea of, but which is not the Case of some other Poisons. *K.*

should be rubbed a Quarter of an Ounce of the Ointment N°. 28; and the Wound should be dressed twice daily, with the soft lenient Ointment N° 29, to promote Suppuration; but that of N°. 28 is to be used only once a Day.

In point of Regimen, the Quantity of Nourishment should be less than usual, particularly in the Article of * Flesh: he should abstain from Wine, spirituous Liquors, all Sorts of Spices and hot inflaming Food. He should drink only Barley-Water, or an Infusion of the Flowers of the Lime-tree. He should be guarded against Costiveness by a soft relaxing Diet, or by Glysters, and bathe his Legs once a Day in warm Water. Every third Day one Dose of the Medicine N° 30 should be taken, which is compounded of Mercury, that counterworks the Poison, and of Musk which prevents the Spasms, or convulsive Motions. I confess at the same Time that I have less Dependance on the Mercury given in this Form, and think the rubbing in of its Ointment considerably more efficacious, which I should hope may

---

* It seems not amiss to try the Effects of a solely vegetable Diet, and that perhaps consisting more of the acescent than alcalescent Herbs and Roots, in this Disease, commencing immediately from the Bite of a mad Dog. These carnivorous Animals, who never rely on a vegetable Food, are the only primary Harbingers or Breeders of it, though they are capable of transmitting it by a Bite to graminivorous and granivorous ones. The Virtue of Vinegar in this Disease, said to have been accidentally discovered on the Continent, seems not to have been hitherto experienced amongst us, yet in Case of such a morbid Accident may require Trial, tho' not so far as to occasion the Omission of more certain experienced Remedies, with some of which it might be also proper.

may always prevent the Fatality of this dreadful, surprizing Disease. (a)

§ 196 If the raging Symptom, the Dread of Water, has already appeared, and the Patient is strong, and abounds with Blood, he should, 1, be bled to a considerable Quantity, and this may be repeated twice, thrice, or even a fourth Time, if Circumstances require it.

2, The Patient should be put, if possible, into a warm Bath, and this should be used twice daily

3, He should every Day receive two, or even three of the emollient Glysters N°. 5.

4, The Wound and the Parts adjoining to it should be rubbed with the Ointment N°. 28, twice a Day.

5, The whole Limb which contains the Wound should be rubbed with Oil, and be wrapped up in an oily Flanel.

6, Every

(a) The great Usefulness of mercurial Frictions, we may even say, the certain Security which they procure for the Patients, in these Cases, provided they are applied very soon after the Bite, have been demonstrated by their Success in *Provence*, at *Lyons*, at *Montpelier*, at *Pondicherry*, and in many other Places Neither have these happy Events been invalidated by any Observations or Instances to the contrary It cannot therefore be too strongly inculcated to those who have been bitten by venomous Animals, to comply with the Use of them They ought to be used in such a Quantity, and after such a Manner, as to excite a moderate Salivation, for fifteen, twenty, or even thirty Days *E L* Though this Practice may justly be pursued from great Caution, when no Caustic had been speedily applied to, and no such Discharge had been obtained from the bitten Part, yet wherever it had, this long and depressing Salivation, I conceive, would be very seldom necessary, and might be hurtful to weak Constitutions K

6, Every three Hours a Dose of the Powder Nº. 30, should be taken in a Cup of the Infusion of Lime-tree and Elder Flowers.

7, The Prescription Nº. 31, is to be given every Night, and to be repeated in the Morning, if the Patient is not easy, washing it down with the same Infusion.

8, If there be a great Nauseousness at Stomach, with a Bitterness in the Mouth, give the Powder Nº. 35, which brings up a copious Discharge of glewy and bilious Humours.

9, There is very little Occasion to say any thing relating to the Patient's Food, in such a Situation. Should he ask for any, he may be allowed Panada, light Soup, Bread, Soups made of farinaceous or mealy Vegetables, or a little Milk.

§ 197. By the Use of these Remedies the Symptoms will be observed to lessen, and to disappear by Degrees; and finally Health will be re-established. But if the Patient should long continue weak, and subject to Terrors, he may take a Dose of the Powder Nº. 14, thrice a Day.

§ 198. It is certain that a Boy, in whom the raging Symptom of this Disease had just appeared, was perfectly cured, by bathing all about the wounded Part with Sallad-Oil, in which some Camphire and Opium were dissolved, with the Addition of repeated Frictions of the Ointment Nº. 28, and making him take some *Eau de luce* with a little Wine. This Medicine, a Coffee-Cup of which may be given every four Hours, allayed

allayed the great Inquietude and Agitation of the Patient; and brought on a very plentiful Sweat, on which all the Symptoms vanished.

§ 199. Dogs may be cured by rubbing in a triple Quantity of the same Ointment directed for Men, and by giving them the Bolus N°. 33. But both these Means should be used as soon as ever they are bit. When the great Symptom is manifest, there would be too much Danger in attempting to apply one, or to give the other; and they should be immediately killed. It might be well however to try if they would swallow down the Bolus, on its being thrown to them.

As soon as ever Dogs are bit, they should be safely tied up, and not let loose again, before the Expiration of three or four Months.

§ 200. A false and dangerous Prejudice has prevailed with Regard to the Bites from Dogs, and it is this—That if a Dog who had bit any Person, without being mad at the Time of his biting, should become mad afterwards, the Person so formerly bitten, would prove mad too at the same Time. Such a Notion is full as absurd, as it would be to affirm, that if two Persons had slept in the same Bed, and that one of them should take the Itch, the Small-Pocks, or any other contagious Disease, ten or twelve Years afterwards, that the other should also be infected with that he took, and at the same Time too.

Of two Circumstances, whenever a Person is bit, one must certainly be. Either the Dog which gives the Bite, is about to be mad himself, in which

which Case this would be evident in a few Days; and then it must be said the Person was bitten by a mad Dog: Or else, that the Dog was absolutely sound, having neither conceived, or bred in himself, nor received from without the Cause, the Principle, of Madness: in which last Case I ask any Man in his Senses, if he could communicate it. No Person, no Thing imparts what it has not. This false and crude Notion excites those who are possessed with it to a dangerous Action: they exercise that Liberty the Laws unhappily allow them of killing the Dog; by which Means they are left uncertain of his State, and of their own Chance. This is a dreadful Uncertainty, and may be attended with embarrassing and troublesome Consequences, independant of the Poison itself. The reasonable Conduct would be to secure and observe the Dog very closely, in Order to know certainly whether he is, or is not, mad.

§ 201. It is no longer necessary to represent the Horror, the Barbarity and Guilt of that cruel Practice, which prevailed, not very long since, of suffocating Persons in the Height of this Disease, with the Bed-cloaths, or between Matrasses. It is now prohibited in most Countries; and doubtless will be punished, or, at least ought to be, even in those where as yet it is not.

Another Cruelty, of which we hope to see no repeated Instance, is that of abandoning those miserable Patients to themselves, without the least Resource or Assistance: a most detestable Custom

Custom even in those Times, when there was not the least Hope of saving them; and still more criminal in our Days, when they may be recovered effectually. I do again affirm, that it is not very often these afflicted Patients are disposed to bite, and that even when they are, they are afraid of doing it, and request the By-standers to keep out of their Reach: So that no Danger is incurred; or where there is any, it may easily be avoided by a few Precautions.

Chapter XIII.

Of the Small-Pocks.

Sect. 202.

THE Small-Pocks is the most frequent, the most extensive of all Diseases, since out of a hundred Persons there are not more than * four or five exempted from it. It is equally true however, that if it attacks almost every Person, it attacks them but once, so that having escaped through it, they are always secure

---

* As far as the Number of inoculated Persons, who remained entirely uninfected (some very few after a second Inoculation) has enabled me, I have calculated the Proportion naturally exempted from this Disease, though residing within the Influence of it, to be full 25 in 1000. See Analysis of Inoculation, Ed 2d P 157 Note *. K

secure from (a) it. It must be acknowleged, at the same Time, to be one of the most destructive Diseases; for if in some Years or Seasons, it proves to be of a very mild and gentle Sort, in others it is almost as fatal as the Plague: it being demonstrated, by calculating the Consequences of its most raging, and its gentlest Prevalence, that it kills one seventh of the Number it attacks.

§ 203 People generally take the Small-Pocks in their Infancy, or in their Childhood. It is very seldom known to attack only one Person in one Place. Its Invasions being very generally epidemical, and seizing a large Proportion of those who

---

(a) It has sometimes been observed (and the Observation has been such as not to be doubted) that a very mild distinct Small-Pocks has sometimes invaded the same Person twice. But such Instances are so very rare, that we may very generally affirm, those who have once had it, will never have it again. E. L —— In Deference to a few particular Authorities, I have also supposed such a repeated Infection, (Analysis of Inoculation, Ed. 2d P. 43) though I have really never seen any such myself, nor ever heard more than two Physicians affirm it, one at *Versailles*, and another in *London*, the last of whom declared, he took it upon the Credit of a Country Physician, thoroughly acquainted with this Disease, and a Witness to the Repetition of it. Hence we imagine the Editor of this Work at *Lyons* might have only termed this Re-infection *extremely* rare, which would have a Tendency to reconcile the Subjects of the Small Pocks, more generally, to the most salutary Practice of Inoculation. Doubtless some other eruptive Fevers, particularly, the Chicken Pocks, Crystals &c. have been often mistaken for the real Small Pocks by incompetent Judges, and sometimes even by Persons better qualified, yet who were less attentive to the Symptoms and Progress of the former. But whoever will be at the Pains to read Dr *Baux* Praité de la petite verole naturelle avec l'artificiele, or a practical Abstract of Part of it in the Monthly Review Vol. XXV p. 30 to 31, will find such a just, clear and useful Distinction of them as may prevent many future Deceptions on this frequently recurring Subject. K

who have not suffered it. It commonly ceases at the End of some Weeks, or of some Months, and rarely ever appears again in the same Place, until four, five or six Years after.

§ 204. This Malady often gives some Intimation of its Approach, three or four Days before the Appearance of the Fever, by a little Dejection, less Vivacity and Gaiety than usual; a great Propensity to sweat; less Appetite; a slight Alteration of the Countenance, and a kind of pale livid Colour about the Eyes: Notwithstanding which, in Children of a lax and phlegmatic Constitution, I have known a moderate Agitation of their Blood, (before their Shivering approached) give them a * Vivacity, Gaiety, and a rosy Improvement of their Complexion, beyond what Nature had given them.

Certain short Vicissitudes of Heat or Coldness succeed the former introductory Appearances, and at length a considerable Shivering, of the Duration of one, two, three or four Hours: This is succeeded by violent Heat, accompanied with Pains of the Head, Loins, Vomiting, or at least with a frequent Propensity to vomit.

This State continues for some Hours, at the Expiration of which the Fever abates a little in a Sweat, which is sometimes a very large one: the Patient then finds himself better, but is notwithstanding cast down, torpid or heavy, very

O squeamish,

---

* The same Appearances very often occur in such Subjects by Inoculation, before actual Sickening, as I have observed and in Pinced, Ed 1st. P. 62. Ld 2 P 75, -6 K

squeamish, with a Head-ach and Pain in the Back, and a Disposition to be drowsy. The last Symptom indeed is not very common, except in Children, less than seven or eight Years of Age.

The Abatement of the Fever is of small Duration, and some Hours after, commonly towards the Evening, it returns with all its Attendants, and terminates again by Sweats, as before.

This State of the Disease lasts three or four Days, at the End of which Term, and seldom later, the first Eruptions appear among the Sweat, which terminates the Paroxysm or Return of the Fever. I have generally observed the earliest Eruption to appear in the Face, next to that on the Hands, on the fore Part of the Arms, on the Neck, and on the upper Part of the Breast. As soon as this Eruption appears, if the Distemper is of a gentle Kind and Disposition, the Fever almost entirely vanishes: the Patient continues to sweat a little, or transpire; the Number of Eruptions increases, others coming out on the Back, the Sides, the Belly, the Thighs, the Legs, and the Feet. Sometimes they are pushed out very numerously even to the Soles of the Feet, where, as they increase in Size, they often excite very sharp Pain, by Reason of the great Thickness and Hardness of the Skin in these Parts.

Frequently on the first and second Day of Eruption (speaking hitherto always of the mild Kind and Degree of the Disease) there returns upon a very gentle Revival of the Fever about the

the Evening, which, about the Termination of it, is attended with a confiderable and final Eruption: though as often as the Fever terminates perfectly after the earlieft Eruption, a very diftinct and very fmall one is a pretty certain Confequence. For though the Eruption is already, or fhould prove only moderate, the Fever, as I have before faid, does not totally difappear; a fmall Degree of it ftill remaining, and heightening a little every Evening.

Thefe Puftules, or Efflorefcences, on their firft Appearance, are only fo many very little red Spots, confiderably refembling a Flea-bite; but diftinguifhable by a fmall white Point in the Middle, a little raifed above the reft, which gradually increafes in Size, with the Rednefs extended about it. They become whiter, in Proportion as they grow larger, and generally upon the fixth Day, including that of their firft Eruption, they attain their utmoft Magnitude, and are full of *Pus* or Matter. Some of them grow to the Size of a Pea, and fome ftill a little larger, but this never happens to the greateft Number of them. From this Time they begin to look yellowifh, they gradually become dry, and fall off in brown Scales, in ten or eleven Days from their firft Appearance. As their Eruption occurred on different Days, they alfo wither and fall off fucceffively. The Face is fometimes clear of them, while Puftules ftill are feen upon the Legs, not fully ripe, or fuppurated: and thofe in the Soles of the Feet often remain much longer

§ 205.

§ 205. The Skin is of Course extended or stretched out by the Pustules; and after the Appearance of a certain Quantity, all the Interstices, or Parts between the Pustules, are red and bright, as it were, with a proportionable Inflation or Swelling of the Skin. The Face is the first Part that appears bloated, from the Pustules there first attaining their utmost Size: and this Inflation is sometimes so considerable, as to look monstrous, the like happens also to the Neck, and the Eyes are entirely closed up by it. The Swelling of the Face abates in Proportion to the scabbing and drying up of the Pustules; and then the Hands are puffed up prodigiously. This happens successively to the Legs, the Tumour or Swelling being the Consequence of the Pustules attaining their utmost Size, which happens by Succession, in these different Parts.

§ 206. Whenever there is a very considerable Eruption, the Fever is heightened at the Time of Suppuration, which is not to be wondered at; one single Boil excites a Fever: How is it possible then that some hundred, nay some thousand of these little Abscesses should not excite one? This Fever is the most dangerous Period, or Time of the Disease, and occurs between the ninth and the thirteenth Days, as many Circumstances vary the Term of Suppuration, two or three Days. At this painful and perilous Season then, the Patient becomes very hot, and thirsty; he is harrassed with Pain; and finds it very difficult to discover a favourable easy Posture.

If

If the Malady runs very high, he has no Sleep, he raves, becomes greatly oppressed, is seized with a heavy Drowsiness, and when he dies, he dies either suffocated or lethargic, and sometimes in a State compounded of both these Symptoms.

The Pulse, during this Fever of Suppuration, is sometimes of an astonishing Quickness, while the Swelling of the Wrists makes it seem, in some Subjects, to be very small. The most critical and dangerous Time is, when the Swellings of the Face, Head and Neck are in their highest Degree. Whenever the Swelling begins to fall, the Scabs on the Face to dry [*supposing neither of these to be too sudden and premature, for the visible Quantity of the Pustules*] and the Skin to shrivel, as it were, the Quickness of the Pulse abates a little, and the Danger diminishes. When the Pustules are very few, this second Fever is so moderate, that it requires some Attention to discern it, so that the Danger is next to none.

§ 207. Besides those Symptoms, there are some others, which require considerable Attention and Vigilance. One of these is the Soreness of the Throat, with which many Persons in the Small-Pocks are afflicted, as soon as the Fever grows pretty strong. It continues for two or three Days, feels very strait and troublesome in the Action of Swallowing, and whenever the Disease is extremely acute, it entirely prevents Swallowing. It is commonly ascribed to the Eruption of Pustules in the Throat, but this is a

Mistake, such Pustules being almost constantly [*] imaginary. It begins, most frequently, before the Eruption appears; if this Complaint is in a light Degree, it terminates upon the Eruption, and whenever it revives again in the Course of the Disease, it is always in Proportion to the Degree of the Fever. Hence we may infer it does not arise from the Pustules, but is owing to the Inflammation; and as often as it is of any considerable Duration, it is almost ever attended with another Symptom, the Salivation, or a Discharge of a great Quantity of Spittle. This Salivation rarely exists, where the Disease is very gentle, or the Patient very young, and is full as rarely absent, where it is severe, and the Patient is past seven or eight Years old: but when the Eruption is very confluent, and the Patient adult, or grown up, the Discharge is surprizing. Under these Circumstances it flows out incessantly, allowing the afflicted Patient no Rest or Respite, and often incommodes him more than any other Symptom of the Distemper; and so much the more, as after its Continuance for some Days, the

---

[*] As Pustules are, and not very seldom, visible on the Tongue, and sometimes on the Roof, even to its Process called the Palate, which I have plainly seen, it seems not very easy to assign any insuperable Obstacle to the Existence of a few within the Throat, though this scarcely ever occurs, in the distinct Small-Pocks. Doubtless however a considerable Inflammation of that Part will be as likely to produce the great Difficulty of Swallowing, as the Evidence of Pustules there, which our learned Author does not absolutely reject, and consequently will forgive this Supposition of them, especially if he credits the ocular Testimony of Dr *Isearts*, cited in the Analysis, Ed 2d p 71. K

the Lips, the Inside of the Cheeks, the Tongue, and the Roof of the Mouth are entirely peeled or flead, as it were. Nevertheless, however painful and embarrassing this Discharge may prove, it is very important and salutary Meer Infants are less subject to it, some of them having a Looseness, in Lieu of it: and yet I have observed even this last Discharge to be considerably less frequent in them, than a Salivation is in grown People

§ 208. Children, to the Age of five or six Years, are liable to Convulsions, before Eruption: these however are not dangerous, if they are not accompanied with other grievous and violent Symptoms. But such Convulsions as supervene, either when Eruption having already occurred, suddenly retreats, or *strikes in*, according to the common Phrase; or during the Course of the Fever of Suppuration, are greatly more terrifying.

Involuntary Discharges of Blood from the Nose often occur, in the first Stage of this Distemper, which are extremely serviceable, and commonly lessen, or carry off, the Head-ach. Meer Infants are less subject to this Discharge, though they have sometimes a little of it: and I have known a considerable *Stupor* or Drowsiness, vanish immediately after this Bleeding.

§ 209 The Small-Pocks is commonly distinguished into two Kinds, the confluent and the distinct, such a Distinction really existing in Nature: but as the Treatment of each of them is the same; and as the Quantity or Dose of the Medicines is only to be varied, in Proportion to the Danger of the Patient (not to enter here into very tedious Details, and such as might exceed the Comprehension of many of our Readers; as well as whatever might relate particularly to the malignant Small-Pocks) I shall limit myself within the Description I have premised, which includes all the Symptoms common to both these Kinds of the Small-Pocks. I content myself with adding here, that we may expect a very confluent and dangerous Pock, if, at the very Time of Seizure, the Patient is immediately attacked with many violent Symptoms; more especially if his Eyes are extremely quick, lively, and even glistening, as it were; if he vomits almost continually, if the Pain of his Loins be violent; and if he suffers at the same Time great Anguish and Inquietude: If in Infants there is great *Stupor* or Heaviness; if Eruption appears on the third Day, and sometimes even on the second: as the hastier Eruptions in this Disease signify the most dangerous Kind and Degree of it, and on the contrary, the slower Eruption is, it is the safer too, supposing this Slowness of the Eruption not to have been the Consequence of great Weakness, or of some violent inward Pain

§ 210 The Disorder is sometimes so very mild and slight, that Eruption appears with scarcely any Suspicion of the Child's having the least Ailment, and the Event is as favourable as the Invasion. The Pustules appear, grow large, suppu-

suppurate and attain their Maturity, without confining the Patient to his Bed, or lessening either his Sleep, or Appetite.

It is very common to see Children in the Country (and they are seldom more than Children who have it so very gently) run about in the open Air, through the whole Course of this Disease, and feeding just as they do in Health. Even those who take it in a somewhat higher Degree, commonly go out when Eruption is finished, and give themselves up, without Reserve, to the Voracity of their Hunger. Notwithstanding all this Neglect, many get perfectly cured; though such a Conduct should never be proposed for Imitation, since Numbers have experienced its pernicious Consequences, and several of these Children have been brought to me, especially from *Jurat*, who after such Neglect, in the Course of the mild and kindly Sort of this Distemper, have contracted Complaints and Infirmities of different Kinds, which have been found very difficult to subdue.

§ 211 This still continues to be one of these Distempers, whose Danger has long been increased by its improper Treatment, and especially by forcing the Patients into Sweats, and it still continues to be increased, particularly among Country People. They have seen Eruption appear, while the Patient sweats, and observed he found himself better after its Appearance: and hence they conclude that, by quickening and forcing out this Eruption, they contribute to his Relief;
and

and suppose, that by increasing the Quantity of his Sweats, and the Number of his Eruptions, the Blood is the better cleared and purified from the Poison. These are mortal Errors, which daily Experience has demonstrated, by their tragical Consequences.

When the Contagion or Poison, which generates this Disease, has been admitted into the Blood, it requires a certain Term to produce its usual Effects: at which Time the Blood being tainted by the Venom it has received, and by that which such Venom has formed or assimilated from it, Nature makes an Effort to free herself of it, and to expell it by the Skin, precisely at the Time when every Thing is predisposed for that Purpose. This Effort pretty generally succeeds, being very often rather too rapid and violent, and very seldom too weak. Hence it is evident, that whenever this Effort is deficient, it ought not to be heightened by hot Medicines or Means, which make it too violent and dangerous: for when it already exceeds in this Respect, a further Increase of such Violence must render it mortal. There are but few Cases in which the Efforts of Nature, on this Occasion, are too languid and feeble, especially in the Country, and whenever such rare Cases do occur, it is very difficult to form a just and proper Estimation of them. for which Reason we should be very reserved and cautious in the Use of heating Medicines, which are so mortally pernicious in this Disease.

Wine, Venice Treacle, cordial Confections, hot

hot Air, and Loads of Bed-cloths, annually sweep off Thousands of Children, who might have recovered, if they had taken nothing but warm Water: and every Person who is interested in the Recovery of Patients in this Distemper, ought carefully to prevent the smallest Use of such Drugs; which, if they should not immediately aggravate it to a fatal Degree, yet will certainly increase the Severity and Torment of it, and annex the most unhappy and tragical Consequences to it.

The Prejudice in this Point is so strongly rooted, that a total Eradication of it must be very difficult: but I only desire People would be convinced by their own Eyes, of the different Success of the hot Regimen, and of that I shall propose. And here indeed I must confess, I found more Attention and Docility, on this Point, among the Inhabitants of the City, and especially in the last epidemical spreading of the Small-Pocks, than I presumed to hope for. Not only as many as consulted me on the Invasion of it, complied exactly with the cooling Regimen I advised them; but their Neighbours also had Recourse to it, when their Children sickened and being often called in when it had been many Days advanced, I observed with great Pleasure, that in many Houses, not one heating Medicine had been given, and great Care had been taken to keep the Air of the Patient's Chamber refreshingly cool and temperate. This encourages me to expect, that this Method hereafter will become general here.

here. What certainly ought most essentially to conduce to this is, that notwithstanding the Diffusion or spreading of this Disease was as numerous and extensive as any of the former, the Mortality, in Consequence of it, was evidently less.

§ 212. At the very Beginning of the Small-Pocks (which may be reasonably suspected, from the Presence of the Symptoms I have already described; supposing the Person complaining never to have had it, and the Disease to prevail near his Residence) the Patient is immediately to be put on a strict Regimen, and to have his Legs bathed Night and Morning in warm Water. This is the most proper and promising Method to lessen the Quantity of Eruption in the Face and Head, and to facilitate it every where else on the Surface. Glysters also greatly contribute to abate the Head-ach, and to diminish the Reachings to vomit, and the actual Vomitings, which greatly distress the Patient, but which however it is highly absurd and pernicious to stop by any stomachic cordial Confection, or by Venice Treacle, and still more dangerous to attempt removing the Cause of them, by a Vomit or Purge, which are hurtful in the beginning of the Small-Pocks.

If the Fever be moderate, the Bathings of the Legs on the first Day of sickening, and one Glyster may suffice then. The Patient must be restrained to his Regimen; and instead of the Ptisan N°. 1, 2, 4, a very young Child should drink nothing but Milk diluted with two thirds of Elder Flower or Lime-tree Tea, or with Balm Tea,

Tea, if there be no perceivable Fever; and in short, if they have an Aversion to the Taste of them all, with only the same Quantity of good clear * Water. An Apple coddled or baked may be added to it, and if they complain of Hunger, a little Bread may be allowed, but they must be denied any Meat, or Meat Broth, Eggs and strong Drink, since it has appeared from Observations frequently repeated, that Children who had been indulged with such Diet proved the worse for it, and recovered more slowly than others. In this early Stage too, clear Whey alone may serve them instead of every other Drink, the good Effects of which I have frequently been a Witness to, or some Buttermilk may be allowed. When the Distemper is of a mild Species, a perfect Cure ensues, without any other Assistance or Medicine: but we should not neglect to purge the Patient as soon as the Pustules are perfectly scabbed

* A Negro Girl, about five or six Years old, under a coherent Pock, stole by Night out of the Garret where she lay, into a Kitchen out of Doors, where she drank plentifully of cold Water. How often she repeated these nightly cooling Potions I never could certainly learn, though they occurred in my own House in *South-Carolina* in Summer. But it is certain the Child recovered as speedily as others, whose Eruption was more distinct, and who drank Barley-Water, very thin Rice or Indian Corn Gruel, Balm Tea, or the like. In fact, throughout the Course of this Visitation from the Small Pocks in *Carolina* in 1738, we had but too many Demonstrations of the fatal Co-operation of violent Heat with their Contagion, and not a very few surprizing Instances of the salutary Effects of being necessarily and involuntarily exposed to some very cooling Accidents after Infection, and in some Cases after Eruption too, which I then more particularly mentioned in a small controversial Tract printed there. K.

scabbed on the greater Part of his Face, with the Prescription N°. 11, which must be repeated six Days after. He should not be allowed Flesh 'till after this second Purge; though after the first he may be allowed some well-boiled Pulse, or Garden-stuff and Bread, and in such a Quantity, as not to be pinched with Hunger, while he recovers from the Disease.

§ 213. But if the Fever should be strong, the Pulse hard, and the Pain of the Head and Loins should be violent, he must, 1. immediately lose Blood from the Arm, receive a Glyster two Hours after, and, if the Fever continues, the Bleeding must be repeated. I have directed a Repetition of it even to the fourth Time, within the two first Days, to young People under the Age of eighteen; and it is more especially necessary in such Persons as, with a hard and full Pulse, are also affected with a heavy Drowsiness and a *Delirium*, or Raving.

2. As long as the Fever continues violently, two, three, and even four Glysters should be given in the 24 Hours; and the Legs should be bathed twice.

3. The Patient is to be taken out of Bed, and supported in a Chair as long as he can tolerably bear it.

4. The Air of his Chamber should frequently be renewed, and if it be too hot, which it often is in Summer, in Order to refresh it, and the Patient, the Means must be employed which are directed § 36.

5. He

5. He is to be restrained to the Ptisans N°. 2 or 4, and if that does not sufficiently moderate the Fever, he should take every Hour, or every two Hours, according to the Urgency of the Case, a Spoonful of the Mixture N°. 10; mixed with a Cup of Ptisan. After the Eruption, the Fever being then abated, there is less Occasion for Medicine, and should it even entirely disappear, the Patient may be regulated, as directed, § 212.

§ 214. When, after a Calm, a Remission or Intermission of some Days, the Process of Suppuration revives the Fever, we ought first, and especially, to keep the * Body very open. For this

---

* We must remember that Dr Tissot is treating *here* of the higher or confluent Degrees of this Disease, for in the distinct Small-Pocks, it is common to find Persons for several Days without a Stool, and without the least perceivable Disorder for Want of one (their whole Nourishment being very light and liquid) in which Cases, while Matters proceeded well in all other Respects, there seems little Occasion for a great Solicitude about Stools. But if one should be judged necessary after four or five Days Costiveness, accompanied with a Fulness or Hardness of the Belly, doubtless the Glyster should be of the lenient Kind (as those directed by our Author are) and not calculated to produce more than a second Stool at the very most. Indeed, where there is Reason to apprehend a strong secondary Fever, from the Quantity of Eruption, and a previously high Inflammation, it is more prudent to provide for a Mitigation of it, by a moderately open Belly, than to suffer a long Costiveness, yet so as to incur very little Hazard of abating the Salivation, or retarding the Growth or Suppuration of the Pustules, by a Superpurgation, which it may be too easy, to excite in some Habits. If the Discharge by spitting, and the Brightness and Quantity of Suppuration, have been in Proportion to the Number of Eruptions, though the Convulsions from the secondary Fever, where these have been numerous, is often acute and high, and the Patient, who is in great Anguish,

this Purpose, α an Ounce of *Catholicon* should be added to the Glysters; or they might be simply made of Whey, with Honey, Oil and Salt. β Give the Patient three times every Morning, at the Interval of two Hours between each, three Glasses of the Ptisan N°. 32. γ Purge him *after* two Days, with the Potion N°. 23, but on that Day he must not take the Ptisan N°. 32.

2. He must, if the Distemper be very violent, take a double Dose of the Mixture N°. 10.

3 The Patient should be taken out of Bed, and kept up in a Room well aired Day and Night, until the Fever has abated. Many Persons will probably be surprized at this Advice; nevertheless it is that which I have often experienced to be the most efficacious, and without which the others are ineffectual. They will say, how shall the Patient sleep at this Rate? To which it may be answered, Sleep is not necessary, nay, it is hurtful in this State and Stage of the Disease. Besides, he is really unable to sleep: the continual Salivation prevents it, and it is very necessary to keep up the Salivation, which is facilitated by often injecting warm Water and Honey into his Throat. It is also of considerable Service to throw some up his Nostrils, and often thus to cleanse

cleanse the Scabs which form within them. A due Regard to these Circumstances not only contributes to lessen the Patient's Uneasiness, but very effectually also to his Cure.

4. If the Face and Neck are greatly swelled, emollient Cataplasms are to be applied to the Soles of the Feet; and if these should have very little Effect, Sinapisms should be applied. These are a kind of Plaister or Application composed of Yeast, Mustard-flower, and some Vinegar. They sometimes occasion sharp and almost burning Pain; but in Proportion to the Sharpness and Increase of these Pains, the Head and Neck are remarkably relieved.

§ 215. The Eyelids are puffed up and swelled when the Disease runs high, so as to conceal the Eyes, which are closed up fast for several Days. Nothing further should be attempted, with Respect to this Circumstance, but the frequent moistening of them with a little warm Milk and Water. The Precautions which some take to stroke them with Saffron, a gold Ducat, or Rosewater are equally childish and insignificant. What chiefly conduces to prevent the Redness or Inflammation of the Eyes after the Disease, and in general all its other bad Consequences, is to be content for a considerable Time, with a very moderate Quantity of Food, and particularly to abstain from Flesh and Wine. In the very bad Small Pocks, and in little Children, the Eyes are closed up from the Beginning of the Eruption.

§ 216. One extremely ferviceable Affiftance, and which has not been made ufe of for a long Time paft, except as a Means to preferve the Smoothnefs and Beauty of the Face; but yet which has the greateft Tendency to preferve Life itfelf, is the Opening of the Puftules, not only upon the Face, but all over the Body. In the firft Place, by opening them, the Lodgment or Retention of *Pus* is prevented, which may be fuppofed to prevent any Erofion, or eating down, from it; whence Scars, deep Pitts and other Deformities are obviated. Secondly, in giving a Vent to the Poifon, the Retreat of it into the Blood is cut off, which removes a principal Caufe of the Danger of the Small-Pocks. Thirdly, the Skin is relaxed, the Tumour of the Face and Neck diminifh in Proportion to that Relaxtion; and thence the Return of the Blood from the Brain is facilitated, which muft prove a great Advantage. The Puftules fhould be opened every where, fuccefsively as they ripen. The precife Time of doing it is when they are entirely white, when they juft begin to turn but a very little yellowifh, and when the red Circle furrounding them is quite pale. They fhould be opened with very fine fharp-pointed Sciffars, this does not give the Patient the leaft Pain, and when a certain Number of them are opened, a Spunge dipt in a little warm Water is to be repeatedly applied to fuck up and remove that *Pus*, which would foon be dried up up into Scabs. But as the Pustules, when emptied thus, soon fill again, a Discharge of this fresh Matter must be obtained in the same Manner some Hours after, and this must sometimes be repeated five or even six Times successively. Such extraordinary Attention in this Point may probably be considered as minute, and even trivial, by some; and is very unlikely to become a * general Practice: but I do again affirm it to be of much more Importance than many may imagine; and that as often as the Fever attending Suppuration is violent and menacing, a very general, exact and repeated opening, emptying, and absorbing of the ripened Pustules, is a Remedy of the utmost Importance and Efficacy, as it removes two very considerable Causes of the Danger of this Disease, which are the Matter itself,

---

* This Practice which I had heard of, and even suggested to myself but never seen actually enterprized, seems so very rational as highly to deserve a fair Trial in the confluent Degrees of the Small Pocks [for in the distinct it can scarcely be necessary] wherein every probable Assistance should be employed, and in which the most potent Medicines are very often unsuccessful. We have but too many Opportunities of trying it sufficiently, and it certainly has a more promising Aspect than a Practice so highly recommended many Years ago, of covering all the Pustules (which is sometimes the whole Surface of the Patient) in Melilot, or suppose any other suppurating, Plaister, which must effectually prevent all Perspiration, and greatly increase the Soreness, Pain and Embarrassment of the Patient, at the Height of the Disease. I can conceive but one bad Consequence that might possibly sometimes result from the former, but this (besides the Means that may be used to avert it) is rather remote, and so uncertain, until the Trial is repeatedly made, that I think it ought not to be named, in Competition with the Benefits that may arise from it in such Cases, as seem, otherwise, too generally irrecoverable. K

itself, and the great Tension and Stiffness of the Skin.

§ 217. In the Treatment of this Disease, I have said nothing with Respect to Anodynes, or such Medicines as procure Sleep, which I am sensible are pretty generally employed in it, but which I scarcely ever direct in this violent Degree of the Disease, and the Dangers of which Medicine in it I have demonstrated in the Letter to Baron Haller, which I have already mentioned. For which Reason, wherever the Patient is not under the Care and Direction of a Physician, they should very carefully abstain from the Use of Venice Treacle, Laudanum, *Diacodium*, that is the Syrup of white Poppies, or even of the wild red Poppy, Syrup of Amber, Pills of Storax, of Cynoglossum or Hounds-tongue, and, in one Word, of every Medicine which produces Sleep. But still more especially should their Use be entirely banished, throughout the Duration of the secondary Fever, when even natural Sleep itself is dangerous. One Circumstance in which their Use may sometimes be permitted, is in the Case of weakly Children, or such as are liable to Convulsions, where Eruption is effected not without Difficulty. But I must again inculcate the greatest Circumspection, in the Use of such Medicines, whose Effects are fatal, * when the Blood-vessels

are

---

* The Use of Opiates in this Disease undoubtedly requires no small Consideration, the great Sydenham himself not seeming even sufficiently guarded in the Exhibition of them, as far as Experience since his Day has enabled Physicians to judge of this Matter.

are turgid or full; whenever there is Inflammation, Fever, a great Distension of the Skin; whenever the Patient raves, or complains of Heaviness and Oppression; and when it is necessary that the Belly should be open, the Urine plentifully discharged; and the Salivation be freely promoted.

§ 218. If Eruption should suddenly retreat, or strike in, heating, soporific, spirituous and volatile Remedies should carefully be avoided; but the Patient may drink plentifully of the Infusion N°. 12 pretty hot, and should be blistered on the fleshy Part of the Legs. This is a very embarrassing

Matter. In general our Author's Limitations of them seem very just, though we have seen a few clear Instances, in which a light Raving, which evidently arose from Want of Sleep (joined to some Dread of the Event of the Disease by Inoculation) was happily removed, with every other considerable Complaint, by a moderate Opiate. In sore and fretful Children too, under a large or middling Eruption, as the Time gained to Rest is taken from Pain, and from wasting their Spirits in Crying and Clamour, I have seen Suppuration very benignly promoted by *Diacodium*. But in the *Crisis* of the secondary Fever in the confluent or coherent Pock, when there is a morbid Fulness, and Nature is struggling to unload herself by some other Outlets than those of the Skin, which now are totally obstructed (and which seems the only Evacuation, that is not restrained by Opiates) the giving and repeating them then, as has too often been practised, seems importantly erroneous; for I think Dr. SWAN has taken a judicious Liberty of dissenting from the great Author he translates, in forbidding an Opiate, if the Spitting abates, or grows so tough and ropy, as to endanger Suffocation. As the Difference of our Oeconomy in the Administration of Physic from that in *Switserland*, and Dr TISSOT's just Reputation may dispose many Country Practitioners to peruse this Treatise, I take the Liberty of referring such Readers, for a Recollection of some of my Sentiments of Opiates, long before the Appearance of this Work in French, to the second Edition of the Analysis from P. 94 to 97, &c. K

barrassing and difficult Case, and the different Circumstances attending it may require different Means and Applications, the Detail and Discussion of which are beyond my Plan here. Sometimes a single Bleeding has effectually recalled Eruption at once.

§ 219. The only certain Method of surmounting all the Danger of this Malady, is to inoculate. But this most salutary Method, which ought to be regarded as a particular and gracious Dispensation of Providence, can scarcely be attainable by, or serviceable to, the Bulk of the People, except in those Countries, where Hospitals * are destined particularly for Inoculation. In these where as yet there are none, the only Resource that is left for Children who cannot be inoculated at home, is to dispose them happily for the Distemper, by a simple easy Preparation.

§ 220 This Preparation consists, upon the whole, in removing all Want of, and all Obstructions to, the Health of the Person subject to this Disease, if he have any such, and in bringing him into a mild and healthy, but not into a very robust and vigorous, State, as this Distemper is often exceedingly violent in this last.

It is evident, that since the Defects of Health are very different in different Bodies, the Preparations of them must as often vary; and that a
Child

* The Translator long since had the Honour of agreeing with our learned Author, in this Consideration for the Benefit of the People, which is the Benefit of the State, will appear from p 258 of An. of Ed 1st and from p 371, 372 of the second.

Child subject to some habitual Disorder, cannot be prepared in the same Method with another who has a very opposite one. The Detail and Distinctions which are necessary on this important Head, would be improper here, whether it might be owing to their unavoidable Length; or to the Impossibility of giving Persons, who are not Physicians, sufficient Knowlege and Information to qualify them for determining on, and preferring, the most proper Preparation in various Cases. Nevertheless I will point out some such as may be very likely to agree, pretty generally, with Respect to strong and healthy Children. *

The first Step then is an Abatement of their usual Quantity of Food. Children commonly eat too much. Their Limitation should be in Proportion to their Size and Growth, where we could exactly ascertain them: but with Regard to all, or to much the greater Number of them, we may be allowed to make their Supper very light, and very small.

Their

---

* The Substance of this Section flows from the Combination of an excellent Understanding with great Experience, mature Reflection, and real Probity, and fundamentally exposes both the Absurdity of such as universally decry any Preparation of any Subject previous to Inoculation, (which is said to be the Practice of a present very popular Inoculator in *Paris*) and the opposite Absurdity of giving one and the very same Preparation to all Subjects, without Distinction, though this was avowed to have been successfully practised in *Pensylvania*, some Years since, which the Reader may see Analys'd Ed 2d, from p 329 to 331 and the Note there, *K*.

Their second Advantage will consist in the Choice of their Food. This Circumstance is less within the Attainment of, and indeed less necessary for, the common People, who are of Course limited to a very few, than to the Rich, who have Room to make great Retrenchments on this Account. The Diet of Country People being of the simplest Kind, and almost solely consisting of Vegetables and of Milk-meats, is the most proper Diet towards preparing for this Disease. For this Reason, such Persons have little more to attend to in this Respect, but that such Aliments be sound and good in their Kind; that their Bread be well baked; their Pulse dressed without Bacon, or rancid strong Fat of any sort, that their Fruits should be well ripened; that their Children should have no Cakes or Tarts, [But see Note *, P. 40, 41.] and but little Cheese. These simple Regulations may be sufficient, with Regard to this Article of their Preparation.

Some Judgment may be formed of the good Consequences of their Care on these two Points, concerning the Quantity and Quality of the Childrens Diet, by the moderate Shrinking of their Bellies, as they will be rendered more lively and active by this Alteration in their living; and yet, notwithstanding a little less Ruddiness in their Complexion, and some Abatement of their common Plight of Body, their Countenances, upon the whole, will seem improved

The third Article I would recommend, is to bathe their Legs now and then in warm Water, before

before they go to Bed. This promotes Perspiration, cools, dilutes the Blood, and allays the Sharpness of it, as often as it is properly timed.

The fourth Precaution, is the frequent Use of very clear Whey. This agreeable Remedy, which consists of the Juices of Herbs filtred through, and concocted, or as it were, sweetened by the Organs of a healthy Animal, answers every visible Indication (I am still speaking here of sound and hearty Children) It imparts a Flexibility, or Soupleness to the Vessels, it abates the Density, the heavy Consistence and Thickness of the Blood, which being augmented by the Action of the poisonous Cause of the Small-Pocks, would degenerate into a most dangerous inflammatory * Viscidity or Thickness. It removes all Obstructions in the *Viscera*, or Bowels of the lower Cavity, the Belly It opens the Passages which strain off the Bile, sheaths, or blunts, its Sharpness, gives it a proper Fluidity, prevents its Putridity, and sweetens whatever excessive Acrimony may reside throughout the Mass of Humours It likewise promotes Stools, Urine and Perspiration; and, in a Word, it communicates the most favourable Disposition to the Body, not to be too violently impressed and agitated by the Opera-

---

* There may certainly be an inflammatory Acrimony or Thinness, as well as Thickness of the Blood, and many medical Readers may think a morbid Fusion of the red Globules to be a more frequent Effect of this Contagion, than an increased Viscidity of them. See Analys Ed 2d p 75 to 83 But this Translation, conforming to the Spirit of its Original, admits very little Theory, and still less Controversy, into its Plan

Operation of an inflammatory Poison: And with Regard to such Children as I have mentioned, for those who are either sanguine or bilious, it is beyond all Contradiction, the most effectual preparatory Drink, and the most proper to make them amends for the Want of Inocu'ation.

I have already observed, that it may also be used to great Advantage, during the Course of the Disease: but I must also observe, that however salutary it is, in the Cases for which I have directed it, there are many others in which it would be hurtful. It would be extremely pernicious to order it to weak, languishing, scirrhous, pale Children, subject to Vomitings, Purgings, Acidities, and to all Diseases which prove their Bowels to be weak, their Humours to be sharp; so that People must be very cautious not to regard it as an universal and infallible Remedy, towards preparing for the Small-Pocks. Those to whom it is advised, may take a few Glasses every Morning, and even drink it daily, for their common Drink, they may also sup it with Bread for Breakfast, for Supper, and indeed at any Time.

If Country People will pursue these Directions, which are very easy to observe and to comprehend, whenever the Small-Pocks rages, I am persuaded it must lessen the Mortality attending it. Some will certainly experience the Benefit of them; such I mean as are very sensible and discreet, and strongly influenced by the truest Love

Love of their Children. Others there are Alas! who are too stupid to discern the Advantage of them, and too unnatural to take any just Care of their Families.

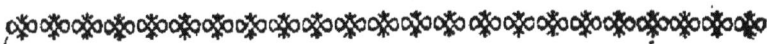

Chapter XIV.

Of the Measles.

Sect. 221.

THE Measles, to which the human Species are as generally liable, as to the Small-Pocks, is a Distemper considerably related to it, though, generally speaking, it is less fatal; notwithstanding which, it is not a little destructive in some Countries. In *Swisserland* we lose much fewer, immediately in the Disease, than from the Consequences of it.

It happens now and then that the Small-Pocks and the Measles rage at the same Time, and in the same Place; though I have more frequently observed, that each of them was epidemical in different Years. Sometimes it also happens that both these Diseases are combined at once in the same Person; and that one supervenes before the other has finished its Course, which makes the Case very perilous.

§ 222 In some Constitutions the Measles gives Notice of its Approach many Days before its evident Invasion, by a small, frequent and dry Cough, without any other sensible Complaint: though more frequently by a general Uneasiness; by Successions of Shivering and of Heat; by a severe Head-ach in grown Persons; a Heaviness in Children; a considerable Complaint of the Throat; and, by what particularly characterizes this Distemper, an Inflammation and a considerable Heat in the Eyes, attended with a Swelling of the Eye-lids, with a Defluxion of sharp Tears, and so acute a Sensation, or Feeling of the Eyes, that they cannot bear the Light, by very frequent Sneezings, and a Dripping from the Nose of the same Humour with that, which trickles from the Eyes.

The Heat and the Fever increases with Rapidity; the Patient is afflicted with a Cough, a Stuffing, with Anguish, and continual Reachings to vomit; with violent Pains in the Loins; and sometimes with a Looseness, under which Circumstance he is less persecuted with Vomiting At other times, and in other Subjects, Sweating chiefly prevails, though in less Abundance than in the Small-Pocks. The Tongue is foul and white; the Thirst is often very high, and the Symptoms are generally more violent than in the mild Small-Pocks.

At length, on the fourth or fifth Day, and sometimes about the End of the third, a sudden Eruption appears and in a very great Quantity, especially about the Face, which in a few Hours is covered with Spots, each of which resembles a

Flea-

Flea-bite; many of them soon joining form red Streakes or Suffusions larger or smaller, which inflame the Skin, and produce a very perceivable Swelling of the Face, whence the very Eyes are sometimes closed. Each small Spot or Suffusion is raised a little above the Surface, especially in the Face, where they are manifest both to the Sight and the Touch. In the other Parts of the Body, this Elevation or Rising is scarcely perceivable by any Circumstance, but the Roughness of the Skin.

The Eruption, having first appeared in the Face, is afterwards extended to the Breast, the Back, the Arms, the Thighs and Legs. It generally spreads very plentifully over the Breast and the Back, and sometimes red Suffusions are found upon the Breast, before any Eruption has appeared in the Face.

The Patient is often relieved, as in the Small-Pocks, by plentiful Discharges of Blood from the Nose, which carry off the Complaints of the Head, of the Eyes, and of the Throat.

Whenever this Distemper appears in its mildest Character, almost every Symptom abates after Eruption, as it happens in the Small-Pocks, though, in general, the Change for the better is not as thoroughly perceivable, as it is in the Small-Pocks. It is certain the Reachings and Vomitings cease almost entirely, but the Fever, the Cough, the Head-ach continue; and I have sometimes observed that a bilious Vomiting, a Day or two after the Eruption, proved a more considerable Relief to the Patient than the Eruption had. On the third or fourth Day of the Eruption, the Redness diminishes; the Spots, or very small Pustules, dry up and fall off in very little branny Scales; the Cuticle, or superficial Skin also shrivels off, and is replaced by one succeeding beneath it. On the ninth Day, when the Progress of the Malady has been speedy, and on the eleventh, when it has been very slow, no Trace of the Redness is to be found; and the Surface immediately resumes its usual Appearance.

§ 223. Notwithstanding all which the Patient is not safe, except, during the Course of the Distemper, or immediately after it, he has had some considerable Evacuation; such as the Vomiting I have just mentioned; or a bilious Looseness; or considerable Discharges by Urine; or very plentiful Sweating. For when any of these Evacuations supervene, the Fever vanishes, the Patient resumes his Strength, and perfectly recovers. It happens sometimes too, and even without any of these perceivable Discharges, that insensible Perspiration expels the Relics of the poisonous Cause of this Disease, and the Patient recovers his Health. Yet it occurs too often, that this Venom not having been entirely expelled (or its internal Effects not having been thoroughly effaced) it is repelled upon the Lungs, where it produces a slight Inflammation. In Consequence of this the Oppression, the Cough, the Anguish, and Fever return, and the Patient's Situation becomes

comes very dangerous. This Outrage is frequently less vehement, but it proves tedious and chronical, leaving a very obstinate Cough behind it, with many Resemblances of the Whooping-Cough. In 1758 there was an epidemic State of the Measles here extremely numerous, which affected great Numbers. Almost all who had it, and who were not very carefully and judiciously attended, were seized in Consequence of it with that Cough, which proved very violent and obstinate.

§ 224. However, notwithstanding this be the frequent Progress and Consequence of this Disease, when left entirely to itself, or erroneously treated, and more particularly when treated with a hot Regimen, yet when proper Care was taken to moderate the Fever at the Beginning, to dilute, and to keep up the Evacuations, such unhappy Consequences have been very rare.

§ 225. The proper Method of conducting this Distemper is much the same with that of the Small-Pocks.

1, If the Fever be high, the Pulse hard, the Load and Oppression heavy, and all the Symptoms violent, the Patient must be bled once or twice.

2, His Legs must be bathed, and he must take some Glysters · the Vehemence of the Symptoms must regulate the Number of each.

3, The Ptisans N°. 3 or 4 must be taken, or a Tea of Elder and Lime-tree Flowers, to which a fifth Part Milk may be added.

4, The

4, The Vapour, the Steam of warm Water, should also be employed, as very conducive to assuage the Cough, the Soreness of the Throat, and the Oppression the Patient labours under.

5, As soon as the Efflorescence, the Redness becomes pale, the Patient is to be purged with the Draught N°. 23.

6, He is still to be kept strictly to his Regimen, for two Days after this Purge, after which he is to be put upon the Diet of those who are in a State of Recovery.

7, If during the Eruption such Symptoms supervene as occur [at the same Term] in the Small-Pocks, they are to be treated in the Manner already directed there.

§ 226. Whenever this Method has not been observed, and the Accidents described § 223 supervene, the Distemper must be treated like an Inflammation in its first State, and all must be done as directed § 225. If the Disease is not vehement, † Bleeding may be omitted. If it is of
some

† Our Author very prudently limits this Discharge, and the Repetition of it, in this Disease (§ 225) as an erroneous Excess of it had sometimes prevailed. I have seen a very epidemical Season of the Measles, where Bleeding was not indicated in one third of the infected. And yet I have known such an Abuse of Bleeding in it, that being repeated more than once in a Case before Eruption (the Measles probably not being suspected) the Eruption was retarded several Days, and the Patient, a young Lady of Condition, remained exceeding low, faint and sickish, 'till after recruiting a very little, the Measles appeared, and she recovered. In a Youth of a lax Fibre, where the Measles had appeared, a seventh or eighth Bleeding was ordered on a Stitch in
the

some standing in gross Children, loaded with Humours, inactive, and pale, we must add to the Medicines already prescribed the Potion N°. 8, and Blisters to the Legs.

§ 227. It often happens from the Distance of proper Advice, that the Relics, the Dregs as it were, of the Disease have been too little regarded, especially the Cough; in which Circumstance it forms a real Suppuration in the Lungs, attended with a slow Fever. I have seen many Children in Country Villages destroyed by this Neglect. Their Case is then of the same Nature with that described § 68 and 82, and terminates in the same Manner in a Looseness, (attended with very little Pain) and sometimes a very fœtid one, which carries off the Patient. In such Cases we must recur to the Remedies prescribed § 74, Article 3, 4, 5; to the Powder N°. 14; and to Milk and Exercise. But it is so very difficult to make Children take the Powder, that it may be sometimes necessary to trust to the Milk without it, which I have often seen in such Situations accomplish a very difficult Cure. I must advise the Reader at the same Time, that it has not so compleat an Effect, as when it is taken solely un-

joined

---

the Side, supervening from their too early Disappearance, and the Case seemed very doubtful. But Nature continued very obstinately favourable in this Youth, who at length, but very slowly, recovered. His Circulation remained so languid, his flesh, with his Juices, so exhausted, that he was many Weeks before he could sit upright in a Chair, being obliged to make Use of a Cord depending from the Ceiling, to raise himself erectly in his Seat *K*.

joined by any other Aliment; and that it is of the last Importance not to join it with any, which has the least Acidity or Sharpness. Persons in easy Circumstances may successfully take, at the same Time, *Pfiffer*, *† Seltzer*, *Peterstal*, or some other light Waters, which are but moderately loaded with mineral Ingredients. These are also successfully employed in all the Cases, in which the Cure I have mentioned is necessary.

§ 228. Sometimes there remains, after the Course of the Measles, a strong dry Cough, with great Heat in the Breast, and throughout the whole Body, with Thirst, an excessive Dryness of the Tongue, and of the whole Surface of the Body. I have cured Persons thus indisposed after this Distemper, by making them breathe in the Vapour of warm Water, by the repeated Use of warm Baths, and by allowing them to take nothing for several Days but Water and Milk.

Before I take leave of this Subject, I assure the Reader again, that the contagious Cause of the Measles is of an extremely sharp and acrid Nature. It appears to have some Resemblance to the bilious Humour, which produces the *Erisipelas*, or St Anthony's Fire, and thence it demands our particular Attention and Vigilance, without which very troublesome and dangerous Consequences may be apprehended. I have seen, not very long since, a young Girl, who was in a very

languid

† *Balaruc water will be no bad substitute for any of these, in such cases.*

languid State after the Measles, which she had undergone three Years before: It was at length attended with an Ulceration in her Neck, which was cured, and her Health finally restored by *Sarsaparilla* with Milk and Water.

§ 229. The Measles have been communicated by * Inoculation in some Countries, where it is of a very malignant Disposition, and that Method might also be very advantageous in this. But what we have already observed, with Respect to the Inoculation of the Small-Pocks, *viz* That it cannot be extended to the general Benefit of the People, without the Foundation of Hospitals for that very Purpose, is equally applicable to the Inoculation of the Measles.

---

* The only Account I have read of this Practice, is in the learned Dr Home's *Medical Facts and Experiments*, published in 1759, which admits, that but nine out of fifteen of the Subjects of this Practice took Cotton dipt in the Blood of a Patient in the Measles was inserted into the Arms of twelve, and three received the Cotton into their Nostrils, after the Chinese Manner of infusing the Small Pocks, but of these last not one took, and one of those who had taken, had the Measles again two Months after We think the sharp hot Lymph distilling from the inflamed Eyes of Persons in this Disease, a likelier Vehicle to communicate it than the Blood, especially the dry Blood, which was sometimes tried, since the human *Serum* seems the Fluid more particularly affected by it, and this must have been evaporated when the Blood grew dry A few practical Strictures on this Work, and particularly on this Practice described in it, appeared in the Monthly Review Vol XXI P 68 to 75 K.

Chapter XV.

Of the ardent or burning Fever.

Sect. 230.

THE much greater Number of the Diseases I have hitherto considered, result from an Inflammation of the Blood, combined with the particular Inflammation of some Part, or occasioned by some Contagion or Poison, which must be evacuated. But when the Blood is solely and strongly inflamed, without an Attack on any particular Part, this Fever, which we term hot or burning, is the Consequence

§ 231 The Signs which make it evident are, a Hardness and Fulness of the Pulse in a higher Degree than happens in any other Malady; an excessive Heat, great Thirst, with an extraordinary Dryness of the Eyes, Nostrils, Lips, of the Tongue, and of the Throat, a violent Headach, and sometimes a Raving at the Height of the Paroxysm, or Increase of the Fever, which rises considerably every Evening. The Respiration is also somewhat oppressed, but especially at the Return of this Paroxysm, with a Cough now and then, though without any Pain in the Breast, and without any Expectoration, or coughing

ing up. The Body is coſtive; the Urine very high coloured, hot, and in a ſmall Quantity. The Sick are alſo liable to ſtart ſometimes, but eſpecially when they ſeem to ſleep; for they have little ſound refreſhing Sleep, but rather a kind of Drowſineſs, that makes them very little attentive to, or ſenſible of, whatever happens about them, or even of their own Condition. They have ſometimes a little Sweat or Moiſture, though commonly a very dry Skin, they are manifeſtly weak, and have either little or no Smell or Taſte.

§ 232. This Diſeaſe, like all other inflammatory ones, is produced by the Cauſes which thicken the Blood, and increaſe its Motion, ſuch as exceſſive Labour, violent Heat, Want of Sleep, the Abuſe of Wine or other ſtrong Liquors, the long Continuance of a dry Conſtitution of the Air, Exceſs of every kind, and heating inflaming Food.

§ 233. The Patient, under theſe Circumſtances, ought, 1, immediately to be put upon a Regimen, to have the Food allowed him given only every eight Hours, and, in ſome Caſes, only twice a Day: and indeed, when the Attack is extremely violent, Nouriſhment may be wholly omitted.

2, Bleeding ſhould be performed and repeated, 'till the Hardneſs of the Pulſe is ſenſibly abated. The firſt Diſcharge ſhould be conſiderable, the ſecond ſhould be made four Hours after. If the Pulſe is ſoftened by the firſt, the ſecond may be ſuſpended, and not repeated before it becomes ſufficiently

sufficiently hard again, to make us apprehensive of Danger: but should it continue strong and hard, the Bleeding may be repeated on the same Day to a third Time, which often happens to be all the Repetitions that are necessary.

3, The Glyster N°. 5 should be given twice, or even thrice, daily.

4, His Legs are to be bathed twice a Day in warm Water: his Hands may be bathed in the same Water. Linen or Flanel Cloths dipt in warm Water may be applied over the Breast, and upon the Belly, and he should regularly drink the Almond Milk N°. 4 and the Ptisan N°. 7. The poorest Patients may content themselves with the last, but should drink very plentifully of it, and after the Bleeding properly repeated, fresh Air and the plentiful Continuance of small diluting Liquors generally establish the Health of the Patient.

5, If notwithstanding the repeated Bleedings, the Fever still rages highly, it may be lessened by giving a Spoonful of the Potion N°. 10 every Hour, till it abates, and afterwards every three Hours, until it becomes very moderate.

§ 234. Hæmorrhages, or Bleedings, from the Nose frequently occur in this Fever, greatly to the Relief and Security of the Patient.

The first Appearances of Amendment are a softening of the Pulse, (which however does not wholly lose all its Hardness, before the Disease entirely terminates) a sensible Abatement of the Heat, a greater Quantity of Urine, and that

less

less high coloured, and a manifestly approaching Moisture of the Tongue. These favourable Signs keep increasing in their Degree, and there frequently ensue between the ninth and the fourteenth Day, and often after a Flurry of some Hours Continuance, very large Evacuations by Stool; a great Quantity of Urine, which lets fall a palely reddish Sediment, the Urine above it being very clear, and of a natural Colour, and these accompanied with Sweats in a less or greater Quantity. At the same Time the Nostrils and the Mouth grow moist: the brown and dry Crust which covered the Tongue, and which was hitherto inseparable from it, peels off of itself, the Thirst is diminished, the Clearness of the Faculties rises, the Drowsiness goes off, it is succeeded by comfortable Sleep, and the natural Strength is restored. When Things are evidently in this Way, the Patient should take the Potion N°. 23, and be put upon the Regimen of those who are in a State of Recovery. It should be repeated at the End of eight or ten Days. Some Patients have perfectly recovered from this Fever, without the least Sediment in their Urine.

§ 235. The augmenting Danger of this Fever may be discerned, from the continued Hardness of the Pulse, though with an Abatement of its Strength, if the Brain becomes more confused, the Breathing more difficult; if the Eyes, Nose, Lips and Tongue become still more dry, and the Voice more altered. If to these Symptoms there be also added a Swelling of the Belly; a Diminution

nution of the Quantity of Urine; a constant Raving; great Anxiety, and a certain Wildness of the Eyes, the Case is in a manner desperate; and the Patient cannot survive many Hours. The Hands and Fingers at this Period are incessantly in Motion, as if feeling for something upon the Bed-Cloths, which is commonly termed, their hunting for Flies.

CHAPTER XVI.

Of putrid Fevers.

SECT. 236.

HAVING treated of such feverish Distempers, as arise from an Inflammation of the Blood, I shall here treat of those produced by corrupt Humours, which stagnate in the Stomach, the Guts, or other Bowels of the lower Cavity, the Belly, or which have already passed from them into the Blood. These are called putrid Fevers, or sometimes bilious Fevers, when a certain Degeneracy or Corruption of the Bile seems chiefly to prevail in the Disease.

§ 237. This Distemper frequently gives Notice of its Approach, several Days before its manifest Attack, by a great Dejection, a Heaviness of the Head, Pains of the Loins and Knees; a

Foulness

Foulness of the Mouth in the Morning, little Appetite, broken Slumber; and sometimes by an excessive Head-ach for many Days, without any other Symptom. After this, or these Disorders, a Shivering comes on, followed by a sharp and dry Heat: the Pulse, which was small and quick during the Shivering, is raised during the Heat, and is often very strong, though it is not attended with the same Hardness, as in the preceding Fever; except the putrid Fever be combined with an inflammatory one, which it sometimes is. During this Time, that is the Duration of the Heat, the Head-ach is commonly extremely violent; the Patient is almost constantly affected with Loathings, and sometimes even with Vomiting, with Thirst, disagreeable Risings, a Bitterness in the Mouth; and very little Urine. This Heat continues for many Hours, frequently the whole Night, it abates a little in the Morning, and the Pulse, though always feverish, is then something less so, while the Patient suffers less, though still greatly dejected.

The Tongue is white and furred, the Teeth are foul, and the Breath smells very disagreeably. The Colour, Quantity and Consistence of the Urine, are very various and changeable. Some Patients are costive, others frequently have small Stools, without the least Relief accruing from them. The Skin is sometimes dry, and at other Times there is some sensible Perspiration, but without any Benefit attending it. The Fever augments every Day, and frequently at unexpected

pected irregular Periods. Besides that *great* Paroxysm or Increase, which is perceivable in all the Subjects of this Fever, some have also other *less* intervening ones.

§ 238. When the Disease is left to itself, or injudiciously treated, or when it proves more powerful than the Remedies against it, which is by no Means seldom the Case, the Aggravations of it become longer, more frequent and irregular. There is scarcely an Interval of Ease. The Patient's Belly is swell'd out like a Foot-ball; a *Delirium* or Raving comes on, he proves insensible of his own Evacuations, which come away involuntarily, he rejects Assistance, and keeps muttering continually, with a quick, small, irregular Pulse. Sometimes little Spots of a brown, or of a livid Colour appear on the Surface, but particularly about the Neck, Back and Breast. All the Discharges from his Body have a most fœtid Smell: convulsive Motions also supervene, especially in the Face, he lies down only on his Back, sinks down insensibly towards the Feet of the Bed, and picks about, as if catching Flies, his Pulse becomes so quick and so small, that it cannot be perceived without Difficulty, and cannot be counted. His Anguish seems inexpressible his Sweats stream down from Agony: his Breast swells out as if distended by Fulness, and he dies miserably.

§ 239. When this Distemper is less violent, or more judiciously treated, and the Medicines succeed well, it continues for some Days in the State described

Of putrid Fevers.

described § 237, without growing worse, though without abating. None of these Symptoms however appear, described § 238, but, on the contrary, all the Symptoms become milder, the Paroxysms, or Aggravations, are shorter and less violent, the Head-ach more supportable; the Discharges by Stool are less frequent, but more at once, and attended with Relief to the Patient. The Quantity of Urine is very considerable, though it varies at different Times in Colour and Consistence, as before. The Patient soon begins to get a little Sleep, and grows more composed and easy. The Tongue disengages itself from its Filth and Furriness, and Health gradually, yet daily, advances.

§ 240. This Fever seems to have no critical Time, either for its Termination in Recovery, or in Death. When it is very violent, or very badly conducted, it proves sometimes fatal on the ninth Day. Persons often die of it from the eighteenth to the twentieth, sometimes only about the fortieth, after having been alternately better and worse.

When it happens but in a light Degree, it is sometimes cured within a few Days, after the earliest Evacuations. When it is of a very different Character, some Patients are not out of Danger before the End of six Weeks, and even still later. Nevertheless it is certain, that these Fevers, extended to this Length of Duration, often depend in a great Measure on the Manner of treating them, and that in general their Course must be

deter-

determined, some time from the fourteenth to the thirtieth Day.

§ 241. The Treatment of this Species of Fevers is comprized in the following Method and Medicines.

1, The Patient must be put into a *Regimen*; and notwithstanding he is far from costive, and sometimes has even a small Purging, he should receive one Glyster daily. His common Drink should be Lemonade, (which is made of the Juice of Lemons, Sugar and Water) or the Ptisan N°. 3. Instead of Juice of Lemons, Vinegar may be occasionally substituted, which, with Sugar and Water, makes an agreeable and very wholesome Drink in these Fevers.

2, If there be an Inflammation also, which may be discovered by the Strength and the Hardness of the Pulse, and by the Temperament and Complexion of the Patient, if he is naturally robust, and has heated himself by any of the Causes described, § 232, he should be bled once, and even a second Time, if necessary, some Hours after. I must observe however, that very frequently there is no such Inflammation, and that in such a Case, Bleeding would be hurtful.

3, When the Patient has drank very plentifully for two Days of these Liquids, if his Mouth still continues in a very foul State, and he has violent Reachings to vomit, he must take the Powder N°. 34, dissolved in half a † Pot of warm

---

† That is about two Ounces more than a Pint and a half of our Measure.

warm Water, a ‖ Glaſs of it being to be drank every half Quarter of an Hour. But as this Medicine vomits, it muſt not be taken, except we are certain the Patient is not under any Circumſtance, which forbids the Uſe of a Vomit: all which Circumſtances ſhall be particularly mentioned in the Chapter, reſpecting the Uſe of ſuch Medicines, as are taken by way of Precaution, or Prevention. If the firſt Glaſſes excite a plentiful Vomiting, we muſt forbear giving another, and be content with obliging the Patient to drink a conſiderable Quantity of warm Water But if the former Glaſſes do not occaſion Vomiting, they muſt be repeated, as already directed until they do. Thoſe who are afraid of taking this Medicine, which is uſually called, the Emetic, may take that of N° 35, alſo drinking warm Water plentifully during its Operation, but the former is preferable, as more prevalent, in dangerous Caſes. We muſt caution our Readers at the ſame Time, that wherever there is an Inflammation of any Part, neither of theſe Medicines muſt be given, which might prove a real Poiſon in ſuch a Circumſtance; and even if the Fever is extremely violent, though there ſhould be no particular Inflammation, they ſhould not be given.

The Time of giving them is ſoon after the End of the Paroxyſm, when the Fever is at the loweſt. The Medicine N°. 34 generally purges, after it ceaſes
to

‖ About three Ounces

to make the Patient vomit: But N°. 35 is seldom attended with the same Effect.

When the Operation of the Vomit is entirely over, the Sick should return to the Use of the Ptisan; and great Care must be taken to prohibit them from the Use of Flesh Broth, under the Pretext of working off a Purging with it. The same Method is to be continued on the following Days as on the first; but as it is of Importance to keep the Body open, he should take every Morning some of the Ptisan N° 32. Such, as this would be too expensive for, may substitute, in the room of it, a fourth Part of the Powder N°. 34 in five or six Glasses of Water, of which they are to take a Cup every two Hours, beginning early in the Morning. Nevertheless, if the Fever be very high, N°. 32 should be preferred to it.

4, After the Operation of the Vomit, if the Fever still continue, if the Stools are remarkably fœtid, and if the Belly is tense and distended as it were, and the Quantity of Urine is small, a Spoonful of the Potion N°. 10 should be given every two Hours, which checks the Putridity and abates the Fever. Should the Distemper become violent, and very pressing, it ought to be taken every Hour.

5, Whenever, notwithstanding the giving all these Medicines as directed, the Fever continues obstinate, the Brain is manifestly disordered, there is a violent Head-ach, or very great Restlessness, two blistering Plaisters N°. 36 must be applied

Of putrid Fevers.

applied to the inside and fleshy Part of the Legs, and their Suppuration and Discharge should be continued as long as possible.

6, If the Fever is extremely violent indeed, there is a Necessity absolutely to prohibit the Patient from receiving the least Nourishment

7, When it is thought improper, or unsafe, to give the Vomit, the Patient should take in the Morning, for two successive Days, three Doses of the Powder Nº. 24, at the Interval of one Hour between each: This Medicine produces some bilious Stools, which greatly abate the Fever, and considerably lessen the Violence of all the other Symptoms of the Disease. This may be done with Success, when the excessive Height of the Fever prevents us from giving the Vomit: and we should limit ourselves to this Medicine, as often as we are uncertain, whether the Circumstances of the Disease and the Patient will admit of the Vomiting; which may also be dispensed with, in many Cases.

8, When the Distemper has manifestly and considerably declined; the Paroxysms are more slight; and the Patient continues without any Fever for several Hours, the daily Use of the purging opening Drinks should be discontinued. The common Ptisans however should be still made Use of, and it will be proper to give every other Day two Doses of the Powder Nº. 24, which sufficiently obviates every ill Consequence from this Disease.

9, If the Fever has been clearly off for a long Part of the Day, if the Tongue appears in a

good

good healthy State; if the Patient has been well purged; and yet one moderate Paroxysm of the Fever returns every Day, he should take four Doses of the Powder N°. 14 between the End of one Return and the Beginning of the next, and continue this Repetition some Days. People who cannot easily procure this Medicine, may substitute, instead of it, the bitter Decoction N°. 37. four Glasses of which may be taken at equal Intervals, between the two Paroxysms or Returns of the Fever.

10, As the Organs of Digestion have been considerably weakened through the Course of this Fever, there is a Necessity for the Patient's conducting himself very prudently and regularly long after it, with Regard both to the Quantity and Quality of his Food. He should also use due Exercise as soon as his Strength will permit, without which he may be liable to fall into some chronical and languishing Disorder, productive of considerable Languor and Weakness.

* As our Jail, Hospital, and often Camp Fevers may often be ranged in this Class, as of the most putrid Kind, and not seldom occasioned by bad Food, bad Air, unclean, unwholesome Lodging, &c. a judicious Use may certainly be made of a small Quantity of genuine, and not dangerous, Wine in such of them, as are not blended with an inflammatory Cause, or inflammable Constitution, or which do not greatly result from a bilious Cause; though in these last, where there is manifest Lowness and Dejection, perhaps a little Rhenish might be properly interposed between the Lemonade and other Drinks directed § 241 Doubtless Dr Tissot was perfectly apprized of this salutary Use of it in some low Fevers, but the Necessity of its being regulated by the Presence of a Physician has probably disposed him rather to omit mentioning it, than to leave the Allowance of it to the Discretion of a simple Country Patient, or his ignorant Assistants. K.

CHAPTER

Chapter XVII.

Of malignant Fevers.

Sect. 242.

THOSE Fevers are termed malignant, in which the Danger is more than the Symptoms would make us apprehensive of: they have frequently a fatal Event without appearing so very perilous; on which Account it has been well said of this Fever, that it is a Dog which bites without barking.

§ 243. The distinguishing *Criterion* or Mark of malignant Fevers is a total Loss of the Patient's Strength, immediately on their first Attack. They arise from a Corruption of the Humours, which is noxious to the very Source and Principle of Strength, the Impairing or Destruction of which is the Cause of the Feebleness of the Symptoms; by Reason none of the Organs are strong enough to exert an Opposition sufficiently vigorous, to subdue the Cause of the Distemper.

If, for Instance or Illustration, we were to suppose, that when two Armies were on the Point of engaging, one of them should be nearly deprived of all their Weapons, the Contest would not appear very violent, nor attended with great Noise or Tumult, though with a horrible Massacre. The Spectator, who, from being ignorant of one of the Armies being disarmed, would not be able to calculate the Carnage of the Battle, but in Proportion to its Noise and Tumult, must be extremely deceived in his Conception of it. The Number of the Slain would be astonishing, which might have been much less (though the Noise and Clangor of it had been greater) if each Army had been equally provided for the Combat.

§ 244. The Causes of this Disease are a long Use of animal Food or Flesh alone, without Pulse, Fruits or Acids, the continued Use of other bad Provisions, such as Bread made of damaged Corn or Grain, or very stale Meat. Eight Persons, who dined together on corrupt Fish, were all seized with a malignant Fever, which killed five of them, notwithstanding the Endeavours of the most able Physicians. These Fevers are also frequently the Consequence of a great Dearth or Famine, of too hot and moist an Air, or an Air, which highly partakes of these two Qualities; so that they happen to spread most in hot Years, in Places abounding with Marshes and standing Waters. They are also the Effect of a very close and stagnant Air, especially if many Persons are crouded together in it, this being a Cause that particularly tends to corrupt the Air. Tedious Grief and Vexation also contribute to generate these Fevers.

§ 245. The Symptoms of malignant Fevers are, as I have already observed, a total and sudden

den Loss of Strength, without any evident preceding Cause, sufficient to produce such a Privation of Strength: at the same Time there is also an utter Dejection of the Mind, which becomes almost insensible and inattentive to every Thing, and even to the Disease itself; a sudden Alteration in the Countenance, especially in the Eyes: some small Shiverings, which are varied throughout the Space of twenty-four Hours, with little Paroxysms or Vicissitudes of Heat; sometimes there is a great Head-ach and a Pain in the Loins; at other Times there is no perceivable Pain in any Part, a kind of Sinkings or Faintings, immediately from the Invasion of the Disease, which is always very unpromising, not the least refreshing Sleep; frequently a kind of half Sleep, or Drowsiness; a light and silent or inward Raving, which discovers itself in the unusual and astonished Look of the Patient, who seems profoundly employed in meditating on something, but really thinks of nothing, or not at all: Some Patients have, however, violent Ravings, most have a Sensation of Weight or Oppression, and at other Times of a Binding or Tightness about, or around, the Pit of the Stomach.

The sick Person seems to labour under great Anguish. he has sometimes slight convulsive Motions and Twitchings in his Face and his Hands, as well as in his Arms and Legs His Senses seem torpid, or as it were benumbed. I have seen many who had lost, to all Appearance, the whole five, and yet some of them recover. It is not uncommon to meet with some, who neither see, understand, nor speak. Their Voices change, become weak, and are sometimes quite lost. Some of them have a fixed Pain in some Part of the Belly: this arises from a Stuffing or Obstruction, and often ends in a Gangrene, whence this Symptom is highly dangerous and perplexing.

The Tongue is sometimes very little altered from its Appearance in Health; at other Times covered over with a yellowish brown Humour; but it is more rarely dry in this Fever than in the others; and yet it sometimes does resemble a Tongue that has been long smoaked.

The Belly is sometimes very soft, and at other Times tense and hard. The Pulse is weak, sometimes pretty regular, but always more quick than in a natural State, and at some Times even very quick, and such I have always found it, when the Belly has been distended.

The Skin is often neither hot, dry, nor moist: it is frequently overspread with petechial or eruptive Spots (which are little Spots of a reddish livid Colour) especially on the Neck, about the Shoulders, and upon the Back. At other Times the Spots are larger and brown, like the Colour of Wheals from the Strokes of a Stick.

The Urine of the Sick is almost constantly crude, that is of a lighter Colour than ordinary. I have seen some, which could not be distinguished, merely by the Eye, from Milk. A black

black and stinking Purging sometimes attends this Fever, which is mortal, except the Sick be evidently relieved by the Discharge.

Some of the Patients are infested with livid Ulcers on the Inside of the Mouth, and on the Palate. At other Times Abscesses are formed in the Glands of the Groin, of the Arm-pit, in those between the Ears and the Jaw, or a Gangrene may appear in some Part, as on the Feet, the Hands, or the Back. The Strength proves entirely spent, the Brain is wholly confused: the miserable Patient stretched out on his Back, frequently expires under Convulsions, an enormous Sweat, and an oppressed Breast and Respiration. Hæmmorrhages also happens sometimes and are mortal, being almost unexceptionably such in this Fever. There is also in this, as in all other Fevers, an Aggravation of the Fever in the Evening

§ 246 The Duration and *Crisis* of these malignant, as well as those of putrid Fevers, are very irregular. Sometimes the Sick die on the seventh or eighth Day, more commonly between the twelfth and the fifteenth, and not infrequently at the End of five or six Weeks. These different Durations result from the different Degree and Strength of the Disease Some of these Fevers at their first Invasion are very slow, and during a few of the first Days, the Patient, though very weak, and with a very different Look and Manner, scarcely thinks himself sick.

The Term or Period of the Cure or the Recovery, is as uncertain as that of Death in this Distemper. Some are out of Danger at the End of fifteen Days, and even sooner; others not before the Expiration of several Weeks.

The Signs which portend a Recovery are, a little more Strength in the Pulse, a more concocted Urine; less Dejection and Discouragement, a less confused Brain; an equal kindly Heat; a pretty warm or hot Sweat in a moderate Quantity, without Inquietude or Anguish; the Revival of the different Senses that were extinguished, or greatly suspended in the Progress of the Disease, though the Deafness is not a very threatening Symptom, if the others amend while it endures.

This Malady commonly leaves the Patient in a very weak Condition; and a long Interval will ensue between the End of it, and their recovering their full Strength.

§ 247. It is, in the first place, of greater Importance in this Distemper than in any other, both for the Benefit of the Patients, and those who attend them, that the Air should be renewed and purified. Vinegar should often be evaporated from a hot Tile or Iron in the Chamber, and one Window kept almost constantly open.

2, The Diet should be light, and the Juice of Sorrel may be mixed with their Water, the Juice of Lemons may be added to Soups prepared from different Grains and Pulse; the Patient may eat

sharp

sharp acid Fruits, such as tart juicy * Cherries, Gooseberries, small black Cherries; and those who can afford them, may be allowed Lemons, Oranges and Pomgranates

3, The Patient's Linen should be changed every two Days.

4, Bleeding is very rarely necessary, or even proper, in this Fever; the Exceptions to which are very few, and cannot be thoroughly ascertained, as fit and proper Exceptions to the Omission of Bleeding, without a Physician, or some other very skilful Person's seeing the Patient

5, There is often very little Occasion for Glysters, which are sometimes dangerous in this Fever

6, The Patient's common Drink should be Barley Water made acid with the Spirit N°. 10, at the Rate of one Quarter of an Ounce to at least full three Pints of the Water, or acidulated agreeably to his Taste. He may also drink Lemonade.

7, It is necessary to open and evacuate the Bowels, where a great Quantity of corrupt Humours is generally lodged. The Powder N°. 35 may be given for this Purpose, after the Operation of which the Patient generally finds himself better, at least for some Hours. It is of Importance not to omit this at the Beginning of the Disease, though if it has been omitted at first, it were

---

* The French Word is *Griottes*, which *Boyer* englishes, *the Agriot, the red or sour Cherry*, and *Chambard, the sweeter large Black Cherry or Mazzerd*—But as Dr Tissot was recommending the Use of Acids, it is more probably the first of these so that our Morellas, which make a pleasant Preserve, may be a good Substitute to them, supposing them not to be the same Our Berbery Jam, and Jelly of Red Currants, may be also employed to answer the same Indication K

were beſt to give it even later, provided no particular Inflammation has ſupervened, and the Patient has ſtill ſome Strength. I have given it, and with remarkable Succeſs, on the twentieth Day.

8. Having by this Medicine expelled a conſiderable Portion of the bad Humours, which contribute to feed and keep up the Fever, the Patient ſhould take every other Day, during the Continuance of the Diſeaſe, and ſometimes even every Day, one Doſe of the Cream of Tartar and Rhubarb N°. 38. This Remedy evacuates the corrupt Humours, prevents the Corruption of the others, expells the Worms that are very common in theſe Fevers, which the Patient ſometimes diſcharges upwards and downwards; and which frequently conduce to many of the odd and extraordinary Symptoms, that are obſerved in malignant Fevers. In ſhort it ſtrengthens the Bowels, and, without checking the neceſſary Evacuations, it moderates the Looſeneſs, when it is hurtful.

9. If the Skin be dry, with a Looſeneſs, and that by checking it, we deſign to increaſe Perſpiration, inſtead of the Rhubarb, the Cream of Tartar may be blended with the Ipecacuana, N°. 39, which, being given in ſmall and frequent Doſes, reſtrains the Purging, and promotes Perſpiration. This Medicine, as the former, is to be taken in the Morning, two Hours after, the Sick muſt begin with the Potion N°. 40, and repeat it regularly every three Hours, until it be inter-

Of malignant Fevers.

interrupted by giving one of the Medicines N°. 38 or 39: After which the Potion is to be repeated again, as already directed, till the Patient grows considerably better.

10, If the Strength of the Sick be very confiderably depreffed, and he is in great Dejection and Anguifh, he fhould take, with every Draught of the Potion, the Bolus, or Morfel N° 41. If the *Diarrhæa*, the Purging is violent, there fhould be added, once or twice a Day to the Bolus, the Weight of twenty Grains, or the Size of a very fmall Bean, of *Diafcordium*; or if that is not readily to be got, as much Venice Treacle.

11, Whenever, notwithftanding all this Affiftance, the Patient continues in a State of Weaknefs and Infenfibility, two large Blifters fhould be applied to the fleſhy Infides of the Legs, or a large one to the Nape of the Neck: and fometimes, if there be a great Drowfinefs, with a manifeft Embarraffment of the Brain, they may be applied with great Succefs over the whole Head Their Suppuration and Difcharge is to be promoted abundantly, and, if they dry up within a few Days, others are to be applied, and their Evacuation is to be kept up for a confiderable Time.

12 As foon as the Diftemper is fufficiently abated, for the Patient to remain fome Hours with very little or no Fever, we muft avail ourfelves of this Interval, to give him fix, or at leaft five Dofes of the Medicine N° 14, and repeat the fame the next Day, which may prevent the

Return

Return of the Fever: * after which it may be sufficient to give daily only two Doses for a few Days.

13, When the Sick continue entirely clear of a Fever, or any Return, they are to be put into the *Regimen* of Persons in a State of Recovery. But if his Strength returns very flowly, or not at all; in Order to the speedier Establishment and Confirmation of it, he may take three Doses a Day of the *Theriaca Pauperum*, or poor Man's Treacle N° 42, the first of them fasting, and the other twelve Hours after. It were to be wished indeed, this Medicine was introduced into all the Apothecaries Shops, as an excellent Stomachic, in which Respect it is much preferable to Venice Treacle, which is an absurd Composition, dear and often dangerous. It is true it does not dispose the Patients to Sleep, but when we would procure them Sleep, there are better Medicines than the Treacle to answer that Purpose. Such as may not think the Expence of the Medicine N° 14, too much, may take three Doses of it daily for some Weeks, instead of the Medicine N° 42, already directed.

§ 248. It is necessary to eradicate a Prejudice that prevails among Country People, with Regard

---

* Observation and Experience have demonstrated the Advantage of the Bark, to obviate a Gangrene and prevent the Putrefaction of animal Substances. We therefore conclude it may be usefully employed in malignant Fevers, as soon as the previous and necessary Evacuations shall have taken Place. *T. L.* — Provided there be very clear and regular Remissions at least. *K*

gard to the Treatment of these Fevers; not only because it is false and ridiculous, but even dangerous too. They imagine that the Application of Animals can draw out the Poison of the Disease, in Consequence of which they apply Poultry, or Pigeons, Cats or sucking Pigs to the Feet, or upon the Head of the Patient, having first split the living Animals open. Some Hours after they remove their strange Applications, corrupted, and stinking very offensively, and then ascribe such Corruption and horrid Stink to the Poison they suppose their Application to be charged with, and which they suppose to be the Cause of this Fever. But in this supposed Extraction of Poison, they are grossly mistaken, since the Flesh does not stink in Consequence of any such Extraction, but from its being corrupted through Moisture and Heat: and they contract no other Smell but what they would have got, if they had been put in any other Place, as well as on the Patient's Body, that was equally hot and moist. Very far from drawing out the Poison, they augment the Corruption of the Disease, and it would be sufficient to communicate it to a sound Person, if he was to suffer many of these animal Bodies, thus absurdly and uselessly butchered, to be applied to various Parts of his Body in Bed; and to lie still a long Time with their putrified Carcases fastened about him, and corrupting whatever Air he breathed there.

With the same Intention they fasten a living Sheep to the Bed's-foot for several Hours, which, though

though not equally dangerous, is in some Measure hurtful, since the more Animals there are in a Chamber, the Air of it is proportionably corrupted, or altered at least from its natural Simplicity, by their Respiration and Exhalations: but admitting this to be less pernicious, it is equally absurd. It is certain indeed, the Animals who are kept very near the sick Person breathe in the poisonous, or noxious Vapours which exhale from his Body, and may be incommoded with them, as well as his Attendants: But it is ridiculous to suppose their being kept near the Sick causes such Poison to come out of their Bodies. On the very contrary, in contributing still further to the Corruption of the Air, they increase the Disease. They draw a false Consequence, and no Wonder, from a false Principle, saying, if the Sheep dies, the Sick will recover. Now, most frequently the Sheep does not die; notwithstanding which the Sick sometimes recover, and sometimes they both die.

§ 249. The Cause of malignant Fevers is, not infrequently, combined with other Diseases, whose Danger it extremely increases. It is blended for Instance, with the Poison of the Small-Pocks, or of the Measles. This may be known by the Union of those Symptoms, which carry the Marks of Malignity, with the Symptoms of the other Diseases. Such combined Cases are extremely dangerous; they demand the utmost Attention of the Physician, nor is it possible to prescribe their

exact

exact Treatment here; since it consists in general of a Mixture of the Treatment of each Disease; though the Malignity commonly demands the greatest Attention.

Chapter XVIII.

Of intermitting Fevers.

Sect. 250.

INTERMITTING Fevers, commonly called here, Fevers and Agues, are those, which after an Invasion and Continuance for some Hours, abate very perceivably, as well as all the Symptoms attending them, and then entirely cease; nevertheless, not without some periodical or stated Return of them.

They were very frequent with us some Years since; and indeed might even be called epidemical. but for the five or six last Years, they have been much less frequent throughout the greater Part of *Swisserland*: notwithstanding they still continue in no small Number in all Places, where the Inhabitants breathe the Air that prevails in all the marshy Borders of the *Rhone*, and in some other Situations that are exposed to much the same humid Air and Exhalations.

§ 251.

§ 251. There are several Kinds of intermitting Fevers, which take their different Names from the Interval or different Space of Time, in which the Fits return.

If the Paroxysm or Fit returns every Day, it is either a true Quotidian, or a double Tertian Fever: The first of these may be distinguished from the last by this Circumstance, that in the Quotidian, or one Day Fever, the Fits are long; and correspond pretty regularly to each other in Degree and Duration. This however is less frequent in *Switserland*. In the double Tertian, the Fits are shorter, and one is alternately light, and the other more severe.

In the simple Tertian, or third Day's Fever, the Fits return every other Day; so that three Days include one Paroxysm, and the Return of another.

In a Quartan, the Fit returns every fourth Day, including the Day of the first and that of the second Attack. so that the Patient enjoys two clear Days between the two sick ones.

The other kinds of Intermittents are much rarer. I have seen however one true Quintan, or fifth Day Ague, the Patient having three clear Days between two Fits, and one regularly weekly Ague, as it may be called, the Visitation of every Return happening every Sunday

§ 252 The first Attack of an intermittent Fever often happens, when the Patient thought himself in perfect Health. Sometimes however it is preceded by a Sensation of Cold and a kind of of Numbness, which continue some Days before the manifest Invasion of the Fit. It begins with frequent Yawnings, a Lassitude, or Sensation of Weariness, with a general Weakness, with Coldness, Shivering and Shaking: There is also a Paleness of the extreme Parts of the Body, attended with Loathings, and sometimes an actual Vomiting. The Pulse is quick, weak, and small, and there is a considerable Degree of Thirst.

At the End of an Hour or two, and but seldom so long as three or four Hours, a Heat succeeds, which increases insensibly, and becomes violent at its Height. At this Period the whole Body grows red, the Anxiety of the Patient abates; the Pulse is very strong and large, and his Thirst proves excessive. He complains of a violent Head-ach, and of a Pain in all his Limbs, but of a different sort of Pain from that he was sensible of, while his Coldness continued. Finally, having endured this hot State, four, five or six Hours, he falls into a general Sweat for a few more: upon which all the Symptoms already mentioned abate, and sometimes Sleep supervenes.

At the Conclusion of this Nap the Patient often wakes without any sensible Fever; complaining only of Lassitude and Weakness. Sometimes his Pulse returns entirely to its natural State between the two Fits, though it often continues a little quicker than in perfect Health, and does not recover its first Distinctness and Slowness, till some Days after the last Fit.

One

One Symptom, which most particularly characterises these several Species of intermitting Fevers, is the Quality of the Urines which the Sick pass after the Fit. They are of a reddish Colour, and let fall a Sediment, or Settling; which exactly resembles Brick-dust. They are sometimes frothy too, and a Pellicle, or thin filmy Skin, appears on the Top, and adheres to the Sides of the Glass that contains them.

§ 253. The Duration of each Fit is of no fixed Time or Extent, being various according to the particular sort of Intermittents, and through many other Circumstances. Sometimes they return precisely at the very same Hour; at other Times they come one, two, or three Hours sooner, and in other Instances as much later than the former. It has been imagined that those Fevers, whose Paroxysms returned sooner than usual, were sooner finally terminated: but there seems to be no general Rule in this Case.

§ 254. Intermitting Fevers are distinguished into those of Spring and Autumn. The former generally prevail from February to June: the latter are those which reign from July to January. Their essential Nature and Characters are the very same, as they are not different Distempers; though the various Circumstances attending them deserve our Consideration. These Circumstances depend on the Season itself, and the Constitution of the Patients, during such Seasons. The Spring Intermittents are sometimes blended with an inflammatory Disposition, as that is the Disposition fition of Bodies in that Seafon; but as the Weather then advances daily into an improving State, the Spring Fevers are commonly of a fhorter Duration. The autumnal Fevers are frequently combined and aggravated with a Principle of Putrefaction; and as the Air of that Seafon rather degenerates, they are more tedious and obftinate.

§ 255. The autumnal Fevers feldom begin quite fo early as July, but much oftner in Auguft: and the Duration to which they are often extended, has increafed the Terror which the People entertain of Fevers that begin in that Month. But that Prejudice which afcribes their Danger to the Influence of Auguft, is a very abfurd Error; fince it is better they fhould fet in then than in the following Months, becaufe they are obftinate in Proportion to the Tardinefs, the Slownefs of their Approach They fometimes appear at firft confiderably in the Form of putrid Fevers, not affuming that of Intermittents till fome Days after their Appearance: but very happily there is little or no Danger in miftaking them for putrid Fevers, or in treating them like fuch. The Brick-coloured Sediment, and particularly the Pellicle or Film on the Surface of the Urine, are very common in autumnal Intermittents, and are often wanting in the Urine of putrid Fevers. In thefe latter, it is generally lefs high coloured, and leaning rather to a yellow, a kind of Cloudinefs is fufpended in the Middle of it. These also deposite a white Sediment, which affords no bad Prognostic.

§ 256 Generally speaking, intermitting Fevers are not mortal, often terminating in Health of their own Accord (without the Use of any Medicine) after some Fits. In this last Respect Intermittents in the Spring differ considerably from those in the Fall, which continue a long Time, and sometimes even until Spring, if they are not removed by Art, or if they have been improperly treated.

Quartan Fevers are always more obstinate and inveterate than Tertians, the former sometimes persevering in certain Constitutions for whole Years. When these Sorts of Fevers occur in boggy marshy Countries, they are not only very chronical or tedious, but Persons infested with them are liable to frequent Relapses.

§ 257 A few Fits of an Intermittent are not very injurious, and it happens sometimes, that they are attended with a favourable Alteration of the Habit in Point of Health, by their exterminating the Cause or Principle of some languid and tedious Disorder, though it is erroneous to consider them as salutary. If they prove tedious and obstinate, and the Fits are long and violent, they weaken the whole Body, impairing all its Functions, and particularly the Digestions: They make the Humours sharp and unbalmy, and introduce several other Maladies, such as the Jaundice, Dropsy, Asthma and slow wasting Fevers. Nay sometimes old Persons, and those who are

very

very weak, expire in the Fit, though such an Event never happens but in the cold Fit.

§ 258. Very happily Nature has afforded us a Medicine, that infallibly cures these Fevers: this is the *Kinkina*, or Jesuits Bark; and as we are possessed of this certain Remedy, the only remaining Difficulty is to discover, if there be not some other Disease combined with these Fevers, which Disease might be aggravated by the Bark. Should any such exist, it must be removed by Medicines adapted to it, before the Bark is given. *

---

* This admirable Medicine was unknown in Europe, till about one hundred and twenty Years past, we are obliged to the Spaniards for it, who found it in the Province of Quito in Peru; the Countess of Chinchon being the first European who used it in America, whence it was brought to Spain, under the Name of the Countesses Powder. The Jesuits having soon dispensed and distributed it abroad, it became still more publick by the Name of the Jesuits Powder and since it has been known by that of *Kinkina* or the Peruvian Bark. It met with great Opposition at first; some deeming it a Poison, while others considered it as a divine Remedy so that the Prejudices of many being heightened by their Animosity, it was nearly a full Century, before its true Virtue and its Use were agreed to and about twenty Years since the most unfavourable Prejudices against it pretty generally subsided. The Insufficience of other Medicines in several Cases, its great Efficaciousness, and the many and surprizing Cures which it did, and daily does effect, the Number of Distempers, the different kinds of Fevers, in which it proves the sovereign Remedy, its Effects in the most difficult chirurgical Cases, the Comfort, the Strength and Spirits it gives those who need and take it, have at length opened every Persons Eyes, so that it has almost unanimously obtained the first Reputation, among the most efficacious Medicines. The World is no longer amused with Apprehensions of its injuring the Stomach, of its fixing, or *shutting up the Loose* (as the Phrase has been)

§ 259. In the vernal, or Spring-Fevers, if the Fits are not very severe; if the Patient is evidently well in their Intervals; if his Appetite, his Strength, and his Sleep continue as in Health, no Medicine should be given, nor any other Method be taken, but that of putting the Person, under such a gentle Intermittent, upon the Regimen directed for Persons in a State of Recovery. This is such a Regimen as pretty generally agrees with all the Subjects of these Fevers: for if they should be reduced to the Regimen proper in acute Diseases, they would be weakened to no Purpose, and perhaps be the worse for it. But at the same Time if we were not to retrench from the Quantity, nor somewhat to vary the Quality of their usual Food in a State of Health, as there is not the least Digestion made in the Stomach, during the whole Term of the Fit, and as the Stomach is always weakened a little by the Disease, crude and indigested Humours would be produced, which might afford a Fuel to the Disease. Not the least solid Food should be allowed, for at least two Hours before the usual Approach of the Fit.

§ 260.

been) without curing it, that it shuts up the Wolf in the Sheepfold, that it throws those who take it into the Scurvy, the Asthma, the Dropsy, the Jaundice. On the contrary they are persuaded it prevents these very Diseases, and, that if it is ever hurtful, it is only when it is either adulterated, as most great Remedies have been, or has been wrongly prescribed, or improperly taken or last when it meets with some latent, some unknown Particularities in a Constitution, which Physicians term an *Idiosyncrasy*, and which prevent or pervert its very general Effects Tissot.

§ 260. If the Fever extends beyond the sixth, or the seventh Fit; and the Patient seems to have no Occasion for a Purge; which may be learned by attending to the Chapter, which treats of Remedies to be taken by Way of Precaution; * he may take the Bark, that is the Powder N°. 14. If it is a Quotidian, a daily Fever, or a double Tertian, six Doses, containing three Quarters of an Ounce, should be taken between the two Fits; and as these Intermissions commonly consist of but ten or twelve, or at the most of fourteen or fifteen Hours, there should be an Interval of only one Hour and a half between each Dose. During this Interval the Sick may take two of his usual Refreshments or Suppings.

When the Fever is a Tertian, an Ounce should be given between the two Fits: which makes eight Doses, one of which is to be taken every three Hours.

In a Quartan I direct one Ounce and a half, to be taken in the same Manner. It is meer trifling to attempt preventing the Returns with smaller Doses. The frequent Failures of the

Bark

---

* It happens very seldom that intermitting Fevers require † no Purge towards their Cure, especially in Places, which are disposed to generate Putridity. There is always some material Cause essential to these Fevers, of which Nature disembarrasses herself more easily by Stools, than by any other Discharge. And as there is not the least Danger to be apprehended from a gentle Purge, such as those of N° 11 or 23, we think it would be prudent always to premise a Dose or two of either to the Bark. *E. L.*

† Yet I have known many in whom no Purge was necessary, and he is in some rendered more obstinate and chronical by erroneous Purging. But a Vomit is very generally necessary before the Bark is given. *K.*

Bark are owing to over small Doses. On such Occasions the Medicine is cried down, and censured as useless, when the Disappointment is solely the Fault of those who do not employ it properly. The last Dose is to be given two Hours before the usual Return of the Fit.

The Doses, just mentioned, frequently prevent the Return of the Fit, but whether it returns or not, after the Time of its usual Duration is past, repeat the same Quantity, in the same Number of Doses, and Intervals, which certainly keeps off another. For six Days following, half the same Quantity must be continued, in the Intervals that would have occurred between the Fits, if they had returned: and during all this Time the Patient should inure himself to as much Exercise, as he can well bear.

§ 261 Should the Fits be very strong, the Pain of the Head violent, the Visage red, the Pulse full and hard, if there is any Cough, if, even after the Fit is over, the Pulse still is perceivably hard; if the Urine is inflamed, hot and high-coloured, and the Tongue very dry, the Patient must be bled, and drink plentifully of Barley Water Nº 3. These two Remedies generally bring the Patient into the State described § 259. in which State he may take on a Day, when the Fever is entirely off, three or four Doses of the Powder Nº 24, and then leave the Fever to pursue its own Course for the Space of a few Fits. But should it not then terminate of itself, the Bark must be recurred to.

If

If the Patient, even in the Interval of the Returns, has a fœtid, furred Mouth, a Loathing, Pains in the Loins, or in the Knees, much Anxiety, and bad Nights, he should be purged with the Powder N°. 21 or the Potion N°. 23, before he takes the Bark.

§ 262. If Fevers in Autumn appear to be of the continual kind, and very like putrid Fevers, the Patients should drink abundantly of Barley Water, and if at the Expiration of two or three Days, there still appears to be a Load or Oppression at the Stomach, the Powder N°. 34 or that of 35 is to be given (but see § 241) and if, after the Operation of this, the Signs of Putridity continue, the Body is to be opened with repeated Doses of the Powder N°. 24, or, where the Patients are very robust, with N°. 21, and when the Fever becomes quite regular, with distinct *Remissions* at least, the Bark is to be given as directed § 260.

But as autumnal Fevers are more obstinate; after having discontinued the Bark for eight Days, and notwithstanding there has been no Return of the Fever, it is proper to resume the Bark, and to give three Doses of it daily for the succeeding eight Days, more especially if it was a Quartan, in which Species I have ordered it to be repeated, every other eight Days, for six Times.

Many People may find it difficult to comply with this Method of Cure, which is unavoidably expensive, through the Price of the Bark; I thought however this ought not to prevent us

from

from averring it to be the only certain one; since nothing can be an equivalent *Succedaneum* or Substitute to this Remedy, which is the only sure and safe one in all these Cases. The World had long been prepossessed with Prejudices to the contrary: it was supposed to be hurtful to the Stomach; to prevent which it has been usual to make the Sick eat something an Hour after it. Nevertheless, very far from injuring the Stomach, it is the best Medicine in the Universe to strengthen it, and it is a pernicious Custom, when a Patient is obliged to take it often, to eat an Hour after it. It had also been imagined to cause Obstructions, and that it subjected Patients to a Dropsy: but at present we are convinced, it is the obstinate and inveterate Duration of the Intermittent, that causes Obstructions, and paves the Way to a Dropsy. The Bark, in Consequence of its speedily curing the Fever, does not only prevent the former Disease, but when it continues, through an injudicious Omission of the Bark, a proper Use of it is serviceable in the Dropsy. In a Word, if there is any other Malady combined with the Fever, sometimes that indeed prevents the Success of the Bark, yet without rendering it hurtful. But whenever the intermitting Fever is simple and uncombined, it ever has, and ever will render the Patient all possible Service. In another Place I shall mention such Means and Methods as may in some Degree, though but imperfectly, be substituted instead of it

After

After the Patient has begun with the Bark, he muſt take no purging Medicine, as that Evacuation would, with the greateſt Probability, occaſion a Return of the Fever.

§ 263. Bleeding is never, or extremely ſeldom indeed neceſſary in a Quartan Ague, which occurs in the Fall oftner than in the Spring; and with the Symptoms of Putridity rather than of Inflammation.

§ 264. The Patient ought, two Hours before the Invaſion of the Fit, to drink a ſmall Glaſs of warm Elder Flower Tea, ſweetened with Honey, every Quarter of an Hour, and to walk about moderately, this diſpoſes him to a very gentle Sweat, and thence renders the enſuing Coldneſs and the whole Fit milder. He is to continue the ſame Drink throughout the Duration of the cold Fit; and when the hot one approaches, he may either continue the ſame, or ſubſtitute that of N°. 2, which is more cooling. It is not neceſſary however, in this State, to drink it warm, it is ſufficient that it be not over cold. When the Sweat, at the Termination of the hot Fit, is concluded, the Patient ſhould be well wiped and dried, and may get up. If the Fit was very long, he may be allowed a little Gruel, or ſome other ſuch Nouriſhment during the Sweat.

§ 265. Sometimes the firſt, and a few ſucceſſive Doſes of the Bark purge the Patient. This is no otherwiſe an ill Conſequence, than by its retarding the Cure; ſince, when it purges, it does not commonly prevent the Return of the Fever,

Fever; so that these Doses may be considered as to no Purpose, and others should be repeated, which, ceasing to purge, do prevent it. Should the Looseness notwithstanding continue, the Bark must be discontinued for one entire Day, in order to give the Patient half a Quarter of an Ounce of Rhubarb: after which the Bark is to be resumed again, and if the Looseness still perseveres, fifteen Grains of Venice Treacle should be added to each Dose, but not otherwise. All other Medicines which are superadded, very generally serve only to increase the Bulk of the Dose, while they lessen its Virtue.

§ 266. Before our thorough Experience of the Bark, other bitter Medicines were used for the same Purpose: these indeed were not destitute of Virtue in such Cases, though they were considerably less available than the Bark. Under N°. 43, some valuable Prescriptions of that kind may be seen, whose Efficacy I have often experienced: though at other Times I have been obliged to leave them off, and recur to the Bark more successfully. Filings of Iron, which enters into the third Prescription, are an excellent Febrifuge in particular Cases and Circumstances. In the Middle of the Winter 1753, I cured a Patient of a Quartan Ague with it, who would not be prevailed on to take the Bark. It must be confessed he was perfectly regular in observing the *Regimen* directed for him; and that, during the most rigid Severity of the Winter, he got every Day on Horseback, and took such a Degree

gree of other Exercise in the open Air, as disposed him to perspire abundantly.

§ 267. Another very practicable easy Method, of which I have often availed my Patients, under tertian Fevers (but which succeeded with me only twice in Quartans) was to procure the Sufferer a very plentiful Sweat, at the very Time when the Fit was to return, in its usual Course. To effect this he is to drink, three or four Hours before it is expected, an Infusion of Elder Flowers sweetened with Honey, which I have already recommended § 264; and one Hour before the usual Invasion of the Shivering, he is to go into Bed, and take, as hot as he can drink it, the Pre-Precription N°. 44.

I have also cured some Tertians and even Quartans, in 1751 and 1752, by giving them, every four Hours between the Fits, the Powder N°. 45. But I must acknowledge that, besides its having often failed me, and its never succeeding so speedily as the Bark, I have found it weaken some Patients; it disorders, or disagrees with, their Stomach: and in two Cases, where it had removed the Fever, I was obliged to call in the Bark for a thorough Establishment of the Patient's Health. Nevertheless as these Medicines are very cheap and attainable, and often do succeed, I thought I could not properly omit them.

§ 268. A Multitude of other Remedies are cried up for the Cure of Fevers: though none of them are equally efficacious with those I have directed: and as many of them are even dangerous,

gerous, it is prudent to abstain from them. Some Years since certain Powders were sold here, under the Name of the *Berlin* Powders; these are nothing but the Bark masqued or disguised (which has sometimes been publickly discovered) and have always been sold very dear: though the Bark well chosen, and freshly powdered when wanted, is greatly preferable.

§ 269 I have often known Peasants, who had laboured for several Months under intermitting Fevers; having made Use of many bad Medicines and Mixtures for it, and observed no Manner of Regimen. Such I have happily treated by giving them the Remedies N°. 34, or 35; and afterwards, for some Days, that of N°. 38; at the End of which Time, I have ordered them the Bark (See § 260) or other Febrifuges, as at § 266, 267, and then finally ordered them for some Days, to take Morsels of the poor Man's Treacle (See § 247, *Art.* 13) to strengthen and confirm their Digestions, which I have found very weak and irregular.

§ 270. Some Intermittents are distinguished as pernicious or malignant, from every Fit's being attended with the most violent Symptoms. The Pulse is small and irregular, the Patient exceedingly dejected, and frequently swooning, afflicted with inexpressible Anguish, Convulsions, a deep Drowsiness, and continual Efforts to go to Stool, or make Urine, but ineffectually. This Disease is highly pressing and dangerous, the Patient may die in the third Fit, and rarely survives the

the sixth, if he is not very judiciously treated. Not a Moment should be lost, and there is no other Step to be taken, but that of giving the Bark continually, as directed § 260, to prevent the succeeding Fits. These worst Kinds of Intermittents are often combined with a great Load of putrid Humours in the first Passages: and as often as such an aggravating Combination is very evident, we should immediately after the End of one Fit, give a Dose of Ipecacuana N°. 35, and, when its Operation is finished, give the Bark. But I chuse to enter into very few Details on this Species of Intermittents, both as they occur but seldom, and as the Treatment of them is too difficult and important, to be submitted to the Conduct of any one but a Physician. My Intention has only been to represent them sufficiently, that they may be so distinguished when they do occur, as to apprize the People of their great Danger.

§ 271 The same Cause which produces these intermitting Fevers, frequently also occasions Disorders, which return periodically at the same Hour, without Shivering, without Heat, and often without any Quickness of the Pulse. Such Disorders generally preserve the Intermissions of quotidian or tertian Fevers, but much seldomer those of Quartans. I have seen violent Vomittings, and Reachings to vomit, with inexpressible Anxiety; the severest Oppressions, the most racking Cholics, dreadful Palpitations and excessive Tooth-achs. Pains in the Head, and very often an unaccountable Pain over one Eye, the Eyelid, Eyebrow,

Eyebrow and Temple, on the same Side of the Face; with a Redness of that Eye, and a continual, involuntary trickling of Tears. I have also seen such a prodigious Swelling of the affected Part, that the Eye projected, or stood out, above an Inch from the Head, covered by the Eyelid, which was also extremely inflated or puffed up. All these Maladies begin precisely at a certain Hour, last about the usual Time of a Fit; and terminating without any sensible Evacuation, return exactly at the same Hour, the next Day, or the next but one.

There is but one known Medicine that can effectually oppose this Sort, which is the Bark, given as directed § 260. Nothing affords Relief in the Fit, and no other Medicine ever suspends or puts it off. But I have cured some of these Disorders with the Bark, and especially those affecting the Eyes, which happen oftner than the other Symptoms, after their Duration for many Weeks, and after the ineffectual Use of Bleeding, Purging, Baths, Waters, Blisters, and a great Number of other Medicines. If a sufficient Dose of it be given, the next Fit is very mild, the second is prevented, and I never saw a Relapse in these Cases, which sometimes happens after the Fits of common Intermittents seemed cured.

§ 272. In Situations where the Constitution of the Air renders these Fevers very common, the Inhabitants should frequently burn in their Rooms, at least in their lodging Rooms, some aromatic Wood or Herbs. They should daily chew some Juniper

Juniper Berries, and drink a fermented Infusion of them. These two Remedies are very effectual to fortify the weakest Stomachs, to prevent Obstructions, and to promote Perspiration. And as these are the Causes which prolong these Fevers the most obstinately, nothing is a more certain Preservation from them than these cheap and obvious Assistances. *

CHAPTER

---

* I have seen several Cases in very marshy maritime Countries, with little good drinking Water, and far South of *Switzerland*, where intermitting Fevers, with Agues at different Intervals, are annually endemic, very popular, and often so obstinate as to return repeatedly, whenever the weekly precautionary Doses of the Bark have been omitted (through the Patient's nauseating the frequent Swallowing of it) so that the Disease has sometimes been extended beyond the Term of a full Year, and even far into a second, including the temporary Removals of it by the Bark. Nevertheless, in some such obstinate Intermittents, and particularly Quartans there, wherein the Bark alone has had but a short and imperfect Effect, I have known the following Composition, after a good Vomit, attended with speedy and final Success, viz. Take of fresh Sassafras Bark, of Virginia Snake-root, of Roch Allom, of Nutmeg, of diaphoretic Antimony, and of Salt of Wormwood of each one Drachm. To these well rubbed together into fine Powder, add the Weight of the whole, of the best and freshest Bark; then drop in three Drops of the chemical Oil of Mint, and with Syrup of Cloves make it into the Consistence of an Electuary or Bolus, for 12 Doses for a grown Person, to be taken at the Distance of three or four Hours from each other, while the Patient is awake, according to the longer or shorter Intermission of the Fever.

I have also known, particularly in obstinate autumnal Agues here, an Infusion of two Ounces of the best Bark in fine Powder, or two Ounces and a half in gross Powder, in a Quart of the best Brandy, for three or four Days (a small Wine Glass to be taken by grown Persons at the Distance of from four to six Hours) effectually and speedily terminate such inveterate Agues, as had given but little Way to the Bark in Substance. This was certainly most suitable for those who were not of a light delicate Habit and Temperament, and who had not been remarkable for their Abstinence

Chapter XIX.

Of the Erisipelas, and the Bites of Animals.

Sect. 273.

THE Erisipelas, commonly called in English, St. Anthony's Fire, and in Swisserland *the Violet*, is sometimes but a very slight Indisposition which appears on the Skin, without the Person's being sensible of any other Disorder; and it most commonly breaks out either in the Face, or on the Legs. The Skin becomes tense, or stiff, rough and red; but this Redness disappears on pressing the Spot with a Finger, and returns on removing it. The Patient feels in the Part affected a burning Heat, which makes him uneasy, and sometimes hinders him from sleeping. The Disorder increases for the Space of two or three Days; continues at its Height one or two, and then abates. Soon after this, that Part of the Skin that was affected, falls off in pretty large Scales, and the Disorder entirely terminates.

§ 274.

stinence from strong Liquors the inebriating Force of the Brandy being remarkably lessened by the Addition and long Infusion of the Bark. These Facts which I saw, are the less to be wondered at, as in such inveterate but perfectly clear and distinct Intermittents, both the State of the Fluids and Solids seem very opposite to their State in an acutely inflammatory Disease. *K*

§ 274 But sometimes this Malady is considerably more severe, beginning with a violent Shivering, which is succeeded by a burning Heat, a vehement Head-ach, a Sickness at Heart, as it is commonly termed, or Reachings to vomit, which continue till the *Erisipelas* appears, which sometimes does not happen before the second, or even the third Day. The Fever then abates, and the Sickness goes off, though frequently a less Degree of Fever, and of Sickness or Loathing remain, during the whole Time, in which the Disease is in its increasing State. When the Eruption and Inflammation happen in the Face, the Head-ach continues, until the Decline, or going off, of the Disease. The Eyelid swells, the Eye is closed, and the Patient has not the least Ease or Tranquillity. It often passes from one Cheek to the other, and extends successively over the Forehead, the Neck, and the Nape of the Neck, under which Circumstance the Disease is of a more than ordinary Duration. Sometimes also when it exists in a very high Degree, the Fever continues, the Brain is obstructed and oppressed, the Patient raves; his Case becomes extremely dangerous, whence sometimes, if he is not very judiciously assisted, he dies, especially if of an advanced Age. A violent *Erisipelas* on the Neck brings on a Quinsey, which may prove very grievous, or even fatal

When it attacks the Leg, the whole Leg swells up, and the Heat and Irritation from it is extended up to the Thigh.

Whenever this Tumour is confiderable, the Part it feizes is covered with fmall Puftules filled with a clear watery Humour, refembling thofe which appear after a Burn, and drying afterwards and fcaling off. I have fometimes obferved, efpecially when this Diftemper affected the Face, that the Humour, which iffued from thefe little Puftules, was extremely thick or glewy, and formed a thick Scurf, or Scabs nearly refembling thofe of fucking Children: they have continued faft on the Face many Days before they fell off.

When the Difeafe may be termed violent, it fometimes continues eight, ten, twelve Days at the fame Height, and is at laft terminated by a very plentiful Sweat, that may fometimes be predicted by a Reftleffnefs attended with Shiverings, and a little Anxiety of fome Hours Duration. Throughout the Progrefs of the Difeafe, the whole Skin is very dry, and even the Infide of the Mouth.

§ 275. An *Erifipelas* rarely comes to Suppuration, and when it does, the Suppuration is always unkindly, and much difpofed to degenerate into an Ulcer. Sometimes a malignant kind of *Erifipelas* is epidemical, feizing a great Number of Perfons, and frequently terminating in Gangrenes.

§ 276 This Diftemper often fhifts its Situation, it fometimes retires fuddenly; but the Patient is uneafy and difordered, he has a Propenfity to vomit, with a fenfible Anxiety and Heat: the *Erifipelas* appears again in a different Part, and

and he feels himself quite relieved from the preceding Symptoms. But if instead of re-appearing on some other Part of the Surface, the Humour is thrown upon the Brain, or the Breast, he dies within a few Hours; and these fatal Changes and Translations sometimes occur, without the least Reason or Colour for ascribing them either to any Error of the Patient, or of his Physician.

If the Humour has been transferred to the Brain, the Patient immediately becomes delirious, with a highly flushed Visage, and very quick sparkling Eyes: very soon after he proves downright frantic, and goes off in a Lethargy.

If the Lungs are attacked, the Oppression, Anxiety, and Heat are inexpressible.

§ 277 There are some Constitutions subject to a very frequent, and, as it were, to an habitual *Erysipelas*. If it often affects the Face, it is generally repeated on the same Side of it, and that Eye is, at length, considerably weakened by it.

§ 278. This Distemper results from two Causes; the one, an acrid sharp Humour, which is commonly bilious, diffused through the Mass of Blood, the other consists in that Humour's not being sufficiently discharged by Perspiration.

§ 279 When this Disease is of a gentle Nature, such as it is described § 273, it will be sufficient to keep up a very free Perspiration, but without heating the Patient, and the best Method to answer this Purpose is putting him upon the Regimen so often already referred to, with a plentiful Use of Nitre in Elder Tea. Flesh, Eggs and Wine are prohibited of Course, allowing the Patient a little Pulse and ripe Fruits. He should drink Elder Flower Tea abundantly, and take half a Drachm of Nitre every three Hours; or, which amounts to the same Thing, let three Drachms of Nitre be dissolved in as much Infusion of Elder Flowers, as he can drink in twenty-four Hours. Nitre may be given too in a Bolus with Conserve of Elder-berries. These Medicines keep the Body open, and increase Urine and Perspiration.

§ 280. When the Distemper prevails in a severer Degree, if the Fever is very high, and the Pulse, at the same Time, strong or hard, it may be necessary to bleed once: but this should never be permitted in a large Quantity at a Time in this Disease, it being more adviseable, if a sufficient Quantity has not been taken at once, to bleed a second Time, and even a third, if the Fever should prove very high, as it often does, and that sometimes in so violent a Degree, as to render it extremely dangerous: and in some such Cases Nature has sometimes saved the Patients by effecting a large Hæmorrhage, or Bleeding, to the Quantity of four or five Pounds. This Conduct a very intelligent and prudent Physician may presume to imitate, but I dare not advise the same Conduct to that Class of Physicians, for which only I write, it being safer for them to use repeated Bleedings in such Cases, than one in an excessive Quantity. These erisipelatous Fevers are

are often excited by a Person's being too long over-heated.

After Bleeding the Patient is to be restrained to his Regimen; Glysters are to be given until there is a sensible Abatement of the Fever; and he should drink the Barley Water freely, N°. 3.

When the Fever is somewhat diminished, either the Purge N°. 23 should be given, or a few Doses every Morning of Cream of Tartar N° 24. Purging is absolutely necessary to carry off the stagnant Bile, which is generally the first Cause of the violent Degrees of this Distemper. It may sometimes be really necessary too, if the Disease is very tedious, if the Loathing and Sickness at Stomach is obstinate; the Mouth ill-favoured, and the Tongue foul, (provided there be only a slight Fever, and no Fear of an Inflammation) to give the Medicines N°. 34 or 35, which, in Consequence of the Agitation, the Shaking they occasion, remove these Impediments still better than Purges.

It commonly happens that this Disease is more favourable after these Evacuations; nevertheless it is sometimes necessary to repeat them the next Day, or the next but one, especially if the Malady affects the Head. Purging is the true Evacuation for curing it, whenever it attacks this Part. By carrying off the Cause of the Disease, they diminish it, and prevent its worst Events.

Whenever, even after these Evacuations, the Fever still continues to be very severe, the Patient should take every two Hours, or occasionally,

ally, oftner, two Spoonfuls of the Prescription N° 10, added to a Glass of Ptisan.

It will be very useful, when this Disease is seated in the Head or Face, to bathe the Legs frequently in warm Water; and where it is violent there, also to apply Sinapisms to the Soles of the Feet. I have seen this Application, in about four Hours attract, or draw down an *Erysipelas* to the Legs, which had spread over the Nose, and both the Eyes. When the Distemper once begins to go off by Sweating, this should be promoted by Elder-flower Tea and Nitre (See § 279) and the Sweating may be encouraged to Advantage for some Hours.

§ 281. The best Applications that can be made to the affected Part are 1st, The Herb Robert, a Kind of *Geranium*, or Crane's-Bill; or Chervil, or Parsley, or Elder Flowers; and if the Complaint be of a very mild Disposition, it may be sufficient to apply a very soft smooth Linen over it, which some People dust over with a little dry Meal.

2, If there is a very considerable Inflammation, and the Patient is so circumstanced as to be very tractable and regularly attended, Flanels wrung out of a strong Decoction of Elder-flowers and applied warm, afford him the speediest Ease and Relief. By this simple Application I have appeased the most violent Pains of a St. Anthony's Fire, which is the most cruel Species of an Erysipelas, and has some peculiar Marks or Symptoms extraordinary.

3, The

3, The Plaister of Smalt, and Smalt itself N° 46, are also very successfully employed in this Disease. This Powder, the farinaceous, or mealy ones, or others cried up for it, agree best when a thin watery Humour distills or weeps from the little Vesications attending it, which it is convenient to absorb by such Applications, without which Precaution it might gall, or even ulcerate the Part.

All other Plaisters, which are partly compounded of greasy, or of resinous Substances, are very dangerous: they often repel, or strike in the *Erisipelas*, occasioning it to ulcerate, or even to gangrene. If People who are naturally subject to this Disease should apply any such Plaister to their Skin, even in its soundest State, an *Erisipelas* is the speedy Consequence.

§ 282. Whenever the Humour occasioning the Distemper is repelled, and thrown upon the Brain, the Throat, the Lungs, or any internal Part, the Patient should be bled, Blisters must be applied to the Legs; and Elder Tea, with Nitre dissolved in it, should be plentifully drank.

§ 283. People who are liable to frequent Returns of an Erisipelas, should very carefully avoid using Milk, Cream, and all fat and viscid, or clammy Food, Pies, brown Meat, Spices, thick and heady Liquors, a sedentary Life, the more active Passions, especially Rage, and, if possible, all Chagrin too. Their Food should chiefly consist of Herbage, Fruits, of Substances inclining to Acidity, and which tend to keep the Body open; they should drink Water, and some of the light white Wines; by no Means omitting the frequent Use of Cream of Tartar. A careful Conformity to these Regulations is of real Importance, as, besides the Danger of the frequent Visitations of this Disease, they denote some slight Indispositions of the Liver and the Gallbladder; which, if too little attended to, might in Time prove very troublesome and pernicious.

Such mineral Waters as are gently opening are very proper for these Constitutions, as well as the Juice of Succory, and clarified Whey, of which they should take about three Pints every Morning, during the five or six Summer Months. This becomes still more efficacious, if a little Cream of Tartar and Honey be added to it.

Of the Stings, or little Wounds, by Animals.

§ 284 The Stings or little Bites of Animals, frequently producing a kind of *Erisipelas*, I shall add a very few Words concerning them in this Place

Of the Serpents in this Country none but the Vipers are poisonous, and none of these are found except at *Baume*, where there is a *Viperary*, if we may be allowed that Word. We have no Scorpions, which are somewhat poisonous; our Toads are not in the least so; whence the only Stings we are exposed to are those of Bees, Wasps, Hornets, Musketoes or Gnats, and Dragon * Flies:

all

---

* to Hawks.

all of which are sometimes attended with severe Pain, a Swelling, and a very considerable erisipelatous Redness, which, if it happens in the Face, sometimes entirely closes the Eyes up; occasioning also a Fever, Pains of the Head, Restlessness, and Sickness at Heart, and, when the Pains are in a violent Degree, Faintings and Convulsions, though always without any mortal Consequence. These Symptoms go off naturally within a few Days, without any Assistance: Nevertheless they may either be prevented, diminished in Degree, or shortned in Duration.

1, By extracting the Sting of the Animal, if it is left behind.

2, By a continual Application of one of the Remedies directed § 281, Article 1 and 2, particularly the Infusion of Elder-flowers, to which a little Venice Treacle is added; or by covering the Part affected with a Pultice, made of Crum of Bread, Milk, Honey, and a little Venice Treacle.*

3, By bathing the Legs of the Person stung repeatedly in warm Water

4, By retrenching a little of their customary Food, especially at Night, and by making them drink an Infusion of Elder-flowers, with the Addition of a little Nitre. Oil, if applied very quickly after the Sting, sometimes prevents the Appearance of any Swelling, and from thence the Pains that attend it.

CHAPTER

---

* Pounded Parsley is one of the most availing Applications in such Accidents *E. L.*

Chapter XX.

Of spurious, or false Inflammations of the Breast, and of spurious, bilious, Pleurisies.

Sect. 285.

THE Inflammation of the Breast and that Pleurisy, which is called *bilious*, are the same Disease. It is properly a putrid Fever, attended with an Infarction or Stuffing of the Lungs, though without Pain, in which Circumstance it is called a putrid or bilious Peripneumony: but when attended with a Pain of the Side, a Stitch, it is called a spurious or bastard Pleurisy.

§ 286. The Signs which distinguish these Diseases from the inflammatory ones of the same Name, described Chap. IV and V, are a less hard and less strong, but a quicker Pulse, though unaccompanied with the same Symptoms which constitute the inflammatory ones (See § 47 and 9c) The Mouth is foul, and has a Sensation of Bitterness, the Patient is infested with a sharp and dry Heat, he has a Feeling of Heaviness and Anxiety all about his Stomach, with Loathings: he is less flushed and red in these, than in the inflammatory Diseases, but rather a little yellow. He has a dejected wan Look, his Urine resembles

sembles that in putrid Fevers, and not that of inflammatory ones; and he has very often a small bilious Looseness, which is extremely offensive. The Skin is commonly very dry in this Disease; the Humour spit up is less thick, less reddish, and rather more yellow than in the inflammatory Diseases of the same Names.

§ 287. They must be treated after the manner of putrid Fevers, as in § 241. Supposing some little Degree of Inflammation to be combined with the Disease, it may be removed by a single Bleeding. After this the Patient is to drink Barley Water N°. 3, to make Use of Glysters; and as soon as all Symptoms of any Inflammation wholly disappear, he is to take the vomiting and purging Draught N°. 34. But the utmost Caution must be taken not to give it, before every Appearance of any Inflammation is totally removed, as giving it sooner would be certain Death to the Sick: and it is dreadful but to think of agitating, by a Vomit, Lungs that are inflamed, and overloaded with Blood, whose Vessels burst and discharge themselves, only from the Force of Expectoration. After an Interval of some Days, he may be purged again with the Medicine N°. 23. The Prescription N°. 25 succeeds also very well as a Vomit. If the Fever is violent, he must drink plentifully of the Potion N°. 10.

Blisters to the Legs are very serviceable, when the Load and Oppression are not considerably abated after general Evacuations.

§ 288.

§ 288. The false Inflammation of the Breast is an Overfulness or Obstruction in the Lungs, accompanied with a Fever, and it is caused by extremely thick and tenacious Humours; and not by a really inflammatory Blood, or by any putrid or bilious Humour

§ 289. This Distemper happens more frequently in the Spring, than in any other Season. Old Men, puny, ill-constitutioned Children, languid Women, feeble young Men, and particularly such as have worn their Constitutions out by drinking, are the Subjects most frequently attacked by it, especially if they have used but little Exercise throughout the Winter; if they have fed on viscid, mealy and fat Aliments, as Pastry, Chesnuts, thick Milk or Pap, and Cheese. All their Humours have contracted a thick glutinous Quality, they are circulated with Difficulty, and when Heat or Exercise in the Spring increases their Motion at once, the Humours, already stuffing up the Lungs, still more augment that Plenitude, whence these vital Organs are fatally extended, and the Patient dies

§ 290. This Distemper is known to exist,

1, By the previous Existence of the Causes already mentioned

2, By the Symptoms which precede and usher it in. For Example, the Patient many Days before-hand has a slight Cough, a small Oppression when he moves about, a little Restlessness, and is sometimes a little choleric or fretful. His Countenance is higher coloured than in Health, he he has a Propensity to sleep, but attended with Confusion and without Refreshment, and has sometimes an extraordinary Appetite.

3, When this State has continued for some Days, there comes on a cold Shivering, though more considerable for its Duration than its Violence, it is succeeded by a moderate Degree of Heat, but that attended with much Inquietude and Oppression. The sick Person cannot confine himself to the Bed, but walks to and fro in his Chamber, and is greatly dejected. The Pulse is weak and pretty quick, the Urine is sometimes but little changed from that in Health, at other Times it is discharged but in a small Quantity, and is higher coloured: he coughs but moderately, and does not expectorate, or cough up, but with Difficulty. The Visage becomes very red, and even almost livid, he can neither keep awake, nor sleep well, he raves for some Moments, and then his Head grows clear again. Sometimes it happens, especially to Persons of advanced Age, that this State suddenly terminates in a mortal Swoon or Fainting. at other Times and in other Cases, the Oppression and Anguish increase, the Patient cannot breathe but when sitting up, and that with great Difficulty and Agony. the Brain is utterly disturbed and embarrassed; this State lasts for some Hours, and then terminates of a sudden.

§ 291. This is a very dangerous Distemper; because, in the first Place, it chiefly attacks those Persons whose Temperament and Constitution are deprived of the ordinary Resources for Health and Recovery: in the second Place, because it is of a precipitate Nature, the Patient sometimes dying on the third Day, and but seldom surviving the seventh; while the Cause of it requires a more considerable Term for its Removal or Mitigation. Besides which, if some Indications present for the Employment of a Remedy, there are frequently others which forbid it, and all that seems to be done is, as follows,

1, If the Patient has still a pretty good Share of Health; if he is not of too advanced an Age; if the Pulse has a perceivable Hardness, and yet at the same Time some Strength; if the Weather is dry, and the Wind blows from the North, he should be bled once, to a moderate Quantity. But if the greater Part of these Circumstances are wanting, Bleeding would be very prejudicial. Were we obliged to establish some general and positive Rule in this Case, it were better to exclude Bleeding, than to admit it.

2, The Stomach and the Bowels should be unloaded from their viscid glutinous Contents; and the Medicines which succeed the best in this Respect are N°. 35, when the Symptoms shew there is a great Necessity for vomiting, and there is no Inflammation; or the Prescription N°. 25, which after vomiting, purges by Stool, promotes Urine, breaks down and divides the viscid Humours that occasion the Disease, and increase Perspiration. When we are afraid of hazarding the Agitation of a Vomit and its Consequences, the

the Potion, N°. 11 may be given; but we must be very cautious, in Regard to old Men, even with this, as such may expire during the Operation of it.

3, They should, from the Beginning of the Disease, drink plentifully of the Ptisan N°. 26, which is the best Drink in this Disease, or that of N°. 12, adding half a Dram of Nitre to every Pint of it.

4, A Cup of the Mixture N°. 8 must be taken every two Hours.

5. Blisters are to be applied to the Insides of the Legs.

When the Case is very doubtful and perplexing, it were best to confine ourselves to the three last-mentioned Remedies, which have often been successful in severe Degrees of this Disease; and which can occasion no ill Consequence.

§ 292. When this Malady invades old People, though they partly recover, they never recover perfectly, entirely, from it: and if due Precaution is not taken, they are very liable to fall into a Dropsy of the Breast after it.

§ 293. The spurious or false Pleurisy is a Distemper that does not affect the Lungs, but only the Teguments, the Skin, and the Muscles which cover the Ribs. It is the Effect of a rheumatic Humour thrown upon these Parts, in which, as it produces very sharp Pains resembling that which is called a *Stitch*, it has from this Circumstance, been termed a Pleurisy.

It is generally supposed by the meer Multitude, and even by some of a different Rank, that a false Pleurisy is more dangerous than a genuine, a true one, but this is a Mistake. It is often ushered in by a Shivering, and almost ever attended with a little Fever, a small Cough, and a slight Difficulty of breathing; which, as well as the Cough, is occasioned from the Circumstance of a Patient's (who feels Pain in Respiration, or Breathing) checking Breathing as much as he can; this accumulates a little too much Blood in the Lungs; but yet he has no Anguish, nor the other Symptoms of acute true Pleurisies. In some Patients this Pain is extended, almost over the whole Breast, and to the Nape of the Neck. The sick Person cannot repose himself on the Side affected.

This Disorder is not more dangerous than a Rheumatism, except in two Cases; 1, When the Pain is so very severe, that the Patient strongly endeavours not to breathe at all, which brings on a great Infarction or Stoppage in the Lungs. 2, When this Humour, like any other rheumatic one, is transferred to some internal Part.

§ 294 It must be treated exactly like a Rheumatism See § 168 and 169

After bleeding once or more, a Blister applied to the affected Part is often attended with a very good Effect. This being indeed the Kind of * Pleurisy, in which it particularly agrees.

§ 295.

* The Seneka Rattle Snake root, already recommended in true Pleurisies, will, with the greatest Probability, be found not less effectual

§ 295. This Malady sometimes gives Way to the first Bleeding; often terminating on the third, fourth or fifth Day, by a very plentiful Sweat, and rarely lasting beyond the seventh. Sometimes it attacks a Person very suddenly, after a Stoppage of Perspiration; and then, if at once before the Fever commences, and has had Time to inflame the Blood, the Patient takes some *Faltrank*, it effects a speedy Cure by restoring Perspiration. They are such Cases as these, or that mentioned § 96, which have given this Composition the Reputation it has obtained in this Disease: a Reputation nevertheless, which has every Year proved tragical in its Consequences to many Peasants, who being deceived by some misleading Resemblances in this Distemper, have rashly and ignorantly made Use of it in true inflammatory Pleurisies

---

effectual in these false ones, in which the Inflammation of the Blood is less. The Method of giving it may be seen P. 118, N (ª.) By Dr Tissot's having never mentioned this valuable Simple throughout his Work, it may be presumed, that when he wrote it, this Remedy had not been admitted into the Apothecaries Shops in *Swisserland*. K.

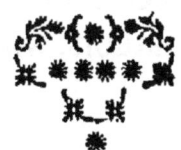

Chapter XXI.

Of the Cholic and its different Kinds.

Sect. 296.

THE Appellation of a Cholic is commonly given to all Pains of the Belly indiscriminately; but I apply it in this Place only to such as attack the Stomach, or the Intestines, the Guts.

Cholics may and do result from very many Causes; and the greater Number of Cholics are chronical or tedious Complaints, being more common among the inactive Inhabitants of Cities, and Workmen in sedentary Trades, than among Country People. Hence I shall treat here only of the small Variety of Cholics, which happen the most usually in Villages. I have already proved that the fatal Events of some Distempers were occasioned by endeavouring to force the Patients into Sweats; and the same unhappy Consequences have attended Cholics, from accustoming the Subjects of this Disease to Drams, and hot inflaming spirituous Liquors, with an Intention to expel the Wind.

Of the inflammatory Cholic.

§ 297. The most violent and dangerous kind of Cholic is that, which arises from an Inflammation of the Stomach, or of the Intestines. It begins most commonly without any Shivering, by a vehement Pain in the Belly, which gradually becomes still more so. The Pulse grows quick and hard; a burning Pain is felt through the whole Region of the Belly; sometimes there is a watery *Diarrhæa*, or Purging; at other Times the Belly is rather costive, which is attended with Vomiting, a very embarrassing and dangerous Symptom: the Countenance becomes highly flushed; the Belly tense and hard; neither can it be touched scarcely without a cruel Augmentation of the Patient's Pain, who is also afflicted with extreme Restlessness, his Thirst is very great, being unquenchable by Drink; the Pain often extends to the Loins, where it proves very sharp, and severe; little Urine is made, and that very red, and with a kind of burning Heat. The tormented Patient has not a Moment's Rest, and now and then raves a little. If the Disease is not removed or moderated, before the Pains rise to their utmost Height and Violence, the Patient begins at length to complain less, the Pulse becomes less strong and less hard than before, but quicker: his Face first abates of its Flush and Redness, and soon after looks pale, the Parts under the Eyes become livid, the Patient sinks into a low stupid Kind of *Delirium*, or Raving; his Strength entirely deserts him; the Face, Hands, Feet, and the whole Body, the Belly only excepted, become cold: the Surface of the Belly appears bluish; extreme Weakness follows, and the Patient dies. There frequently occurs, just a Moment before he expires, an abundant Discharge of excessively fœtid Matter by Stool; and during this Evacuation he dies with his Intestines quite gangrened, or mortified.

When the Distemper assaults the Stomach, the Symptoms are the very same, but the Pain is felt higher up, at the Pit of the Stomach. Almost every thing that is swallowed is cast up again; the Anguish of the tortured Patient is terrible, and the Raving comes on very speedily. This Disease proves mortal in a few Hours.

§ 298. The only Method of succeeding in the Cure of it is as follows:

1, Take a very large Quantity of Blood from the Arm; this almost immediately diminishes the Violence of the Pains, and allays the Vomiting: besides its contributing to the greater Success of the other Remedies. It is often necessary to repeat this Bleeding within the Space of two Hours.

2, Whether the Patient has a Looseness, or has not, a Glyster of a Decoction of Mallows, or of Barley Water and Oil, should be given every two Hours

3, The Patient should drink very plentifully of Almond Milk N°. 4; or a Ptisan of Mallow Flowers,

Flowers, or of Barley, all which should be warm.

4, Flanels dipt in hot, or very warm Water should be continually applied over the Belly, shifting them every Hour, or rather oftner; for in this Case they very quickly grow dry.

5, If the Disease, notwithstanding all this, continues very obstinate and violent, the Patient should be put into a warm Water Bath, the extraordinary Success of which I have observed.

When the Distemper is over, that is to say, when the Pains have terminated, and the Fever has ceased, so that the Patient recovers a little Strength, and gets a little Sleep, it will be proper to give him a Purge, but a very gentle one. Two Ounces of Manna, and a Quarter of an Ounce of Sedlitz * Salt dissolved in a Glass of clear Whey is generally sufficient, at this Period, to purge the most robust and hardy Bodies. Manna alone may suffice for more delicate Constitutions: as all acrid sharp Purges would be highly dangerous, with Regard to the great Sensibility and tender Condition of the Stomach, and of the Intestines after this Disease.

§ 299. It is sometimes the Effect of a general Inflammation of the Blood, and is produced, like other inflammatory Diseases, by extraordinary Labour, very great Heat, heating Meats or Drinks, &c. It is often the Consequence of

---

* Glauber or Epsom Salt may be substituted, where the other is not to be readily procured *K.*

other Cholics which have been injudiciously treated, and which otherwife would not have degenerated into inflammatory ones; as I have many Times feen thefe Cholics introduced after the Ufe of heating Medicines; one Inftance of which may be feen § 164.

§ 300 Ten Days after I had recovered a Woman out of a fevere Cholic, the Pains returned violently in the Night. She, fuppofing them to arife only from Wind, hoped to appeafe them by drinking a deal of diftilled Walnut Water; which, far from producing any fuch Effect, rendered them more outrageous. They foon were heightened to a furpifing Degree, which might reafonably be expected. Being fent for very early in the Morning, I found her Pulfe hard, quick, fhort; her Belly was tenfe and hard; fhe complained greatly of her Loins: her Urine was almoft entirely ftopt. She paft but a few Drops, which felt as it were fcalding hot, and thefe with exceffive Pain. She went very frequently to the Clofe-ftool, with fcarcely any Effect, her Anguifh, Heat, Thirft, and the Drynefs of her Tongue were even terrifying: and her wretched State, the Effect of the ftrong hot Liquor fhe had taken, made me very apprehenfive for her. One Bleeding, to the Quantity of fourteen Ounces, fomewhat abated all the Pains, fhe took feveral Glyfters, and drank off a few Pots of *Orgeat* in a few Hours. By thefe Means the Difeafe was a little mitigated, by continuing the fame Drink and the Glyfters the Loofenefs abated, the Pain of the Loins went off, and she passed a considerable Quantity of Urine, which proved turbid, and then let fall a Sediment, and the Patient recovered. Nevertheless I verily believe, if the Bleeding had been delayed two Hours longer, this spirituous Walnut Water would have been the Death of her. During the Progress of this violent Disease, no Food is to be allowed, and we should never be too inattentive to such Degrees of Pain, as sometimes remain after their Severity is over; lest a *Scirrhus*, an inward hard Tumour, should be generated, which may occasion the most inveterate and tedious Maladies.

§ 301. An Inflammation of the Intestines, and one of the Stomach, may also terminate in an Abscess, like an Inflammation of any other Part, and it may be apprehended, that one is forming, when, though the Violence of the Pains abate, there still remains a slow, obtuse, heavy Pain, with general Inquietude, little Appetite, frequent Shiverings, the Patient at the same Time not recovering any Strength. In such Cases the Patient should be allowed no other Drinks, but what are already directed in this Chapter, and some Soops made of Pulse, or other farinaceous Food.

The Breaking of the Abscess may sometimes be discovered by a slight Swoon or fainting Fit, attended with a perceivable Cessation of a Weight or Heaviness in the Part, where it was lately felt. and when the *Pus*, or ripe Matter, is effused into the Gut, the Patient sometimes has

Reachings to vomit, a *Vertigo*, or Swimming in the Head, and the Matter appears in the next Stools. In this Case there remains an Ulcer within the Gut, which, if either neglected, or improperly treated, may pave the Way to a slow wasting Fever, and even to Death. Yet this I have cured by making the Patient live solely upon skimmed Milk, diluted with one third Part Water, and by giving every other Day a Glyster, consisting of equal Parts of Milk and Water, with the Addition of a little Honey.

When the Abscess breaks on the Outside of the Gut, and discharges its Contents into the Cavity of the Belly, it becomes a very miserable Case, and demands such further Assistance as cannot be particularized here.

Of the bilious Cholic

§ 502. The bilious Cholic discovers itself by very acute Pains, but is seldom accompanied with a Fever, at least not until it has lasted a Day or two. And even if there should be some Degree of a Fever, yet the Pulse, though quick, is neither strong nor hard the Belly is neither tense or stretched as it were, nor burning hot, as in the former Cholic. the Urine comes away with more Ease, and is less high-coloured: Nevertheless the inward Heat and Thirst are considerable; the Mouth is bitter, the Vomiting or Purging, when either of them attend it, discharge a yellowish

lowish Humour or Excrement; and the Patient's Head is often vertiginous or dizzy.

§ 303. The Method of curing this is,

1, By injecting Glysters of Whey and Honey; or, if Whey is not readily procurable, by repeating the Glyster, N°. 5.

2, By making the Sick drink considerably of the same Whey, or of a Ptisan made of the Root of Dog's-Grass (the common Grass) and a little Juice of Lemon, for want of which, a little Vinegar and Honey may be substituted instead of it. *

3, By giving every Hour one Cup of the Medicine N°. 32, or where this is not to be had, half a Drachm of Cream of Tartar at the same short Intervals.

4, Fomentations of warm Water and Half-baths are also very proper.

5, If the Pains are sharp and violent, in a robust strong Person, and the Pulse is strong and tense, Bleeding should be used to prevent an Inflammation.

6, No other Nourishment should be given, except some maigre Soops, made from Vegetables, and particularly of Sorrel.

7, After plentiful Dilution with the proper Drink, if no Fever supervenes; if the Pains still continue, and the Patient discharges but little by Stool, he should take a moderate Purge. That directed N°. 47 is a very proper one.

§ 304.

* Pullet, or rather Chicken Water, but very weak, may often do instead of Ptisan, or serve for a little Variety of Drink to some Patients *E L*—K

§ 304. This bilious Cholic is habitual to many Persons; and may be prevented or greatly mitigated by an habitual Use of the Powder N°. 24; by submitting to a moderate Retrenchment in the Article of Flesh-meat; and by avoiding heating and greasy Food, and the Use of Milk.

Of Cholics from Indigestions, and of Indigestion.

§ 305. Under this Appellation I comprehend all those Cholics, which are either owing to any overloading Quantity of Food taken at once; or to a Mass or Accumulation of Aliments formed by Degrees in such Stomachs, as digest but very imperfectly; or which result from noxious Mixtures of Aliment in the Stomach, such as that of Milk and Acids, or from Food either not wholesome in its self, or degenerated into an unwholesome Condition.

This kind of Cholic may be known from any of these Causes having preceded it; by its Pains, which are accompanied with great Restlessness, and come on by Degrees, being less fixed than in the Cholics before treated of. These Cholics are also without any Fever, Heat or Thirst, but accompanied with a Giddiness of the Head, and Efforts to vomit, and rather with a pale, than a high-coloured Visage.

§ 306 These Disorders, from these last Causes, are scarcely ever dangerous in themselves; but may be made such by injudicious Management, and doing more than is necessary or proper: as the

the only Thing to be done is to promote the Discharges by warm Drinks. There are a considerable Variety of them, which seem equally good, such as warm Water, or even cold Water with a Toast, with the Addition either of a little Sugar, or a little Salt: a light Infusion of Chamomile, or of Elder-flowers, common Tea, or Baum, it imports little which, provided the Patient drink plentifully of them: in Consequence of which the offending Matter is discharged, either by vomiting, or a considerable purging; and the speedier and more in Quantity these Discharges are, the sooner the Patient is relieved.

If the Belly is remarkably full and costive, Glysters of warm Water and Salt should be injected:

The Expulsion of the obstructing Matter is also facilitated, by rubbing the Belly heartily with hot Cloths.

Sometimes the Humours, or other retained Contents of the Belly, are more pernicious from their Quality, than their Quantity, and then the Malady may be dissipated without the former Discharges, by the irritating sharp Humour being diluted, or even drowned, as it were, in the Abundance of small watery Drinks. When the Pains invade first in the Stomach, they become less sharp, and the Patient feels less Inquietude, as soon as the Cause of the Pain has descended out of the Stomach into the Intestines, whose Sensations are something less acute than, or somewhat different from, those of the Stomach.

It

It is often found that after these plentiful Discharges, and when the Pains are over, there remains a very disagreeable Taste in the Mouth, resembling the Savour of rotten Eggs. This may be removed by giving some Doses of the Powder N°. 24, and drinking largely of good Water:

It is an essential Point in these Cases, to take no Food before a perfect Recovery.

§ 307. Some have been absurd enough in them, to fly at once to some heating Cordial Confection, to Venice Treacle, Aniseed Water, Geneva, or red Wine to stop these Evacuations; but there cannot be a more fatal Practice: since these Evacuations are the only Thing which can cure the Complaint, and to stop them is to deprive the Person, who was in Danger of drowning, of the Plank which might save him. Nay should this Endeavour of stopping them unhappily succeed, the Patient is either thrown into a putrid Fever, or some chronical tedious Malady; unless Nature, much wiser than such a miserable Assistant, should prevail over the Obstacles opposed to her Recovery, and restore the obstructed Evacuations by her own Oeconomy, in the Space of a few Days.

§ 308. Sometimes an Indigestion happens, with very little Pain or Cholic, but with violent Reachings to vomit, inexpressible Anguish, Faintings, and cold Sweats: and not seldom also the Malady begins, only with a very sudden and unexpected Fainting; the Patient immediately loses

all

Of the Cholic and its different Kinds.

all his Senses, his Face is pale and wan. he has some Hickups rather than Reachings to vomit, which joined to the Smallness of his Pulse, to the Easiness of his respiring, or breathing, and to the Circumstance of his being attacked immediately, or very soon, after a Meal, makes this Disorder distinguishable from a real Apoplexy. Nevertheless, when it rises to this Height, with these terrible Symptoms, it sometimes kills in a few Hours. The first thing to be done is to throw up a sharp Glyster, in which Salt and Soap are to be dissolved; next to get down as much Salt and Water as he can swallow; and if that is ineffectual, the Powder N°. 34 is to be dissolved in three Cups of Water, one half of which is to be given directly, and, if it does not operate in a Quarter of an Hour, the other half. Generally speaking the Patient's Sense begins to return, as soon as he begins to vomit.

Of the flatulent or windy Cholic.

§ 309. Every Particular which constitutes our Food, whether solid or liquid, contains much Air, but some of them more than others. If they do not digest soon enough, or but badly, which occasions a sensible Escape of such Air, if they are such as contain an extraordinary Quantity of Air, or if the Guts being straitened or compressed any where in the Course of their Extent, prevent that Air from being equally diffused (which must occasion a greater Proportion

tion of it in some Places) then the Stomach and the Guts are distended by this Wind; and this Distention occasions these Pains, which are called flatulent, or windy.

This Sort of Cholic rarely appears alone and simple, but is often complicated with, or added, as it were, to the other Sorts, of which it is a Consequence; and is more especially joined with the Cholic from Indigestions, whose Symptoms it multiplies and heightens. It may be known, like that, by the Causes which have preceded it, by its not being accompanied either with Fever, Heat, or Thirst; the Belly's being large and full, though without Hardness, being unequal in its Largeness, which prevails more in one Part of it than in another, forming something like Pockets of Wind, sometimes in one Part, sometimes in another; and by the Patient's feeling some Ease merely from the rubbing of his Belly, as it moves the Wind about, which escaping either upwards or downwards affords him still a greater Relief.

§ 310. When it is combined with any different Species of the Cholic, it requires no distinct Treatment from that Species, and it is removed or dissipated by the Medicines which cure the principal Disease.

Sometimes however it does happen to exist alone, and then it depends on the Windiness of the solid and liquid Food of the Person affected with it, such as the *Must* or new Wine, Beer, especially very new Beer, certain Fruits and Garden-den-stuff. It may be cured by a Glyster; by chaffing the Belly with hot Cloths, by the Use of Drink moderately spiced, and especially by Camomile Tea, to which a little cordial Confection, or even Venice Treacle, may be added. When the Pains are almost entirely vanished, and there is no Fever, nor any unhealthy Degree of Heat; and if the Patient is sensible of a Weakness at Stomach, he may take a little aromatic, or spiced Wine, or even a small cordial stomachic Dram. It should be observed, that these are not to be allowed in any other Kind of Cholic.

§ 311. When any Person is frequently subject to cholic-like Pains, it is a Proof that the digestive Faculty is impaired; the restoring of which should be carefully attended to; without which the Health of the Patient must suffer considerably, and he must be very likely to contract many tedious and troublesome Disorders.

Of Cholics from Cold.

§ 312. When any Person has been very cold, and especially in his Feet, it is not uncommon for him to be attacked, within a few Hours after it, with violent Cholic Pains, in which heating and spirituous Medicines are very pernicious: but which are easily cured by rubbing the Legs well with hot Cloths; and keeping them afterwards for a considerable Time in warm Water; advising them at the same Time to drink freely of a light Infusion of Chamomile or Elder-flowers.

The

The Cure will be effected the sooner, if the Patient is put to Bed and sweats a little; especially in the Legs and Feet.

A Woman who had put her Legs into a pretty cool Spring, after travelling in the Height of Summer, was very quickly after attacked with a most violent Cholic. She took different hot Medicines; she became still worse; she was purged, but the Distemper was still further aggravated. I was called in on the third Day, a few Hours before her Decease.

In such Cases, if the Pain be excessive, it may be necessary to bleed; * to give a Glyster of warm Water; to keep the Legs several Hours over the Steam of hot Water, and afterwards in the Water, to drink plentifully of an Infusion of the Flowers of the Lime-tree, with a little Milk; and if the Distemper is not subdued by these Means, Blisters should be applied to the Legs, which I have known to be highly efficacious.

§ 313. It appears, through the Course of this Chapter, that it is necessary to be extremely on our Guard, against permitting the Use of heating and spirituous Medicines in Cholics, as they may not only aggravate, but even render them mortal.

In

---

* Bleeding should not be determined on too hastily in this Sort of Cholic, but rather be omitted, or deferred at least, till there be an evident Tendency to an Inflammation E L

The Propriety, or Impropriety of Bleeding in a Cholic from th Cause should be determined, I think, from the State of the Person it happens to. So that Bleeding a strong Person with a firm Fibre, and a hard Pulse, may be very prudent and precautionary. But if it be a weakly lax Subject with a soft and low Pulse, there may be Room either for omitting, or for suspending it K

In short they should never be given, and when it is difficult to discover the real Cause of the Cholic, I advise Country People to confine themselves to the three following Remedies, which cannot be hurtful in any Sort of Cholic, and may remove as many as are not of a violent Nature. First then, let Glysters be frequently repeated. 2, Let the Patient drink warm Water plentifully, or Elder Tea. 3, Let the Belly be often fomented in pretty warm Water, which is the most preferable Fomentation of any.

§ 314. I have said nothing here of the Use of any Oils in this Disease, as they agree but in very few Species of Cholics, and not at all in those of which I have been treating. For this Reason I advise a total Disuse of them, since they may be of bad Consequence in many Respects.

§ 315. Chronical Diseases not coming within the Plan of this Work, I purposely forbear treating of any Kind of those tedious Cholics, which afflict some People for many Years: but I think it my Duty to admonish such, that their Torments being very generally occasioned by Obstructions in the *Viscera*, or different Bowels of the Belly, or by some other Fault, and more particularly in those Organs, which are intended to prepare the Bile, they should, 1, avoid with the greatest Care, the Use of sharp, hot, violent Medicines, Vomits, strong Purges, Elixirs, &c. 2, They should be thoroughly on their Guard against all those, who promise them a very speedy Cure, by the Assistance of some specific Remedy; and ought to look upon them as Mountebanks, into whose Hands it is highly dangerous to trust themselves. 3, They should be persuaded, or rather convinced, that they can entertain no reasonable Hope of being cured, without an exact Conformity to a proper and judicious Regimen, and a long Perseverance in a Course of mild and safe Remedies. 4, They should continually reflect with themselves, that there is little Difficulty in doing them great Mischief; and that their Complaints are of that Sort, which require the greatest Knowledge and Prudence in those Persons, to whom the Treatment and Cure of them are confided.

Chapter XXII.

Of the Iliac Passion, and of the Cholera-morbus.

Sect 316.

THESE violent Diseases are fatal to many Country People, while their Neighbours are frequently so ignorant of the Cause of their Death, that Superstition has ascribed it to Poison, or to Witchcraft

§ 317. The first of these, the *Miserere*, or Iliac Passion, is one of the most excruciating Distempers. If any Part of the Intestines, the Cavity of the Guts is closed up, whatever may have

have occasioned it, the Course or Descent of the Food they contain is necessarily stopped; in which Case it frequently happens, that that continual Motion observed in the Guts of a living Animal dissected, and which was intended to detrude, or force their Contents downwards, is propagated in a directly contrary Manner, from the Guts towards the Mouth.

This Disease sometimes begins after a Constipation, or Costiveness, of some Days, at other Times without that Costiveness having been preceded by Pains in any Part of the Belly, especially around the Navel, but which Pains, gradually increasing after their Commencement, at length become extremely violent, and throw the Patient into excessive Anguish. In some of these Cases a hard Tumour may be felt, which surrounds the Belly like a Cord. The Flatulences within become very audible, some of them are discharged upwards, in a little Time after, Vomitings come on, which increase till the Patient has thrown up all he had taken in, with a still further Augmentation of the excessive Pain. With the first of his Vomitings he only brings up the last Food he had taken, with his Drink and some yellowish Humour: but what comes up afterwards proves stinking; and when the Disease is greatly heightened, they have what is called the Smell of Excrement or Dung; but which rather resembles that of a putrid dead Body. It happens too sometimes, that if the Sick have taken Glysters composed of Materials of a strong Smell, the same Smell is discernible in the Matter they vomit up. I confess however I never saw either real Excrements, or the Substance of their Glysters, brought up, much less the Suppositories that were introduced into the Fundament: and were it credible that Instances of this Kind had occurred, they must be allowed very difficult to account for. Throughout this whole Term of the Disease, the Patient has not a single Discharge by Stool; the Belly is greatly distended; the Urine not seldom suppressed, and at other Times thick and fœtid. The Pulse, which at first was pretty hard, becomes quick and small; the Strength entirely vanishes; a Raving comes on; a Hiccup almost constantly supervenes, and sometimes general Convulsions, the Extremities grow cold, the Pulse scarcely perceivable, the Pain and the Vomiting cease, and the Patient dies very quickly after.

§ 318. As this Disease is highly dangerous, the Moment it is strongly apprehended, it is necessary to oppose it by proper Means and Remedies: the smallest Error may be of fatal Consequence, and hot inflaming Liquids have been known to kill the Patient in a few Hours. I was called in the second Day of the Disease to a young Person, who had taken a good deal of Venice Treacle. Nothing could afford her any Relief, and she died early on the third Day.

This Disease should be treated precisely in the same Manner as an inflammatory Cholic; the principal Difference being, that in the former there are no Stools, but continual Vomitings.

1, First

Of the Iliac Passion.

1, First of all then the Patient should be plentifully bled, if the Physician has been called in early enough, and before the Sick has lost his Strength.

2, He should receive opening Glysters made of a Decoction of Barley Water, with five or six Ounces of Oil in each.

3, We should endeavour to allay the violent Efforts to vomit, by giving every two Hours a Spoonful of the Mixture N°. 48.

4, The Sick should drink plentifully, in very small Quantities, very often repeated, of an appeasing, diluting, refreshing Drink, which tends at the same Time to promote both Stools and Urine. Nothing is preferable to the Whey N°. 49, if it can be had immediately: if not, give simple clear Whey sweetened with Honey, and the Drinks prescribed § 298, Art. 3.

5, The Patient is to be put into a warm Bath, and kept as long as he can bear it, repeating it as often daily too, as his Strength will permit.

6, After Bleeding, warm Bathing, repeated Glysters and Fomentations, if each and all of these have availed nothing; the Fume or Smoak of Tobacco may be introduced in the Manner of a Glyster, of which I shall speak further, in the Chapter on Persons drowned.

I cured a Person of this Disease, by conveying him into a Bath, immediately after bleeding him, and giving him a Purge on his going into the Bath.

§ 319. If the Pain abates before the Patient has quite lost his Strength; if the Pulse improves at the same Time; if the Vomitings are less in Number, and in the Quantity of the Matter brought up, if that Matter seems in a less putrid offensive State; if he feels some Commotion and Rumbling in his Bowels; if he has some little Discharge by Stool; and if at the same Time he feels himself a little stronger than before, his Cure may reasonably be expected; but if he is otherwise circumstanced he will soon depart. It frequently happens, a single Hour before Death, that the Pain seems to vanish, and a surprising Quantity of extremely fœtid Matter is discharged by Stool: the Patient is suddenly seized with a great Weakness and Sinking, falls into a cold Sweat, and immediately expires.

§ 320. This is the Disease which the common People attribute to, and term, the *Twisting of the Guts*, and in which they make the Patients swallow Bullets, or large Quantities of Quick-silver. This twisting, tangling, or Knotting of the Guts is an utter, an impossible Chimera; for how can they admit of such a Circumstance, as one of their Extremities, their Ends, is connected to the Stomach, and the other irremoveably fastened to the Skin of the Fork or Cleft of the Buttocks? In Fact this Disease results from a Variety of Causes, which have been discovered on a Dissection of those who have died of it. It were to be wish'd indeed this prudent Custom, so extremely conducive to enrich, and to perfect, the

the Art of Physick, were to prevail more generally; and which we ought rather to consider as a Duty to comply with, than a Difficulty to submit to; as it is our Duty to contribute to the Perfection of a Science, on which the Happiness of Mankind so considerably depends. I shall not enter into a Detail of these Causes, but whatever they are, the Practice of swallowing Bullets in the Disease is always pernicious, and the like Use of Mercury must be often so. Each of these pretended Remedies may aggravate the Disease, and contribute an insurmountable Obstacle to the Cure——Of that Iliac Passion, which is sometimes a Consequence of Ruptures, I shall treat in another Place.

Of the Cholera-morbus.

§ 321. This Disease is a sudden, abundant, and painful Evacuation by vomiting and by Stool.

It begins with much Flatulence, or Wind, with Swelling and slight Pains in the Belly, accompanied with great Dejection, and followed with large Evacuations either by Stool or by Vomit at first, but whenever either of them has begun, the other quickly follows. The Matter evacuated is either yellowish, green, brown, whitish, or black; the Pains in the Belly violent, the Pulse, almost constantly feverish, is sometimes strong at first, but soon sinks into Weakness, in Consequence of the prodigious Discharge. Some Patients purge a hundred Times in the Compass of a few Hours: they may even be seen to fall away, and if the Disease exists in a violent Degree, they are scarcely to be known within three or four Hours from the Commencement of these Discharges. After a great Number of them they are afflicted with Spasms, or Cramps, in their Legs, Thighs, and Arms, which torment them as much as the Pains in the Belly. When the Disease rages too highly to be assuaged, Hiccups, Convulsions and a Coldness of the Extremities approach, there is a scarcely intermitting Succession of fainting, or swooning Fits, the Patient dying either in one of them, or in Convulsions.

§ 322. This Disease, which constantly depends on a Bile raised to the highest Acrimony, commonly prevails towards the End of July and in August: especially if the Heats have been very violent, and there have been little or no Summer Fruits, which greatly conduce to attemper and allay the putrescent Acrimony of the Bile.

§ 323. Nevertheless, however violent this Distemper may be, it is less dangerous, and also less tormenting than the former, many Persons recovering from it.

1, Our first Endeavour should be to dilute, or even to drown this acrid Bile, by Draughts, by Deluges, of the most mitigating Drinks, the Irritation being so very great, that every Thing having the least Sharpness is injurious. Wherefore the Patient should continually take in, by Drink, and by Way of Glyster, either Barley-Water, Almond-Milk, or pure Water, with one eighth

Part

Part Milk, which has succeeded very well in my Practice. Or he may use a very light Decoction, or Ptisan, as it were, of Bread, which is made by gently boiling a Pound of toasted Bread, in three or four Pots of Water for half an Hour. In *Swisserland* we prefer Oat-bread. We also successfully use pounded Rye, making a light Ptisan of it.

A very light thin Soup made of a Pullet, a Chicken, or of one Pound of lean Veal, in three Pots of Water, is very proper too in this Disease. Whey is also employed to good Purpose; and in those Places, where it can easily be had, Buttermilk is the best Drink of any. But, whichever of these Drinks shall be thought preferable, it is a necessary Point to drink very plentifully of it; and the Glysters should be given every two Hours.

2, If the Patient is of a robust Constitution, and sanguine Complexion, with a strong Pulse at the Time of the Attack, and the Pains are very severe, a first, and in some Cases, a second Bleeding, very early in the Invasion, asswages the Violence of the Malady, and allows more Leisure for the Assistance of other Remedies. I have seen the Vomiting cease almost entirely, after the first Bleeding.

The Rage of this Disease abates a little after a Duration of five or six Hours: we must not however, during this Remission or Abatement, forbear to throw in proper Remedies, since it returns soon after with great Force, which

which Return however indicates no Alteration of the Method already entered upon.

3, In general the warm Bath refreshes the Patient while he continues in it; but the Pains frequently return soon after he is taken out, which, however, is no Reason for omitting it, since it has frequently been found to give a more durable Relief. The Patient should continue in it a considerable Time, and, during that Time, he should take six or seven Glasses of the Potion N°. 32, which has been very efficacious in this Disease. By these Means the Vomiting has been stopt, and the Patient, upon going out of the Bath, has had several large Stools, which very considerably diminished the Violence of the Disease.

4, If the Patient's Attendants are terrified by these great Evacuations, and determine to check them (however prematurely) by Venice Treacle, Mint Water, Syrup of white Poppies, called Diacodium, by Opium or Mithridate, it either happens, that the Disease and all its Symptoms are heightened, to which I have been a Witness; or, if the Evacuations should actually be stopt, the Patient, in Consequence of it, is thrown into a more dangerous Condition. I have been obliged to give a Purge, in order to renew the Discharges, to a Man, who had been thrown into a violent Fever, attended with a raging *Delirium*, by a Medicine composed of Venice Treacle, Mithridate and Oil. Such Medicines ought not to be employed, until the Smallness of the Pulse, great Weakness,

Of the Cholera-morbus.   331

Weakness, violent and almost continual Cramps, and even the Insufficience of the Patient's Efforts to vomit, make us apprehensive of his sinking irrecoverably. In such Circumstances indeed he should take, every Quarter or half Quarter of an Hour, a Spoonful of the Mixture N°. 50, still continuing the diluting Drinks. After the first Hour, they should only be given every Hour, and that only to the Extent of eight Doses. But I desire to insist upon it here, that this Medicine should not be given too early in this Distemper.

§ 324 If the Patient is likely to recover, the Pains and the Evacuations gradually abate; the Thirst is less, the Pulse continues very quick, but it becomes regular. There have been Instances of their Propensity to a heavy kind of Drowsiness at this Time; for perfect refreshing Sleep advances but slowly after this Disease. It will still be proper to persevere in the Medicines already directed, though somewhat less frequently. And now we may begin to allow the Patient a few Soups from farinaceous mealy Substances; and as soon as the Evacuations accompanying this Disease are evidently ceased, and the Pains are vanished, though an acute Sensibility and great Weakness continues, beside such Soups, he may be allowed some new-laid Eggs, very lightly boiled, or even raw, for some Days After this he must be referred to the Regimen so frequently recommended to Persons in a State of Recovery: when the concurring Use of the Powder N°. 24, taken twice a Day, will greatly assist to hasten and to establish his Health.

Chapter XXIII.

Of a Diarrhœa, or Looseness.

Sect. 325.

EVERY one knows what is meant by a Looseness or Purging, which the Populace frequently call a Flux, and sometimes a Cholic.

There are certain very chronical, or tedious and obstinate ones, which arise from some essential Fault in the Constitution. Of such, as foreign to my Plan, I shall say nothing.

Those which come on suddenly, without any preceding Disorder, except sometimes a slight Qualm or short Loathing, and a Pain in the Loins and Knees; which are not attended with smart Pains nor a Fever (and frequently without any Pain, or any other Complaint) are oftener of Service than prejudicial. They carry off a Heap of Matter that may have been long amassed and corrupted in the Body, which, if not discharged, might have produced some Distemper; and, far from weakening the Body, such Purgings as these render it more strong, light and active

§ 326.

§ 326. Such therefore ought by no Means to be stopped, nor even speedily checked: they generally cease of themselves, as soon as all the noxious Matter is discharged, and as they require no Medicine, it is only necessary to retrench considerably from the ordinary Quantity of Nourishment; to abstain from Flesh, Eggs and Wine or other strong Drink, to live only on some Soups, on Pulse, or on a little Fruit, whether raw or baked, and to drink rather less than usual. A simple Ptisan with a little Syrup of *Capillaire*, or Maiden-hair, is sufficient in these Purgings, which require no Venice Treacle, Confection, nor any Drug whatever.

§ 327 But should it continue more than five or six Days, and manifestly weaken the Patient, if the Pain attending it grows a little severe, and especially if the Irritation, the urging to Stool, proves more frequent, it becomes seasonable to check, or to stop, it. For this Purpose the Patient is to be put into a Regimen; and if the Looseness has been accompanied with a great Loathing, with Risings or Wamblings at Stomach, with a foul furred Tongue, and a bad Taste in the Mouth, he must take the Powder N°. 35. But if these Symptoms do not appear, give him that of N°. 51. and during the three following Hours, let him take, every half Hour, a Cup of weak light Broth, without any Fat on it.

If the Purging, after being restrained by this Medicine, should return within a few Days, it would

would strongly infer, there was still some tough viscid Matter within, that required Evacuation. To effect this he should take the Medicines N°. 21, 25 or 27; and afterwards take fasting, for two successive Mornings, half the Powder, N°. 51.

On the Evening of that Day when the Patient took N°. 35, or N°. 51, or any other Purge, he may take a small Dose of Venice Treacle.

§ 328 A Purging is often neglected for a long Time, without observing the least Regimen, from which Neglect they degenerate into tedious and as it were habitual, perpetual ones, and entirely weaken the Patient In such Cases, the Medicine N°. 35 should be given first; then, every other Day for four Times successively, he should take N°. 51: during all which Time he should live on nothing but Panada (See § 57) or on Rice boiled in weak Chicken-broth. A strengtning stomachic Plaister has sometimes been successfully applied, which may be often moistened in a Decoction of Herbs boiled in Wine. Cold and Moisture should be carefully avoided in these Cases, which frequently occasion immediate Relapses, even after the Looseness had ceased for many Days

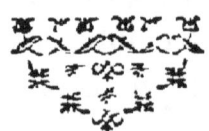

Chapter XXIV.

Of the Dysentery, or Bloody-flux.

Sect. 329.

THE Dysentery is a Flux or Looseness of the Belly, attended with great Restlessness and Anguish, with severe Gripings, and frequent Propensities to go to Stool. There is generally a little Blood in the Stools, though this is not a constant Symptom, and is not essential to the Existence of a Dysentery; notwithstanding it may not be much less dangerous, for the Absence of this Symptom

§ 330. The Dysentery is often epidemical; beginning sometimes at the End of July, though oftner in August, and going off when the Frosts set in. The great preceding Heats render the Blood and the Bile acrid or sharp, and though, during the Continuance of the Heat, Perspiration is kept up (See Introduct. P. 28) yet as soon as the Heat abates, especially in the Mornings and Evenings, that Discharge is diminished; and by how much the more Viscidity or Thickness the Humours have acquired, in Consequence of the violent Heats, the Discharge of the sharp Humour by Perspiration being now checked, it is thrown

upon

upon the Bowels which it irritates, producing Pains in, and Evacuations from them.

This Kind of Dysentery may happen at all Times, and in all Countries; but if other Causes, capable of producing a Putridity of the Humours, be complicated with it; such as the crouding up a great Number of People into very little Room, and very close Quarters, as in Hospitals, Camps, or Prisons, this introduces a malignant Principle into the Humours, which, co-operating with the simpler Cause, of the Dysentery, renders it the more difficult and dangerous.

§ 331. This Disease begins with a general Coldness rather than a Shivering, which lasts some Hours, the Patient's Strength soon abates, and he feels sharp Pains in his Belly, which sometimes continue for several Hours, before the Flux begins. He is affected with *Vertigos,* or Swimmings in the Head, with Reachings to vomit, and grows pale; his Pulse at the same Time being very little, if at all, feverish, but commonly small, and at length the Purging begins. The first Stools are often thin, and yellowish; but in a little Time they are mixt with a viscid ropy Matter, which is often tinged with Blood. Their Colour and Consistence are various too, being either brown, greenish or black, thinner or thicker, and fœtid: The Pains increase before each of the Discharges, which grow very frequent, to the Number of eight, ten, twelve or fifteen in an Hour: then the Fundament

ment becomes considerably irritated, and the *Tenesmus* (which is a great Urgency to go to Stool, though without any Effect) is joined to the Dysentery or Flux, and often brings on a Protrusion or falling down of the Fundament, the Patient being now most severely afflicted. Worms are sometimes voided, and glary hairy Humours, resembling Pieces or Peelings of Guts, and sometimes Clots of Blood.

If the Distemper rises to a violent Height, the Guts become inflamed, which terminates either in Suppuration or in Mortification; the miserable Patient discharges *Pus*, or black and fœtid watery Stools: the Hiccup supervenes; he grows delirious; his Pulse sinks; and he falls into cold Sweats and Faintings which terminate in Death.

A kind of Phrenzy, or raging *Delirium*, sometimes comes on before the Minute of Expiration. I have seen a very unusual Symptom accompany this Disease in two Persons, which was an Impossibility of swallowing, for three Days before Death.

But in general this Distemper is not so extremely violent; the Discharges are less frequent, being from twenty-five to forty within a Day and Night. Their Contents are less various and uncommon, and mixed with very little Blood; the Patient retains more Strength, the Number of Stools gradually decrease, the Blood disappears, the Consistence of the Discharges improves, Sleep and Appetite return, and the Sick recovers.

Many of the Sick have not the least Degree of Fever, nor of Thirst, which perhaps is less common in this Disease, than in a simple Purging or Looseness.

Their Urine sometimes is but in a small Quantity; and many Patients have ineffectual Endeavours to pass it, to their no small Affliction and Restlessness.

§ 332 The most efficacious Remedy for this Disease is a Vomit. That of N°. 34, (when there is no present Circumstance that forbids the giving a Vomit) if taken immediately on the first Invasion of it, often removes it at once; and always shortens its Duration. That of N°. 35 is not less effectual; it has been considered for a long Time, even as a certain Specific, which it is not, though a very useful Medicine. If the Stools prove less frequent after the Operation of either of them, it is a good Sign; if they are no Ways diminished, we may apprehend the Disease is like to be tedious and obstinate.

The Patient is to be ordered to a Regimen, abstaining from all Flesh-meat with the strictest Attention, until the perfect Cure of the Disease. The Ptisan N°. 3 is the best Drink for him.

The Day after the Vomit, he must take the Powder N° 51 divided into two Doses: the next Day he should take no other Medicine but his Ptisan; on the fourth the Rhubarb must be repeated, after which the Violence of the Disease commonly abates. His Diet during the Disease is nevertheless to be continued exactly for some

Of the Dysentery, or Bloody-flux.

some Days; after which he may be allowed to enter upon that of Persons in a State of Recovery.

§ 333. The Dysentery sometimes commences with an inflammatory Fever; a feverish, hard, full Pulse, with a violent Pain in the Head and Loins, and a stiff distended Belly. In such a Case the Patient must be bled once; and daily receive three or even four of the Glysters N°. 6, drinking plentifully of the Drink N°. 3.

When all Dread of an Inflammation is entirely over, the Patient is to be treated in the Manner just related; though often there is no Necessity for the Vomit: and if the inflammatory Symptoms have run high, his first Purge should be that of N°. 11, and the Use of the Rhubarb may be postponed, till about the manifest Conclusion of the Disease

I have cured many Dysenteries, by ordering the Sick no other Remedy, but a Cup of warm Water every Quarter of an Hour, and it were better to rely only on this simple Remedy, which must be of some Utility, than to employ those, of whose Effects Country People are ignorant, and which are often productive of very dangerous ones.

§ 334. It sometimes happens that the Dysentery is combined with a putrid Fever, which makes it necessary, after the Vomit, to give the Purges N°. 23 or 47, and several Doses of N°. 24, before the Rhubarb is given. N°. 32 is excellent in this combined Case.

There was in *Swifferland* in the Autumn of 1755, after a very numerous Prevalence of epidemical putrid Fevers had ceased, a Multitude of Dysenteries, which had no small Affinity with, or Relation to, such Fevers. I treated them first, with the Prescription N°. 34, giving afterwards N° 32, and I directed the Rhubarb only to very few, and that towards the Conclusion of the Disease. By much the greater Number of them were cured at the End of four or five Days. A small Proportion of them, to whom I could not give the Vomit, or whose Cases were more complicated, remained languid a considerable Time, though without Fatality or Danger.

§ 335. When the Dysentery is blended with Symptoms of Malignity (See § 245) after premising the Prescription N° 35, those of N°. 38 and 39 may be called in successfully.

§ 336. When the Disease has already been of many Days standing, without the Patient's having taken any Medicines, or only such as were injurious to him, he must be treated as if the Distemper had but just commenced; unless some Symptoms, foreign to the Nature of the Dysentery, had supervened upon it.

§ 337. Relapses sometimes occur in Dysenteries, some few Days after the Patients appeared well, much the greater Number of which are occasioned either by some Error in Diet, by cold Air, or by being considerably over-heated. They are to be prevented by avoiding these Causes of them, and may be removed by putting the Patient

Of the Dysentery, or Bloody-flux. 341

tient on his Regimen, and giving him one Dose of the Prescription N°. 51. Should it return even without any such discoverable Causes, and if it manifests itself to be the same Distemper renewed, it must be treated as such.

§ 338. This Disease is sometimes combined too with an intermitting Fever; in which Case the Dysentery must be removed first, and the intermittent afterwards. Nevertheless if the Access, the Fits of the Fever have been very strong, the Bark must be given as directed § 259.

§ 339. One pernicious Prejudice, which still generally prevails is, that Fruits are noxious in a Dysentery, that they even give it, and aggravate it; and this perhaps is an extremely ill-grounded one. In truth bad Fruits, and such as have not ripened well, in unseasonable Years, may really occasion Cholics, a Looseness (though oftner a Costiveness) and Disorders of the Nerves, and of the Skin; but never can occasion an epidemical Dysentery or Flux. Ripe Fruits, of whatever Species, and especially Summer Fruits, are the real Preservatives from this Disease. The greatest Mischief they can effect, must result from their thinning and washing down the Humours, especially the thick glutinous Bile, if they are in such a State; good ripe Fruits being the true Dissolvents of such, by which indeed they may bring on a Purging, but such a one, as is rather a Guard against a Dysentery

We had a great, an extraordinary Abundance of Fruit in 1759 and 1760, but scarcely any

Dysenteries. It has been even observed to be more rare, and less dangerous than formerly; and if the Fact is certain, it cannot be attributed to any thing more probably, than to the very numerous Plantations of Trees, which have rendered Fruit very plenty, cheap and common. Whenever I have observed Dysenteries to prevail, I made it a Rule to eat less Flesh, and Plenty of Fruit; I have never had the slightest Attack of one; and several Physicians use the same Caution with the same Success.

I have seen eleven Patients in a Dysentery in one House, of whom nine were very tractable; they eat Fruit and recovered. The Grandmother and one Child, whom she loved more than the rest, were carried off. She managed the Child after her own Fashion, with burnt Wine, Oil, and some Spices, but no Fruit. She conducted herself in the very same Manner, and both died.

In a Country Seat near *Berne*, in the Year 1751, when these Fluxes made great Havock, and People were severely warned against the Use of Fruits, out of eleven Persons in the Family, ten eat plentifully of Prunes, and not one of them was seized with it: The poor Coachman alone rigidly observed that Abstinence from Fruit injoined by this Prejudice, and took a terrible Dysentery.

This same Distemper had nearly destroyed a Swiss Regiment in Garrison in the South of *France*, the Captains purchased the whole Crop of
several

several Acres of Vineyard; there they carried the sick Soldiers, and gathered the Grapes for such as could not bear being carried into the Vineyard; those who were well eating nothing else: after this not one more died, nor were any more even attacked with the Dysentery.

A Clergyman was seized with a Dysentery, which was not in the least mitigated by any Medicines he had taken. By meer Chance he saw some red Currans; he longed for them, and eat three Pounds of them between seven and nine o'Clock in the Morning, that very Day he became better, and was entirely well on the next.

I could greatly enlarge the Number of such Instances; but these may suffice to convince the most incredulous, whom I thought it might be of some Importance to convince. Far from forbidding good Fruit, when Dysenteries rage, the Patients should be encouraged to eat them freely; and the Directors of the Police, instead of prohibiting them, ought to see the Markets well provided with them. It is a Fact of which Persons, who have carefully informed themselves, do not in the least doubt. Experience demonstrates it, and it is founded in Reason, as good Fruit counter-operates all the Causes of Dysenteries. *

§. 340.

---

* The Experience of all Countries and Times so strongly confirms these important Truths, that they cannot be too often repeated, too generally published, whenever and wherever this Disease rages. The Succession of cold Showers to violent Heats, too moist a Constitution of the Air, an Excess of animal Food; Uncleanliness and Contagion, are the frequent Causes of epidemical Fluxes *E L*

§ 340. It is important and even necessary, that each Subject of this Disease should have a Close-stool or Convenience apart to himself, as the Matter discharged is extremely infectious: and if they make Use of Bed-pans, they should be carried immediately out of the Chamber, the Air of which should be continually renewed, burning Vinegar frequently in it

It is also very necessary to change the Patient's Linen frequently; without all which Precautions the Distemper becomes more violent, and attacks others who live in the same House. Hence it is greatly to be wished the People in general were convinced of these Truths.

It was BOERHAAVE's Opinion, that all the Water which was drank, while Dysenteries were epidemical, should be *stummed*, as we term it, or sulphurized. †

§ 341.

I have retained the preceding Note, abridged from this Gentleman, as it contains the Suffrage of another experienced Physician, against that Prejudice of ripe Fruits occasioning Fluxes, which is too popular among ourselves, and probably more so in the Country than in *Lorcon*. I have been also very credibly assured, that the Son of a learned Physician was perfectly cured of a very obstinate Purging, of a Year's Continuance (in Spite of all the usual officinal Remedies) by his devouring large Quantities of ripe Mulberries, for which he ardently longed, and drinking very freely of their expressed Juice. The Fact occurred after his Father's Decease, and was affirmed to me by a Gentleman intimately acquainted with them both   K

† Our learned Author, or his medical Editor at *Lyons*, observes here, ' that in the Edition of this Treatise at *Paris*, there was an essential Mistake, by making *Boerhaave* recommend the Addition of Brandy *Eau de vie*, instead of stumming or sulphurizing it, for which this Note, and the Text too use the Verb *braxter*, which
Word

Of the Dysentery, or Bloody-flux.

§ 341. It has happened, by some unaccountable Fatality, that there is no Disease, for which a greater Number of Remedies are advised, than for the Dysentery. There is scarcely any Person but what boasts of his own Prescription, in Preference to all the rest, and who does not boldly engage to cure, and that within a few Hours, a tedious severe Disease, of which he has formed no just Notion, with some Medicine or Composition, of whose Operation he is totally ignorant: while the poor Sufferer, restless and impatient, swallows every Body's Recommendation, and gets poisoned either through Fear, downright Disgust or Weariness, or through entire Complaisance. Of these many boasted Compositions, some are only indifferent, but others pernicious. I shall not pretend to detail all I know myself, but after repeatedly affirming, that the only true Method of Cure is that I have advised here, the Purpose of which is evacuating the offending Matter, I also affirm that all those Methods, which have a different Scope or Drift, are pernicious; but shall particularly observe, that the Method most generally followed, which is that of stopping the Stools by Astringents, or by Opiates, is the worst of all, and even so mortal a one, as to destroy a Multitude of People annually, and which

Word we do not find in any Dictionary. We are told however, it means to impregnate the Casks in which the Water is reserved, with the Vapour of Sulphur, and then stopping them, in the same Manner that Vessels are in some Countries, for the keeping of Wine. He observes the Purpose of this is to oppose Corruption by the acid Steams of the Sulphur. *K.*

which throws others into incurable Diseases. By preventing the Discharge of these Stools, and inclosing the Wolf in the Fold, it either follows, 1, that this * retained Matter irritates and inflames the Bowels, from which Inflammation excruciating Pains arise, an acute inflammatory Cholic, and finally a Mortification and Death; or a *Schirrhus*, which degenerates into a *Cancer*, (of which I have seen a dreadful Instance) or else an Abscess, Suppuration and Ulcer. Or 2, this arrested Humour is repelled elsewhere, producing a *Scirrhus* in the Liver, or Asthmas, Apoplexy, Epilepsy, or Falling Sickness; horrible rheumatic Pains, or incurable Disorders of the Eyes, or of the Teguments, the Skin and Surface.

Such are the Consequences of all the astringent Medicines, and of those which are given to procure Sleep in this Disease, as Venice Treacle, Mithridate and Diascordium, when given two early in Dysenteries.

I have been consulted on Account of a terrible Rheumatism, which ensued immediately after taking a Mixture of Venice Treacle and Plantain, on the second Day of a Dysentery.

As those who advise such Medicines, are certainly unaware of their Consequences, I hope
this

---

* A first or second Dose of Glauber Salt has been known to succeed in the epidemical Summer Fluxes of the hotter Climates, when repeated Doses of Rhubarb and Opiates had failed. Such Instances seems a collateral Confirmation of Dr Tissot's rational and succesful Use of cooling opening Fruits in them. K

this Account of them will be sufficient, to prevent their Repetition.

§ 342. Neither are Purges without their Abuse and Danger; they determine the Course of all the Humours more violently to the tender afflicted Parts; the Body becomes exhausted; the Digestions fail; the Bowels are weakened, and sometimes even lightly ulcerated, whence incurable *Diarrhæas* or Purgings ensue, and prove fatal after many Years Affliction.

§ 343 If the Evacuations prove excessive, and the Distemper tedious, the Patient is likely to fall into a Dropsy; but if this is immediately opposed, it may be removed by a regular and drying Diet, by Strengthners, by Friction and proper Exercise.

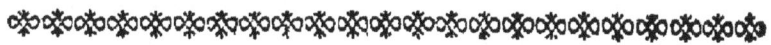

Chapter XXV.

Of the Itch.

Sect. 344.

THE Itch is an infectious Disorder contracted by touching infected Persons or Cloaths, but not imbibed from the Air: So that by carefully avoiding the *Medium*, or Means of Contagion, the Disorder may be certainly escaped.

Though

Though any Part of the Body may be infested with the Itch, it commonly shews itself on the Hands, and chiefly between the Fingers. At first one or two little Pimples or Pustules appear, filled with a kind of clear Water, and excite a very disagreeable Itching. If these Pustules are broke by scratching them, the Water oozing from them infects the neighbouring Parts. At the Beginning of this Infection it can scarcely be distinguished, if a Person is not well apprized of its Nature; but in the Progress of it, the little Pustules increase both in Number and Size; and when they are opened by scratching, a loathsome kind of Scab is formed, and the Malady extends over the whole Surface. Where they continue long, they produce small Ulcers, and are at that Time highly contagious.

§ 345. Bad Diet, particularly the Use of Salt Meat, bad unripe Fruit, and Uncleanliness occasion this Disease, though it is oftnest taken by Contagion. Some very good Physicians suppose it is never contracted otherwise; but I must take Leave to dissent, as I have certainly seen it exist without Contagion.

When it happens to a Person, who cannot suspect he has received it by Contact, his Cure should commence with a total Abstinence from all Salt, sour, fat and spicy Food. He should drink a Ptisan of wild and bitter Succory, or that of N°. 26, five or six Glasses of which may be daily taken, at the End of four or five Days, he may be purged with N°. 21, or with an Ounce of
Sedlitz

Sedlitz [or *Epsom*] Salt. His Abstinence, his Regimen is to be continued; the Purge to be repeated after six or seven Days; and then all the Parts affected, and those very near them, are to be rubbed in the Morning fasting, with a fourth Part of the Ointment N° 52. The three following Days the same Fuction is to be repeated, after which the same Quantity of Ointment is to be procured, and used in the same Proportion; but only every other Day. It happens but seldom that this Method fails to remove this disagreeable Malady, sometimes however it will return, in which Case, the Patient must be purged again, and then recur to the Ointment, whose good Effects I have experienced, and continually do.

If the Disease has been very lately contracted, and most certainly by Contact, the Ointment may be fearlessly employed, as soon as it is discovered, without taking any Purge before it. But if, on the contrary, the Disease has been long neglected, and has rose to a high Degree, it will be necessary to restrain the Patient a long Time to the Regimen I have directed, he must be repeatedly purged, and then drink plentifully of the Ptisan N° 26, before the Ointment is rubbed in. When the Malady is thus circumstanced, I have always begun with the Ointment N°. 28, half a Quarter of which is to be used every Morning. I have also frequently omitted the Use of that N°. 52, having always found the former as certain; but a little slower in its Effects.

§ 346. While these Medicines are employed,

the Patient muſt avoid all Cold and Wet, eſpecially if he makes Uſe of N°. 28, * in which there is Quick-ſilver; which, if ſuch Precautions were neglected, might bring on a Swelling of the Throat and Gums, and even riſe to a Salivation. Yet this Ointment has one Advantage in its having no Smell, and being ſuſceptible of an agreeable one; while it is very difficult to diſguiſe the diſagreeable Odour of the other.

The Linen of a Perſon in this Diſeaſe ought to be often changed; but his upper Cloaths muſt not be changed: becauſe theſe having been infected, might, when worn again, communicate the Itch to the Wearer again, after he had been cured.

Shirts, Breeches and Stockings may be fumigated with Sulphur, before they are put on; and this Fumigation ſhould be made in the open Air.

§ 347.

---

* I have ſeen a pretty ſingular Conſequence from the Abuſe of merſcurial Unction for the Itch, whether it happened from the Strength or Quantity of the Ointment, or from taking Cold after applying it, as this Subject, a healthy Youth of about fifteen, probably did, by riding three or four Miles through the Rain. But without any other previous Complaint, he awoke quite blind one Morning, wondering, as he ſaid, when it would be Day. His Eyes were very clear, and free from Inflammation, but the Pupil was wholly immoveable, as in a *Gutta ſerena*. I effected the Cure by ſome moderate Purges repeated a few Times, by diſpoſing him to ſweat by lying pretty much in Bed (it being towards Winter) and by promoting his Perſpiration chiefly with Sulphur; after which the ſhaved Scalp was embrocated with a warm nervous Mixture, in which Balſam of *Peru* was a conſiderable Ingredient. In ſomething leſs than three Weeks he could diſcern a glowing Fire, or the bright Flame of a Candle. As his Sight increaſed, he diſcerned other Objects, which appeared for ſome Days inverted to him, with their Colours confuſed, but Red was moſt diſtinguiſhable. He diſcovered the Aces ſooner than other Cards, and in about ſix or ſeven Weeks recovered his full Sight in all its natural Strength, which he now enjoys. K.

§ 347. If this Disorder becomes very inveterate and tedious, it exhausts the Patient, in Consequence of its not suffering him to sleep at Nights, as well as by his restless Irritation; and sometimes even brings on a Fever, so that he falls away in Flesh, and his Strength abates.

In such a Case he must take, 1, a gentle Purge.

2, Make Use frequently of warm Baths.

3, He must be put on the Regimen of Persons in a State of Recovery.

4, He must take Morning and Evening, fifteen Days successively, the Powder N°. 53, with the Ptisan N°. 26.

This Malady is often very obstinate, and then the Medicines must be varied according to the Circumstances, the Detail of which I avoid here.

§ 348. After giving repeated Purges in such obstinate Cases, mineral Waters abounding with Sulphur, such as * those of *Yverdun*, &c. often effect a Cure; and simple cold Bathings in Rivers or Lakes have sometimes succeeded in very inveterate Cases of this Disorder.

Nothing conduces more to the long Continuance of this Malady, than the Abuse of hot Waters.

§ 349. I shall conclude this Chapter, with a repeated Injunction not to be too free or rash in the Use of the Ointment N°. 52, and other outward Remedies for extinguishing the Itch. There is hardly any Complaint, but what has been found

to

---

* Sea Water, and those of *Dulwich, Harrigate Shadwell*, &c. will be full as effectual. *K.*

to be the Consequence of too sudden a Removal of this Disorder by outward Applications, before due Evacuations have been made, and a moderate Abatement of the Sharpness of the Humours has been effected.

Chapter XXVI.

The Treatment of Diseases peculiar to Women.

Sect. 350.

BESIDES all the preceding Diseases, to which Women are liable in common with Men, their Sex also exposes them to others peculiar to it, and which depend upon four principal Sources; which are their monthly Discharges, their Pregnancy, their Labours in Child-birth, and the Consequences of their Labours. It is not my present Design to treat professedly on each of the Diseases arising from these Causes, which would require a larger Volume than I have proposed; but I shall confine myself to certain general Directions on these four Heads.

§ 351. Nature, who intended Women for the Increase, and the Nourishment of the human Race at the Breast, has subjected them to a periodical Efflux, or Discharge, of Blood: which stance constitutes the Source, from whence the Infant is afterwards to receive his Nutrition and Growth.

This Discharge generally commences, with us, between the Age of sixteen and eighteen. Young Maidens, before the Appearance of this Discharge, are frequently, and many for a long Time, in a State of Weakness, attended with various Complaints, which is termed the *Chlorosis*, or Green Sickness, and Obstructions. and when their Appearance is extremely slow and backward, it occasions very grievous, and sometimes even mortal Diseases. Nevertheless it is too usual, though very improper, to ascribe all the Evils, to which they are subject at this Term of Life, solely to this Cause; while they really often result from a different Cause, of which the Obstructions themselves are sometimes only the Effect, and this is the natural, and, in some Degree, even necessary Feebleness of the Sex. The Fibres of Women which are intended to be relaxed, and to give Way, when they are unavoidably extended by the Growth of the Child, and its inclosing Membranes (which frequently arise to a very considerable Size) should necessarily be less stiff and rigid, less strong, and more lax and yielding than the Fibres of Men. Hence the Circulation of their Blood is more slow and languid than in Males, their Blood is less compact and dense, and more watery, their Fluids are more liable to stagnate in their different Bowels, and to form Infarctions and Obstructions.

§ 352.

§ 352. The Diforders to which fuch a Conftitution fubjects them might, in fome Meafure, be prevented, by affifting that Languor or Feeblenefs of their natural Movements, by fuch an Increafe of their Force, as Exercife might contribute to: But this Affiftance, which in fome Manner is more neceffary for Females than Males, they are partly deprived of, by the general Education and Habitude of the Sex; as they are ufually employed in managing Houfehold Bufinefs, and fuch light fedentary Work, as afford them lefs Exercife and Motion, than the more active Occupations of Men. They ftir about but little, whence their natural Tendency to Weaknefs increafes from Habit, and thence becomes morbid and fickly. Their Blood circulates imperfectly; its Qualities become impaired, the Humours tend to a pretty general Stagnation; and none of the vital Functions are completely difcharged.

From fuch Caufes and Circumftances they begin to fink into a State of Weaknefs, fometimes while they are very young, and many Years before this periodical Difcharge could be expected. This State of Languor difpofes them to be inactive; a little Exercife foon fatigues them, whence they take none at all. It might prove a Remedy, and even effect a Cure, at the Beginning of their Complaint; but as it is a Remedy, that is painful and difagreeable to them, they reject it, and thus increafe their Diforders.

Their Appetite declines with the other vital Functions, and gradually becomes ftill lefs; the ufual usual salutary Kinds of Food never exciting it; instead of which they indulge themselves in whimsical Cravings, and often of the oddest and most improper Substances for Nutrition, which entirely impair the Stomach with its digestive Functions, and consequently Health itself.

But sometimes after the Duration of this State for a few Years, the ordinary Time of their monthly Evacuations approaches, which however make not the least Appearance, for two Reasons. The first is, that their Health is too much impaired to accomplish this new Function, at a Time when all the others are so languid: and the second is, that under such Circumstances, the Evacuations themselves are unnecessary; since their final Purpose is to discharge (when the Sex are not pregant) that superfluous Blood, which they were intended to produce, and whose Retention would be unhealthy, when not applied to the Growth of the Fœtus, or Nourishment of the Child: and this Superfluity of Blood does not exist in Women, who have been long in a very low and languishing State.

§ 353. Their Disorder however continues to increase, as every one daily must, which does not terminate. This Increase of it is attributed to the Suppression or Non-appearance of their monthly Efflux, which is often erroneous, since the Disorder is not always owing to that Suppression, which is often the Effect of their Distemperature. This is so true, that even when the Efflux happens, if their Weakness still continues, the Patients are far from being the better for it, but the reverse. Neither is it unusual to see young Lads, who have received from Nature, and from their Parents, a sort of feminine Constitution, Education and Habitude, infested with much the same Symptoms, as obstructed young Women.

Country Girls, who are generally more accustomed to such hardy Work and Exercise as Country Men, are less subject to these Complaints, than Women who live in Cities.

§ 354. Let People then be careful not to deceive themselves on this important Account; since all the Complaints of young Maidens are not owing to the Want of their Customs. Nevertheless it is certain there are some of them, who are really afflicted from this Cause. For Instance, when a strong young Virgin in full Health, who is nearly arrived to her full Growth, and who manifestly abounds with Blood, does not obtain this Discharge at the usual Time of Life, then indeed this superfluous Blood is the Fountain of very many Disorders, and greatly more violent ones than those, which result from the contrary Causes already mentioned.

If the lazy inactive City Girls are more subject to the Obstructions, which either arise from the Weakness and Languor I have formerly taken Notice of, or which accompany it; Country Girls are more subject to Complaints from this latter Cause (too great a Retention of superfluous Blood) than Women who live in Cities: and it is

this

this laſt Cauſe that excites thoſe ſingular Diſorders, which appear ſo ſupernatural to the common People, that they aſcribe them to Sorcery.

§ 355. And even after theſe periodical Diſcharges have appeared, it is known that they have often been ſuppreſſed, without the leaſt unhealthy Conſequence reſulting from that Suppreſſion. They are often ſuppreſſed, in the Circumſtances mentioned § 351, by a Continuance of the Diſeaſe, which was firſt an Obſtacle or Retardment to their Appearance; and in other Caſes, they have been ſuppreſſed by other Cauſes, ſuch as Cold, Moiſture, violent Fear, any very ſtrong Paſſion; by too chilly a Courſe of Diet, with Indigeſtion, or too hot and irritating Diet; by Drinks cooled with Ice, by Exerciſe too long continued, and by unuſual Watching. The Symptoms, occaſioned by ſuch Suppreſſions, are ſometimes more violent than thoſe, which preceded the firſt Appearance of the Diſcharge.

§ 356. The great Facility with which this Evacuation may be ſuppreſſed, diminiſhed, or diſordered, by the Cauſes already aſſigned, the terrible Evils which are the Conſequences of ſuch Interruptions and Irregularities of them, ſeem to me very cogent Reaſons to engage the Sex to uſe all poſſible Care, in every Reſpect, to preſerve the Regularity of them; by avoiding, during their Approach and Continuance, every Cauſe that may prevent or leſſen them. Would they be thoroughly perſuaded, not ſolely by my Advice, but by that of their Mothers, their Relations, their Friends, and by their own Experience, of what great Importance it is to be very attentive to themselves, at those critical Times, I think there is not one Woman, who from the first, to the very last Appearance of them, would not conduct herself with the most scrupulous Regularity.

Their Demeanour, in these Circumstances, very fundamentally interests their own Health, as well as that of their Children; and consequently their own Happiness, as well as that of their Husbands and Families.

The younger and more delicate they are, Caution becomes the more necessary for them. I am very sensible a strong Country Girl is too negligent in regulating herself at those critical Seasons, and sometimes without any ill Consequence; but at another Time she may suffer severely for it: and I could produce a long List of many, who, by their Imprudence on such Occasions, have thrown themselves into the most terrible Condition.

Besides the Caution with which Females should avoid these general Causes, just mentioned in the preceding Section, every Person ought to remember what has most particularly disagreed with her during that Term, and for ever constantly to reject it.

§ 357. There are many Women whose Customs visit them without the slightest Impeachment of their Health: others are sensibly disordered on every Return of them, and to others again they are very tormenting, by the violent Cholics,

Cholics, of a longer or a shorter Duration, which precede or accompany them. I have known some of these violent Attacks last but some Minutes, and others which continued a few Hours. Nay some indeed have persisted for many Days, attended with Vomiting, Fainting, with Convulsions from excessive Pain, with Vomiting of Blood, Bleedings from the Nose, &c. which, in short, have brought them to the very Jaws of Death. So very dangerous a Situation requires the closest Attention; though, as it results from several and frequently very opposite Causes, it is impossible within the present Plan, to direct the Treatment that may be proper for each Individual. Some Women have the Unhappiness to be subject to these Symptoms every Month, from the first Appearance, to the final Termination, of these Discharges, except proper Remedies and Regimen, and sometimes a happy Child-birth, remove them. Others complain but now and then, every second, third, or fourth Month; and there are some again, who having suffered very severely during the first Months, or Years, after their first Eruptions, suffer no more afterwards. A fourth Number, after having had their Customs for a long Time, without the least Complaint, find themselves afflicted with cruel Pains, at every Return of them; if by Imprudence, or some inevitable Fatality, they have incurred any Cause, that has suppressed, diminished, or delayed them. This Consideration ought to suggest a proper Caution even to such, as generally undergo these Discharges

Discharges, without Pain or Complaint; since all may be assured, that though they suffer no sensible Disorder at that Time, they are nevertheless more delicate, more impressible by extraneous Substances, more easily affected by the Passions of the Mind, and have also weaker Stomachs at these particular Periods.

§ 358 These Discharges may also be sometimes too profuse in Quantity, in which Case the Patients become obnoxious to very grievous Maladies, into the Discussion of which however I shall not enter here, as they are much less frequent than those, arising from a Suppression of them. Besides which, in such Cases, Recourse may be had to the Directions I shall give hereafter, when I treat of that Loss of Blood, which may be expedient, during the Course of Gravidation or Pregnancy. See § 365.

§ 359. Finally, even when they are the most regular, after their Continuance for a pretty certain Number of Years (rarely exceeding thirty-five) they go off of their own Accord, and necessarily, between the Age of forty-five and fifty; sometimes even sooner, but seldom continuing longer: and this *Crisis* of their ceasing is generally a very troublesome, and often a very dangerous, one for the Sex.

§ 360. The Evils mentioned § 352 may be prevented, by avoiding the Causes producing them, and, 1, by obliging young Maidens to use considerable Exercise, especially as soon as

there

there is the least Reason to suspect the Approach of this Disorder, the *Chlorosis*, or Green Sickness.

2, By watching them carefully, that they eat nothing unwholsome or improper; as there are scarcely any natural Substances, even among such as are most improper for them, and the most distasteful, which have not sometimes been the Objects of their sickly, their unaccountable Cravings. Fat Aliments, Pastry, farinaceous or mealy, and sour and watery Foods are pernicious to them. Herb-Teas, which are frequently directed as a Medicine for them, are sufficient to throw them into the Disorder, by increasing that Relaxation of their Fibres, which is a principal Cause of it. If they must drink any such Infusions, as medicated Drinks, let them be taken cold. but the best Drink for them is Water, in which red hot Iron has been extinguished.

3, They must avoid hot sharp Medicines, and such as are solely intended to force down their Terms, which are frequently attended with very pernicious Consequences, and never do any good: and they are still the more hurtful, as the Patient is the younger.

4, If the Malady increases, it will be necessary to give them some Remedies, but these should not be Purges, nor consist of Diluters, and Decoctions of Herbs, of Salts, and a Heap of other useless and noxious Ingredients, but they should take Filings of Iron, which is the most certain Remedy in such Cases. These Filings should be of true simple Iron, and not from Steel; and Care should be taken that it be not rusty, in which State it has very little Effect.

At the Beginning of this Distemper, and to young Girls, it is sufficient to give twenty Grains daily, enjoining due Exercise and a suitable Diet. When it prevails in a severer Degree, and the Patient is not so young, a Quarter of an Ounce may be safely ventured on: Certain Bitters or Aromatics may be advantageously joined to the Filings, which are numbered in the Appendix, 54, 55, 56, and constitute the most effectual Remedies in this Distemper, to be taken in the Form of Powder, of vinous Infusion, or of Electary.* When there is a just Indication to bring down the Discharge, the vinous Infusion N°. 55 must be given, and generally succeeds: but I must again repeat it (as it should carefully be considered) that the Stoppage or Obstruction of this Discharge is frequently the Effect, not the Cause, of this Disease; and that there should be no Attempt to force it down, which in such a Case, may sometimes prove more hurtful than beneficial; since it would naturally return of its own Accord, on the Recovery, and with the Strength, of the Patient: as their Return should follow that of perfect Health, and neither can precede Health, nor introduce it. There are some

---

* The *French* Word here, *Opiat*, is sometimes used by them for a compound Medicine of the Consistence of an Electary, and cannot be supposed, in this Place, to mean any Preparation, into which *Opium* enters. *K*

some Cases particularly, in which it would be highly dangerous to use hot and active Medicines, such Cases for Instance, as are attended with some Degree of Fever, a frequent Coughing, a Hæmorrhage, or Bleeding, with great Leanness and considerable Thirst: all which Complaints should be removed, before any hot Medicines are given to force this Evacuation, which many very ignorantly imagine cures all other female Disorders; an Error, that has prematurely occasioned the Loss of many Womens' Lives.

§ 361. While the Patient is under a Course of these Medicines, she should not take any of those I have forbidden in the preceding Sections; and the Efficacy of these should also be furthered with proper Exercise. That in a Carriage is very healthy; Dancing is so too, provided it be not extended to an Excess. In Case of a Relapse in these Disorders, the Patient is to be treated, as if it were an original Attack.

§ 362. The other Sort of Obstructions described § 354 requires a very different Treatment. Bleeding, which is hurtful in the former Sort, and the Use, or rather Abuse, of which has thrown several young Women into irrecoverable Weaknesses, has often removed this latter Species, as it were, in a Moment. Bathing of the Feet, the Powders N°. 20, and Whey have frequently succeeded: but at other Times it is necessary to accommodate the Remedies and the Method to each particular Case, and to judge of it

from

from its own peculiar Circumstances and Appearances.

§ 363. When these Evacuations naturally cease through Age (See § 359) if they stop suddenly and all at once, and had formerly flowed very largely, Bleeding must, 1, necessarily be directed, and repeated every six, every four, or even every three Months.

2, The usual Quantity of Food should be somewhat diminished, especially of Flesh, of Eggs and of strong Drink.

3, Exercise should be increased.

4, The Patient should frequently take, in a Morning fasting, the Powder N°. 24, which is very beneficial in such Cases, as it moderately increases the natural Excretions by Stool, Urine and Perspiration; and thence lessens that Quantity of Blood, which would otherwise superabound.

Nevertheless, should this total Cessation of the monthly Discharge be preceded by, or attended with, any extraordinary Loss of Blood, which is frequently the Case, Bleeding is not so necessary; but the Regimen and Powder just directed are very much so, to which the Purge N°. 23 should now and then be joined, at moderate Intervals. The Use of astringent Medicines at this critical Time might dispose the Patient to a Cancer of the Womb.

Many Women die about this Age, as it is but too easy a Matter to injure them then; a Circumstance

cumstance that should make them very cautious and prudent in the Medicines they recur to. On the other Hand it also frequently happens, that their Constitutions alter for the better, after this critical Time of Life; their Fibres grow stronger; they find themselves sensibly more hearty and hardy; many former slight Infirmities disappear, and they enjoy a healthy and happy old Age. I have known several who threw away their Spectacles at the Age of fifty-two, or fifty-three, which they had used five or six Years before.

The Regimen I have just directed, the Powder N°. 24, and the Potion N°. 32, agree very well in almost all inveterate Discharges (I speak of the female Peasantry) at whatever Time of Life.

Of Disorders attending Gravidation, or the Term of going with Child.

§ 364. Gravidation is generally a less ailing or unhealthy State in the Country, than in very populous Towns. Nevertheless Country Women are subject, as well as Citizens, to Pains of the Stomach, to vomiting in a Morning, to Headach and Tooth-ach; but these Complaints very commonly yield to Bleeding, which is almost the only Remedy necessary * for pregnant Women.

§ 365.

---

* Too great a Fulness of Blood is undoubtedly the Cause of all these Complaints, but as there are different Methods of opposing this Cause, the gentlest should always be preferred, nor should the Constitution become habituated to such Remedies, as might either impair the Strength of the Mother, or of her Fruit. Some Expedients

§ 365. Sometimes after carrying too heavy Burthens; after too much or too violent Work; after receiving excessive Jolts, or having had a Fall, they are subject to violent Pains of the Loins, which extend down to their Thighs, and terminate quite at the Bottom of the Belly; and which commonly import, that they are in Danger of an Abortion, or Miscarrying

To prevent this Consequence, which is always dangerous, they should, 1, immediately go to Bed; and if they have not a Mattrass, they should lie upon a Bed stuffed with Straw, a Feather-bed being very improper in such Cases. They should repose, or keep themselves quite still in this Situation for several Days, not stirring, and speaking as little as possible.

2, They should directly lose eight or nine Ounces of Blood from the Arm

3, They should not eat Flesh, Flesh-broth, nor Eggs; but live solely on Soups made of farinaceous or mealy Substances.

4.

dients therefore should be thought of, that may compensate for the Want of Bleeding, by enjoining proper Exercise in a clear Air, with a less nourishing, and a less juicy Diet *E L*

This Note might have its Use sometimes, in the Cases of such delicate and hysterical, yet pregnant Women, as are apt to suffer from Bleeding, or any other Evacuation, though no ways immoderate But it should have been considered, that Dr Tissot was professedly writing here to hearty active Country Wives, who are very rarely thus constituted, and whom he might be unwilling to confuse with such multiplied Distinctions and Directions, as would very seldom be necessary, and might sometimes prevent them from doing what was to Besides which, this Editor might have seen, our Author has hinted at such Cases very soon after *K*

peculiar to Women.

4, They should take every two Hours half a Paper of the Powder N°. 20; and should drink nothing but the Ptisan N°. 2.

Some sanguine robust Women are very liable to miscarry at a certain Time, or Stage, of their Pregnancy. This may be obviated by their bleeding some Days before that Time approaches, and by their observing the Regimen I have advised. But this Method would avail very little for delicate Citizens, who miscarry from a very different Cause; and whose Abortions are to be prevented by a very different Treatment.

Of Delivery, or Child-birth.

§ 366. It has been observed that a greater Proportion of Women die in the Country in, or very speedily after, their Delivery, and that from the Scarcity of good Assistance, and the great Plenty of what is bad; and that a greater Proportion of those in Cities die after their Labours are effected, by a Continuance of their former bad Health.

The Necessity there is for better instructed, better qualified Midwives, through a great Part of *Swisserland*, is but too manifest an Unhappiness, which is attended with the most fatal Consequences, and which merits the utmost Attention of the Government.

The Errors which are incurred, during actual Labour, are numberless, and too often indeed are also irremediable. It would require a whole Book,

Book, expressly for that Purpose (and in some Countries there are such) to give all the Directions that are necessary, to prevent so many Fatalities: and it would be as necessary to form a sufficient Number of well-qualified Midwives to comprehend, and to observe them; which exceeds the Plan of the Work I have proposed. I shall only mark out one of the Causes, and the most injurious one on this Occasion: This is the Custom of giving hot irritating Things, whenever the Labour is very painful, or is slow; such as Castor, or its Tincture, Saffron, Sage, Rue, Savin, Oil of Amber, Wine, Venice Treacle, Wine burnt with Spices, Coffee, Brandy, Aniseed-Water, Walnut-Water, Fennel-Water, and other Drams or strong Liquors. All these Things are so many Poisons in this Respect, which, very far from promoting the Woman's Delivery, render it more difficult by inflaming the Womb (which cannot then so well contract itself) and the Parts, through which the Birth is to pass, in Consequence of which they swell, become more straitened, and cannot yield or be dilated. Sometimes these stimulating hot Medicines also bring on Hæmorrhages, which prove mortal in a few Hours.

§ 367. A considerable Number, both of Mothers and Infants, might be preserved by the directly opposite Method. As soon as a Woman who was in very good Health, just before the Approach of her Labour, being robust and well made, finds her Travail come on, and that it is

painful

painful and difficult, far from encouraging those premature Efforts, which are always destructive; and from furthering them by the pernicious Medicines I have just enumerated, the Patient should be bled in the Arm, which will prevent the Swelling and Inflammation; aſſwage the Pains; relax the Parts, and diſpoſe every thing to a favourable Iſſue.

During actual Labour no other Nouriſhment ſhould be allowed, except a little Panada every three Hours, and as much Toaſt and Water, as the Woman chuſes.

Every fourth Hour a Glyſter ſhould be given, conſiſting of a Decoction of Mallows and a little Oil. In the Intervals between theſe Glyſters ſhe ſhould be ſet over a kind of Stove, or in a pierced eaſy Chair, containing a Veſſel in which there is ſome hot Water: the Paſſage ſhould be gently rubbed with a little Butter; and Stupes wrung out of a Fomentation of ſimple hot Water, which is the moſt efficacious of any, ſhould be applied over the Belly.

The Midwives, by taking this Method, are not only certain of doing no Miſchief, but they alſo allow Nature an Opportunity of doing Good: as a great many Labours, which ſeem difficult at firſt, terminate happily; and this ſafe and unprecipitate Manner of proceeding at leaſt affords Time to call in further Aſſiſtance. Beſides, the Conſequences of ſuch Deliveries are healthy and happy, when by purſuing the heating oppreſſing Practice, even though the Delivery be effected, both

Mother and Infant have been so cruelly, though undesignedly, tormented, that both of them frequently perish.

§ 368. I acknowledge these Means are insufficient, when the Child is unhappily situated in the Womb; or when there is an embarrassing Conformation in the Mother: though at least they prevent the Case from proving worse, and leave Time for calling in Men-Midwives, or other female ones, who may be better qualified.

I beg leave again to remind the Midwives, that they should be very cautious of urging their Women to make any forced Efforts to forward the Birth, which are extremely injurious to them, and which may render a Delivery very dangerous and embarrassing, that might otherwise have been happily effected: and I insist the more freely on the Danger attending these unseasonable Efforts, and on the very great Importance of Patience, as the other very pernicious Practice is become next to universal amongst us.

The Weakness, in which the labouring Woman appears, makes the By-standers fearful that she will not have Strength enough to be delivered; which they think abundantly justifies them in giving her Cordials; but this Way of Reasoning is very weak and chimerical. Their Strength, on such Occasions, is not so very speedily dissipated: the small light Pains sink them, but in Proportion as the Pains become stronger, their Strength arises; being never deficient, when there is no extraordinary and uncommon Symptom;
and

peculiar to Women.

and we may reasonably be assured, that in a healthy, well formed Woman, meer Weakness never prevents a Delivery.

Of the Consequences of Labour, or Child-birth.

§ 369. The most usual Consequences of Child-birth in the Country are, 1, An excessive Hæmorrhage. 2. An Inflammation of the Womb. 3, A sudden Suppression of the *Lochia,* or usual Discharges after Delivery. And, 4, the Fever and other Accidents, resulting from the Milk.

Excessive Bleedings or Floodings, should be treated according to the Manner directed § 365: and if they are very excessive, Folds of Linen, which have been wrung out of a Mixture of equal Parts of Water and Vinegar, should be applied to the Belly, the Loins, and the Thighs: these should be changed for fresh moist ones, as they dry; and should be omitted, as soon as the Bleeding abates.

§ 370. The Inflammation of the Womb is discoverable by Pains in all the lower Parts of the Belly; by a Tension or Tightness of the whole; by a sensible Increase of Pain upon touching it; a kind of red Stain or Spot, that mounts to the Middle of the Belly, as high as the Navel; which Spot, as the Disease increases, turns black, and then is always a mortal Symptom; by a very extraordinary Degree of Weakness; an astonishing Change of Countenance; a light *Delirium* or Raving, a continual Fever with a weak and hard Pulse;

Pulse; sometimes incessant Vomitings; a frequent Hiccup; a moderate Discharge of a reddish, stinking, sharp Water, frequent Urgings to go to Stool, a burning kind of Heat of Urine; and sometimes an entire Suppression of it.

§ 371. This most dangerous and frequently mortal Disease should be treated like inflammatory ones. After Bleeding, frequent Glysters of warm Water must by no Means be omitted; some shou'd also be injected into the Womb, and applied continually over the Belly. The Patient may also drink continually, either of simple Barley-Water, with a Quarter of an Ounce of Nitre in every Pot of it, or of Almond Milk N°. 4.

§ 372 The total Suppression of the *Lochia*, the Discharges after Labour, which proves a Cause of the most violent Disorders, should be treated exactly in the same Manner: but if unhappily hot Medicines have been given, in order to force them down, the Case will very generally prove a most hopeless one.

§ 373. If the Milk-fever run very high, the Barley Ptisan directed § 371, and Glysters, with a very light Diet, consisting only of Panada, or made of some other farinaceous Substances, and very thin, very generally remove it.

§ 374 Delicate infirm Women, who have not all the requisite and necessary Attendance they want, and such as from Indigence are obliged to work too soon, are exposed to many Accidents, which frequently arise from a Want of of due Perspiration, and an insufficient Discharge of the *Lochia*; and hence, the Separation of the Milk in their Breasts being disturbed, there are milky Congestions, or Knots as it were, which are always very painful and troublesome, and especially when they are formed more inwardly. They often happen on the Thighs, in which Case the Ptisan N°. 58 is to be drank, and the Pultices N° 59 must be applied. These two Remedies gradually dissipate and remove the Tumour, if that may be effected without Suppuration. But if that proves impossible, and *Pus*, or Matter, is actually formed, a Surgeon must open the Abscess, and treat it like any other.

§ 375. Should the Milk coagulate, or curdle as it were, in the Breast, it is of the utmost Importance immediately to attenuate or dissolve that Thickness, which would otherwise degenerate into a Hardness and prove a *Scirrhus*, and from a *Scirrhus* in Process of Time a Cancer, that most tormenting and cruel Distemper.

This horrible Evil however may be prevented by an Application to these small Tumours, as soon as ever they appear. For this Purpose nothing is more effectual than the Prescriptions N°. 57 and 60, but under such menacing Circumstances, it is always prudent to take the best Advice, as early as possible.

From the Moment these hard Tumours become excessively and obstinately so, and yet without any Pain, we should abstain from every Application, all are injurious, and greasy, sharp, resinous and spirituous ones speedily change the *Scirrhus* into a Cancer. Whenever it becomes manifestly such, all Applications are also equally pernicious, except that of N°. 60. Cancers have long been thought and found incurable; but within a few Years past some have been cured by the Remedy N°. 57, which nevertheless is not infallible, though it should always be tried.*

§ 376. The Nipples of Women, who give Milk, are often fretted or excoriated, which proves very severely painful to them. One of the best Applications is the most simple Ointment, being a Mixture of Oil and Wax melted together; or the Ointment N°. 66. Should the Complaint prove very obstinate, the Nurse ought to be purged, which generally removes it.

CHAPTER

---

* The Use of Hemlock, which has been tried at *Lyons*, by all who have had cancerous Patients, having been given in very large Doses, has been attended with no Effect there, that merited the serious Attention of Practitioners. Many were careful to obtain the Extract from *Vienna*, and even to procure it from Dr *Storck* himself. But now it appears to have had so little Success, as to become entirely neglected. E L

Having exactly translated in this Place, and in the Table of Remedies, our learned Author's considerable Recommendation of the Extract of Hemlock in Cancers, we think it but fair, on the other Hand, to publish this Note of his Editor's against it; that the real Efficacy or Inefficacy of this Medicine may at length be ascertained, on the most extensive Evidence and Experience. As far as my own Opportunities and Reflections, and the Experience of many others have instructed me on this Subject, it appears clear to myself, that though the Consequences of it have not been constantly unsuccessful with us, yet its Successes have come very short of its Failures. Nevertheless, as in all such Cancers, every other internal Medicine almost universally fails, we think with Dr. Tissot, it should always be tried (from the meer Possibility of its succeeding in some particular Habit and Circumstances) at least till longer Experience shall finally determine against it. K

Chapter XXVII.

Medical Directions concerning Children.

Sect. 377.

THE Diseases of Children, and every Thing relating to their Health, are Objects which generally seem to have been two much neglected by Physicians; and have been too long confided to the Conduct of the most improper Persons for such a Charge. At the same Time it must be admitted their Health is of no little Importance; their Preservation is as necessary as the Continuance of the human Race, and the Application of the Practice of Physick to their Disorders is susceptible of nearer Approaches to Perfection, than is generally conceived. It seems to have even some Advantage over that Practice which regards grown Persons, and it consists in this, that the Diseases of Children are more simple, and less frequently complicated than those of Adults.

It may be said indeed, they cannot make themselves so well understood, and meer Infants certainly not at all. This is true in Fact to a certain Degree, but not rigidly true; for though they do not speak our Language, they have one which we should contrive to understand. Nay every Distemper may be said, in some Sense, to have a Language of its own, which an attentive Physician will learn. He should therefore use his utmost Care to understand that of Infants, and avail himself of it, to increase the Means of rendering them healthy and vigorous, and to cure them of the different Distempers to which they are liable. I do not propose actually to compleat this Task myself, in all that Extent it may justly demand; but I shall set forth the principal Causes of their Distempers, and the general Method of treating them. By this Means I shall at least preserve them from some of the Mischiefs which are too frequently done them; and the lessening such Evils as Ignorance, or erroneous Practice, occasions, is one of the most important Purposes of the present Work

§ 378. Nearly all the Children who die before they are one Year, and even two Years, old, die *with* Convulsions. People say they died *of* them, which is partly true, as it is in Effect, the Convulsions that have destroyed them. But then these very Convulsions are the Consequences, the Effects, of other Diseases, which require the utmost Attention of those, who are entrusted with the Care and Health of the little Innocents: as an effectual Opposition to these Diseases, these morbid Causes, is the only Means of removing the Convulsions. The four principal known Causes are, the *Meconium*; the Excrements contained in the Body of the Infant, at the Birth, *Acidities*, or sharp and sour Humours; the

the Cutting of the Teeth, and Worms. I shall treat briefly of each.

Of the Meconium.

§ 379. The Stomach and Guts of the Infant, at its Entrance into the World, are filled with a black Sort of Matter, of a middling Confistence, and very viscid or glutinous, which is called the *Meconium*. It is necessary this Matter should be discharged before the Infant sucks, since it would otherwise corrupt the Milk, and, becoming extremely sharp itself, there would result from their Mixture a double Source of Evils, to the Destruction of the Infant.

The Evacuation of this Excrement is procured, 1, By giving them no Milk at all for the first twenty-four Hours of their Lives. 2, By making them drink during that Time some Water, to which a little Sugar or Honey must be added, which will dilute this *Meconium*, and promote the Discharge of it by Stool, and sometimes by vomiting.

To be the more certain of expelling all this Matter, they should take one Ounce of Compound Syrup * of Succory, which should be diluted

---

* This Method (says the Editor and Annotator of *Lyons*) is useful, whenever the Mother does not suckle her Child. Art is then obliged to prove a Kind of Substitute to Nature, though always a very imperfect one. But when a Mother, attentive to her own true Interest, as well as her Infant's, and, listening to the Voice of Nature and her Duty, suckles it herself, these Remedies

[he

luted with a little Water, drinking up this Quantity within the Space of four or five Hours. This Practice is a very beneficial one, and it is to be wished it were to become general. This Syrup is greatly preferable to all others, given in such Cases, and especially to Oil of Almonds.

Should the great Weakness of the Child seem to call for some Nourishment, there would be no Inconvenience in allowing a little Biscuit well boiled in Water, which is pretty commonly done, or a little very thin light Panada.

Of

[he adds] seem hurtful, or at least, useless. The Mother should give her Child the Breast as soon as she can. The first Milk, the *Colostrum*, or *Strippings*, as it is called in Quadrupeds, which is very serous or watery, will be serviceable as a Purgative, it will forward the Expulsion of the *Meconium*, prove gradually nourishing, and is better than Biscuits, or Panada, which (he thinks) are dangerous in the first Days after the Birth. *E L*

This Syrup of Succory being scarcely ever prepared with us, though sufficiently proper for the Use assigned it here, I have retained the preceding Note, as the Author of it directs these *Strippings*, for the same Purpose, with an Air of certain Experience, and as this Effect of them seems no Ways repugnant to the physical Wisdom and Oeconomy of Nature, on such important Points. Should it in fact be their very general Operation, it cannot be unknown to any Male or Female Practitioner in Midwifery, and may save poor People a little Expence, which was one Object of our humane Author's Plan. The Oil of *Ricinus*, corruptly called *Castor* Oil (being expressed from the Berries of the *Palma Christi*) is particularly recommended by some late medical Writers from *Jamaica*, &c. for this Purpose of expelling the *Meconium*, to the Quantity of a small Spoonful. These Gentlemen also consider it as the most proper, and almost specific Opener, in the dry Belly-ach of that torrid Climate, which tormenting Disease has the closest Affinity to the *Miserere*, or Iliac Passion, of any I have seen. The Annotator's Objection to our Author's very *thin light* Panada, seems to be of little Weight. *K.*

Of Acidities, or sharp Humours.

§ 380. Notwithstanding the Bodies of Children have been properly emptied speedily after their Birth, yet the Milk very often turns sour in their Stomachs, producing Vomitings, violent Cholics, Convulsions, a Looseness, and even terminating in Death. There are but two Purposes to be pursued in such Cases, which are to carry off the sour or sharp Humours, and to prevent the Generation of more. The first of these Intentions is best effected by the Syrup of Succory* just mentioned.

The Generation of further Acidities is prevented, by giving three Doses daily, if the Symptoms are violent, and but two, or even one only, if they are very moderate, of the Powder N°. 61, drinking after it Bawm Tea, or a Tea of Lime-tree Leaves.

§ 381. It has been a Custom to load Children with Oil of Almonds,† as soon as ever they are infested with Gripes: but it is a pernicious Custom, and attended with very dangerous Consequences. It it very true that this Oil sometimes immediately allays the Gripes, by involving, or sheathing up, as it were, the acid Humours, and somewhat blunting the Sensibility of the Nerves. But it proves only a palliative Remedy, or assuaging for a Time, which, far from removing, increases
the

---

* Or, for Want of it, the solutive Syrup of Roses *K*
† The *Magnesia* is an excellent Substitute in Children, for these Oils Dr Tissot so justly condemns here *K*

the Cause, since it becomes sharp and rancid itself, whence the Disorder speedily returns, and the more Oil the Infant takes, it is griped the more. I have cured some Children of such Disorders, without any other Remedy, except abstaining from Oil, which weakens their Stomachs, whence their Milk is less perfectly, and more slowly digested, and becomes more easily soured. Besides this Weakness of the Stomach, which thus commences at that very early Age, has sometimes an unhealthy Influence on the Constitution of the Child, throughout the Remainder of his Life.

A free and open Belly is beneficial to Children; now it is certain that the Oil very often binds them, in Consequence of its diminishing the Force and Action of the Bowels. There is scarcely any Person, who cannot observe this Inconvenience attending it, notwithstanding they all continue to advise and to give it, to obtain a very different Purpose: But such is the Power of Prejudice in this Case, and in so many others; People are so strongly pre-possessed with a Notion, that such a Medicine must produce such an Effect, that its never having produced it avails nothing with them, their Prejudice still prevails, they ascribe its Want of Efficacy to the Smallness of the Doses, these are doubled then, and notwithstanding its bad Effects are augmented, their obstinate Blindness continues.

This Abuse of the Oil also disposes the Child to knotty hard Tumours, and at length often

proves

proves the first Cause of some Diseases of the Skin, whose Cure is extremely difficult.

Hence it is evident, this Oil should be used on such Occasions but very seldom; and that it is always very injudicious to give it in Cholics, which arise from sharp and sour Humours in the Stomach, or in the Bowels.

§ 382 Infants are commonly most subject to such Cholics during their earliest Months; after which they abate, in Proportion as their Stomachs grow stronger. They may be relieved in the Fit by Glysters of a Decoction of Chamomile Flowers, in which a Bit of Soap of the Size of a Hazel Nut is dissolved. A Piece of Flanel wrung out of a Decoction of Chamomile Flowers, with the Addition of some Venice Treacle, and applied hot over the Stomach and on the Belly, is also very beneficial, and relieving.

Children cannot always take Glysters, the Continuance of which Circumstance might be dangerous to them, and every one is acquainted with the common Method of substituting Suppositories to them, whether they are formed of the smooth and supple Stalks of Vines, &c. of Soap, or of Honey boiled up to a proper Consistence

But one of the most certain Means to prevent these Cholics, which are owing to Children's not digesting their Milk, is to move and exercise them as much as possible, having a due Regard however to their tender Time of Life.

§ 383. Before I proceed to the third Cause of the Diseases of Children, which is, the Cutting of their Teeth, I muſt take Notice of the firſt Cares their Birth immediately requires, that is the Waſhing of them the firſt Time, meerly to cleanſe, and afterwards, to ſtrengthen them.

Of waſhing Children.

§ 384. The whole Body of an Infant juſt born is covered with a groſs Humour, which is occaſioned by the Fluids, in which it was ſuſpended in the Womb. There is a Neceſſity to cleanſe it directly from this, for which nothing is ſo proper as a Mixture of one third Wine, and two thirds Water; Wine alone would be dangerous. This Waſhing may be repeated ſome Days ſucceſſively; but it is a bad Cuſtom to continue to waſh them thus warm, the Danger of which is augmented by adding ſome Butter to the Wine and Water, which is done too often. If this groſs Humour, that covers the Child, ſeems more thick and glutinous than ordinary, a Decoction of Chamomile Flowers, with a little Bit of Soap, may be uſed to remove it. The Regularity of Perſpiration is the great Foundation of Health; to procure this Regularity the Teguments, the Skin, muſt be ſtrengthened, but warm Waſhing tends to weaken it. When it is of a proper Strength it always performs its Functions; nor is Perſpiration diſordered ſenſibly by the Alteration of the Weather. For this Reaſon nothing ſhould be omitted, that may fix it in this State; and to attain ſo important an Advantage, Children

dren should be washed, some few Days after their Birth, with cold Water, in the State it is brought from the Spring.

For this Purpose a Spunge is employed, with which they begin, by washing first the Face, the Ears, the back Part of the Head (carefully avoiding the * *Fontanelle*, or Mould of the Head) the Neck, the Loins, the Trunck of the Body, the Thighs, Legs and Arms, and in short every Spot. This Method which has obtained for so many Ages, and which is practised at present by many People, who prove very healthy, will appear shocking to several Mothers; they would be afraid of killing their Children by it; and would particularly fail of Courage enough to endure the Cries, which Children often make, the first Time they are washed. Yet if their Mothers truly love them, they cannot give a more substantial Mark of their Tenderness to them, than by subduing their Fears and their Repugnance, on this important Head.

Weakly Infants † are those who have the greatest Need of being washed: such as are remarkably strong may be excused from it; and it seems scarcely credible (before a Person has frequently

seen

---

* That Part of the Head where a Pulsation may be very plainly felt, where the Bones are less hard, and not as yet firmly joined with those about them

† There is however a certain Degree of Weakness, which may very reasonably deter us from this Washing, as when the Infant manifestly wants Heat, and needs some Cordial and frequent Frictions, to prevent its expiring from downright Feebleness; in which Circumstances Washing must be hurtful to it. Tissot.

seen the Consequences of it) how greatly this Method conduces to give, and to hasten on, their Strength. I have had the Pleasure to observe, since I first endeavoured to introduce the Custom among us, that several of the most affectionate and most sensible Mothers, have used it with the greatest Success. The Midwives, who have been Witnesses of it; the Nurses and the Servants of the Children, whom they have washed, publish it abroad; and should the Custom become as general, as every thing seems to promise it will, I am fully persuaded, that by preserving the Lives of a great Number of Children, it will certainly contribute to check the Progress of Depopulation.

They should be washed very regularly every Day, in every Season, and every Sort of Weather, and in the fine warm Season they should be plunged into a large Pail of Water, into the Basins around Fountains, in a Brook, a River, or a Lake

After a few Days crying, they grow so well accustomed to this Exercise, that it becomes one of their Pleasures; so that they laugh all the Time of their going through it.

The first Benefit of this Practice is, as I have already said, the keeping up their Perspiration, and rendering them less obnoxious to the Impressions of the Air and Weather: and it is also in Consequence of this first Benefit, that they are preserved from a great Number of Maladies, especially from knotty Tumours, often called Kernels;

Kernels; from Obstructions; from Diseases of the Skin, and from Convulsions, its general Consequence being to insure them firm, and even robust Health.

§ 385. But Care should be taken not to prevent, or, as it were to undo, the Benefit this Washing procures them, by the bad Custom of keeping them too hot. There is not a more pernicious one than this, nor one that destroys more Children. They should be accustomed to light Cloathing by Day, and light Covering by Night, to go with their Heads very thinly covered, and not at all in the Day-time, after their attaining the Age of two Years. They should avoid sleeping in Chambers that are too hot, and should live in the open Air, both in Summer and Winter, as much as possible. Children who have been kept too hot in such Respects, are very often liable to Colds; they are weakly, pale, languishing, bloated and melancholy. They are subject to hard knotty Swellings, a Consumption, all Sorts of languid Disorders, and either die in their Infancy, or only grow up into a miserable valetudinary Life, while those who are washed or plunged into cold Water, and habitually exposed to the open Air, are just in the opposite Circumstances.

§ 386. I must further add here, that Infancy is not the only Stage of Life, in which cold Bathing is advantagious. I have advised it with remarkable Success to Persons of every Age, even to that of seventy: and there are two Kinds of Diseases, more frequent indeed in Cities than in the Country, in which cold Baths succeed very greatly; that is, in Debility, or Weakness of the Nerves; and when Perspiration is disordered, when Persons are fearful of every Breath of Air, liable to Defluxions or Colds, feeble and languishing, the cold Bath re-establishes Perspiration; restores Strength to the Nerves; and by that Means dispels all the Disorders, which arise from these two Causes, in the animal Oeconomy. They should be used before Dinner. But in the same Proportion that cold Bathing is beneficial, the habitual Use, or rather Abuse, of warm Bathing is pernicious; they dispose the Persons addicted to them to the Apoplexy; to the Dropsy; to Vapours, and to the hypochondriacal Disease: and Cities, in which they are too frequently used, become, in some Measure, desolate from such Distempers.

Of the Cutting of the Teeth.

§ 387. Cutting of the Teeth is often very tormenting to Children, some dying under the severe Symptoms attending it. If it proves very painful, we should during that Period, 1, Keep their Bellies open by Glysters consisting only of a simple Decoction of Mallows but Glysters are not necessary, if the Child, as it sometimes happens then, has a Purging

2, Their ordinary Quantity of Food should be lessened for two Reasons, first, because the Stomach

mach is then weaker than usual; and next, because a small Fever sometimes accompanies the Cutting.

3, Their usual Quantity of Drink should be increased a little; the best for them certainly is an Infusion of the Leaves or Flowers, of the Lime or Linden-tree, to which a little Milk may be added.

4, Their Gums should frequently be rubbed with a Mixture of equal Parts of Honey, and Mucilage of Quince-seeds; and a Root of March-Mallows, or of Liquorice, may be given them to chew.

It frequently happens, that during Dentition, or the Time of their toothing, Children prove subject to Knots or Kernels.

Of Worms.

§ 388. The *Meconium*, the Acidity of the Milk, and Cutting of the Teeth are the three great Causes of the Diseases of Children. There is also a fourth, Worms, which is likewise very often pernicious to them, but which, nevertheless, is not, at least not near so much, a general Cause of their Disorders, as it is generally supposed, when a Child exceeding two Years of Age proves sick. There are a great Variety of Symptoms, which dispose People to think a Child has Worms, though there is but one that demonstrates it, which is discharging them upwards or downwards. There is great Difference among

Children too in this Respect, some remaining healthy, though having several Worms, and others being really sick with a few.

They prove hurtful, 1, by obstructing the Guts, and compressing the neighbouring Bowels by their Size. 2, By sucking up the Chyle intended to nourish the Patient, and thus depriving him of his very Substance as well as Subsistence; and, 3, by irritating the Guts and even * gnawing them.

§ 389. The Symptoms which make it probable they are infested with Worms, are slight, frequent and irregular Cholics; a great Quantity of Spittle running off while they are fasting; a disagreeable Smell of their Breath, of a particular Kind, especially in the Morning; a frequent Itchiness of their Noses which makes them scratch or rub them often, a very irregular Appetite, being sometimes voracious, and at other Times having none at all: Pains at Stomach and Vomitings: sometimes a costive Belly; but more frequently loose Stools of indigested Matter; the Belly rather larger than ordinary, the rest of the Body

---

* I have seen a Child about three Years old, whose Navel, after swelling and inflaming, suppurated, and through a small Orifice which must have communicated with the Cavity of the Gut or the Belly discharged one of these Worms we call *teretes*, about three Inches long. He had voided several by Stool, after taking some vermifuge medicines. The Fact I perfectly remember, and to the best of my Recollection, the Ulcer healed some Time after, and the Orifice closed; but the Child died the following Year of a ... Fever, which might be caused, or was aggravated, by Worms. A

Body meagre; a Thirst which no Drink allays; often great Weakness, and some Degree of Melancholy. The Countenance has generally an odd unhealthy Look, and varies every Quarter of an Hour; the Eyes often look dull, and are surrounded with a Kind of livid Circle: the White of the Eye is sometimes visible while they sleep, their Sleep being often attended with terrifying Dreams or *Deliriums*, and with continual Startings, and Grindings of their Teeth. Some Children find it impossible to be at Rest for a single Moment. Their Urine is often whitish, I have seen it from some as white as Milk. They are afflicted with Palpitations, Swoonings, Convulsions, long and profound Drowsiness; cold Sweats which come on suddenly, Fevers which have the Appearances of Malignity; Obscurities and even Loss of Sight and of Speech, which continue for a considerable Time; Palsies either of their Hands, their Arms, or their Legs, and Numbnesses. Their Gums are in a bad State, and as though they had been gnawed or corroded: they have often the Hickup, a small and irregular Pulse, Ravings, and, what is one of the least doubtful Symptoms, frequently a small dry Cough, and not seldom a Mucosity or Sliminess in their Stools: sometimes very long and violent Cholics, which terminate in an Abscess on the Outside of the Belly, from whence Worms issue. (See Note * p. 388.)

§ 390. There are a great Multitude of Medicines against Worms. The *Grenette* or Wormseed, which is one of the commonest, is a very good one. The Prescription N°. 62, is also a very successful one; and the Powder N°. 14 is one of the best. Flower of Brimstone, the Juice of *Nasturtium*, or Cresses, Acids and Honey Water have often been very serviceable; but the first three I have mentioned, succeeded by a Purge, are the best. N°. 63 is a purging Medicine, that the most averse and difficult Children may easily take. But when, notwithstanding these Medicines, the Worms are not expelled, it is necessary to take Advice of some Person qualified to prescribe more efficacious ones. This is of considerable Importance, because, notwithstanding a great Proportion of Children may probably have Worms, and yet many of them continue in good Health, there are, nevertheless, some who are really killed by Worms, after having been cruelly tormented by them for several Years.

A Disposition to breed Worms always shews the Digestions are weak and imperfect, for which Reason Children liable to Worms should not be nourished with Food difficult to digest. We should be particularly careful not to stuff them with Oils, which, admitting such Oils should immediately kill some of their Worms, do

---

* This Word occurs in none of the common Dictionaries; but suspecting it for the *Semen Santonici* of the Shops, I find the learned Dr Parker has rendered it so, in his very well received Translation of the valuable Work into Low Dutch. K.

do yet increase that Cause, which disposes them to generate others. A long continued Use of Filings of Iron is the Remedy, that most effectually destroys this Disposition to generate Worms.

Of Convulsions.

§ 391. I have already said, § 378, that the Convulsions of Children are almost constantly the Effect of some other Disease, and especially of some of the four I have mentioned. Some other, though less frequent Causes, sometimes occasion them, and these may be reduced to the following.

The first of them is the corrupted Humours, that often abound in their Stomachs and Intestines; and which, by their Irritation, produce irregular Motions throughout the whole System of the Nerves, or at least through some Parts of them; whence these Convulsions arise, which are merely involuntary Motions of the Muscles. These putrid Humours are the Consequence of too great a Load of Aliments, of unsound ones, or of such, as the Stomachs of Children are incapable of digesting. These Humours are also sometimes the Effect of a Mixture and Confusion of different Aliments, and of a bad Distribution of their Nourishment

It may be known that the Convulsions of a Child are owing to this Cause, by the Circumstances that have preceded them, by a disgusted loathing Stomach; by a certain Heaviness and

Load at it; by a foul Tongue; a great Belly; by its bad Complexion, and its disturbed unrefreshing Sleep.

The Child's proper Diet, that is, a certain Diminution of the Quantity of its Food; some Glysters of warm Water, and one Purge of N°. 63, very generally remove such Convulsions.

§ 392. The second Cause is the bad Quality of their Milk. Whether it be that the Nurse has fallen into a violent Passion, some considerable Disgust, great Fright or frequent Fear: whether she has eat unwholesome Food, drank too much Wine, spirituous Liquors, or any strong Drink: whether she is seized with a Descent of her monthly Discharges, and that has greatly disordered her Health, or finally whether she prove really sick. In all these Cases the Milk is vitiated, and exposes the Infant to violent Symptoms, which sometimes speedily destroy it.

The Remedies for Convulsions, from this Cause, consist, 1, In letting the Child abstain from this corrupted Milk, until the Nurse shall have recovered her State of Health and Tranquillity, the speedy Attainment of which may be forwarded by a few Glysters, by gentle pacific Medicines; by an entire Absence of whatever caused or conduced to her bad Health; and by drawing off all the Milk that had been so vitiated.

2, In giving the Child itself some Glysters: in making it drink plentifully of a light Infusion of the Lime-tree Leaves; in giving it no other
Nourishment

Nourishment for a Day or two, except Panada and other light Spoon-meat, without Milk.

3, In purging the Child (supposing what has been just directed to have been unavailable) with an Ounce, or an Ounce and a Half, of compound Syrup of Succory, or as much Manna. These lenient gentle Purges carry off the Remainder of the corrupted Milk, and remove the Disorders occasioned by it.

§ 393. A third Cause which also produces Convulsions, is the feverish Distempers which attack Children, especially the Small-pocks and the Measles; but in general such Convulsions require no other Treatment, but that proper for the Disease, which has introduced them.

§ 394. It is evident from what has been said in the Course of this Chapter, and it deserves to be attended to, that Convulsions are commonly a Symptom attending some other Disease, rather than an original Disease themselves: that they depend on many different Causes; that from this Consideration there can be no general Remedy for removing or checking them; and that the only Means and Medicines which are suitable in each Case, are those, which are proper to oppose the particular Cause producing them, which I have already pointed out in treating of each Cause.

The greater Part of the pretended Specifics, which are indiscriminately and ignorantly employed in all Sorts of Convulsions, are often useless,

less, and still oftner prejudicial. Of this last Sort and Character are,

1, All sharp and hot Medicines, spirituous Liquors, Oil of Amber, — other hot Oils and Essences, volatile Salts, and such other Medicines, as, by the Violence of their Action on the irritable Organs of Children, are likelier to produce Convulsions, than to allay them.

2, Astringent Medicines, which are highly pernicious, whenever the Convulsions are caused by any sharp Humour, that ought to be discharged from the Body by Stool; or when such Convulsions are the Consequences of an † Effort of Nature, in Order to effect a *Crisis:* And as they almost ever depend on one or the other of these Causes, it follows that Astringents can very rarely, if ever, be beneficial. Besides that there is always some Danger in giving them to Children without a mature, a thorough Consideration of their particular Case and Situation, as they often dispose them to Obstructions.

3, The over early, and too considerable Use of Opiates, either not properly indicated, or continued too long, such as Venice Treacle, Mithridate, Syrup of Poppies (and it is very easy to run upon some of these Sholes) are also attended with the most embarrassing Events, in Regard to Convulsions; and it may be affirmed they are improper, for nine Tenths of those they are advised

---

† This very important Consideration, on which I have treated pretty largely, in the *last*, seems not to be attended to in Practice, as they ought as it ought.

sed to. It is true they often produce an apparent Ease and Tranquillity for some Minutes, and sometimes for some Hours too; but the Disorder returns even with greater Violence for this Suspension, by Reason they have augmented all the Causes producing it; they impair the Stomach; they bind up the Belly; they lessen the usual Quantity of Urine; and besides, by their abating the Sensibility of the Nerves, which ought to be considered as one of the chief Centinels appointed by Nature, for the Discovery of any approaching Danger, they dispose the Patient insensibly to such Infarctions and Obstructions, as tend speedily to produce some violent and mortal Event, or which generate a Disposition to languid and tedious Diseases: and I do again repeat it, that notwithstanding there are some Cases, in which they are absolutely necessary, they ought in general to be employed with great Precaution and Prudence. To mention the principal Indications for them in convulsive Cases, they are proper,

1, When the Convulsions still continue, after the original Cause of them is removed.

2, When they are so extremely violent, as to threaten a great and very speedy Danger of Life; and when they prove an Obstacle to the taking Remedies calculated to extinguish their Cause; and,

3, When the Cause producing them is of such a Nature, as is apt to yield to the Force of Anodynes;

dynes; as when, for Inſtance, they have been the immediate Conſequence of a Fright.

§ 395. There is a very great Difference in different Children, in Reſpect to their being more or leſs liable to Convulſions. There are ſome, in whom very ſtrong and irritating Cauſes cannot excite them; not even excruciating Gripes and Cholics; the moſt painful Cutting of their Teeth, violent Fevers; the Small Pocks, Meaſles, and though they are, as it were, continually corroded by Worms, they have not the ſlighteſt Tendency to be convulſed. On the other Hand, ſome are ſo very obnoxious to Convulſions, or ſo eaſily *convulſible*, if that Expreſſion may be allowed, that they are very often ſeized with them from ſuch very ſlight Cauſes, that the moſt attentive Conſideration cannot inveſtigate them. This Sort of Conſtitution, which is extremely dangerous, and expoſes the unhappy Subject of it, either to a very ſpeedy Death, or to a very low and languid State of Life, requires ſome peculiar Conſiderations; the Detail of which would be the more foreign to the Deſign of this Treatiſe, as they are pretty common in Cities, but much leſs ſo in Country Places. In general cold Bathing and the Powder N°. 14 are ſerviceable in ſuch Circumſtances.

General Directions, with Reſpect to Children.

§. 396. I ſhall conclude this Chapter by ſuch farther Advice, as may contribute to give Children

dren a more vigorous Constitution and Temperament, and to preserve them from many Disorders.

First then, we should be careful not to cram them too much, and to regulate both the Quantity and the set Time of their Meals, which is a very practicable Thing, even in the very earliest Days of their Life, when the Woman who nurses them, will be careful to do it regularly. Perhaps indeed this is the very Age, when such a Regulation may be the most easily attempted and effected, because it is that Stage, when the constant Uniformity of their Way of living should incline us to suppose, that what they have Occasion for is most constantly very much the same.

A Child who has already attained to a few Years, and who is surrendered up more to his own Exercise and Vivacity, feels other Calls; his Way of Life is become a little more various and irregular, whence his Appetite must prove so too. Hence it would be inconvenient to subject him over exactly to one certain Rule, in the Quantity of his Nourishment, or the Distance of his Meals. The Dissipation or passing off of his Nutrition being unequal, the Occasions he has for repairing it cannot be precisely stated and regular. But with Respect to very little Children in Arms, or on the Lap, a Uniformity in the first of these Respects, the Quantity of their Food, very consistently conduces to a useful Regularity with Respect to the second, the Times of feeding them. Sickness is probably the only Circumstance,

stance, that can warrant any Alteration in the Order and Intervals of their Meals; and then this Change should consist in a Diminution of their usual Quantity, notwithstanding a general and fatal Conduct seems to establish the very Reverse; and this pernicious Fashion authorizes the Nurses to cram these poor little Creatures the more, in Proportion as they have real Need of less feeding. They conclude of Course, that all their Cries are the Effects of Hunger, and the Moment an Infant begins, then they immediately stop his Mouth with his Food; without once suspecting, that these Wailings may be occasioned by the Uneasiness an over-loaded Stomach may have introduced; or by Pains whose Cause is neither removed nor mitigated, by making the Children eat, though the meer Action of eating may render them insensible to slight Pains, for a very few Minutes, in the first Place, by calling off their Attention, and secondly, by hushing them to sleep, a common Effect of feeding in Children, being in fact, a very general and constant one, and depending on the same Causes, which dispose so many grown Persons to sleep after Meals.

A Detail of the many Evils Children are exposed to, by thus forcing too much Food upon them, at the very Time when their Complaints are owing to Causes, very different from Hunger, might appear incredible. They are however so numerous and certain, that I seriously wish sensible Mothers would open their Eyes to the Consideration

ration of this Abuse, and agree to put an End to it.

Those who overload them with Victuals, in Hopes of strengthening them, are extremely deceived; there being no one Prejudice equally fatal to such a Number of them. Whatever unnecessary Aliment a Child receives, weakens, instead of strengthening him. The Stomach, when over-distended, suffers in its Force and Functions, and becomes less able to digest thoroughly. The Excess of the Food last received impairs the Concoction of the Quantity, that was really necessary: which, being badly digested, is so far from yielding any Nourishment to the Infant, that it weakens it, and proves a Source of Diseases, and concurs to produce Obstructions, Rickets, the Evil, slow Fevers, a Consumption and Death.

Another unhappy Custom prevails, with Regard to the Diet of Children, when they begin to receive any other Food besides their Nurse's Milk, and that is, to give them such as exceeds the digestive Power of their Stomachs; and to indulge them in a Mixture of such Things in their Meals, as are hurtful in themselves, and more particularly so, with Regard to their feeble and delicate Organs.

To justify this pernicious Indulgence, they affirm it is necessary to accustom their Stomachs to every Kind of Food, but this Notion is highly absurd, since their Stomachs should first be strengthened, in Order to make them capable of digesting every Food, and crouding indigestible,

or

or very difficultly digestible Materials into it, is not the Way to strengthen it. To make a Foal sufficiently strong for future Labour, he is exempted from any, till he is four Years old; which enables him to submit to considerable Work, without being the worse for it. But if, to inure him to Fatigue, he should be accustomed, immediately from his Birth, to submit to Burthens above his Strength, he could never prove any Thing but an utter Jade, incapable of real Service. The Application of this to the Stomach of a Child is very obvious.

I shall add another very important Remark, and it is this, that the too early Work to which the Children of Peasants are forced, becomes of real Prejudice to the Publick. Hence Families themselves are less numerous, and the more Children that are removed from their Parents, while they are very young, those who are left are the more obliged to Work, and very often even at hard Labour, at an Age when they should exercise themselves in the usual Diversions and Sports of Children. Hence they wear out in a Manner, before they attain the ordinary Term of Manhood; they never arrive at their utmost Strength, nor reach their full Stature; and it is too common to see a Countenance with the Look of twenty Years, joined to a Stature of twelve or thirteen. In fact, they often sink under the Weight of such hard involuntary Labour, and fall into a mortal Degree of Wasting and Exhaustion.

§ 397.

§ 397. Secondly, which indeed is but a Repetition of the Advice I have already given, and upon which I cannot infist too much, they must be frequently washed or bathed in cold Water.

§ 398. Thirdly, they should be moved about and exercised as much as they can bear, after they are some Weeks old: the earlier Days of their tender Life seeming consecrated, by Nature herself, to a nearly total Repose, and to sleeping, which seems not to determine, until they have Need of Nourishment: so that, during this very tender Term of Life, too much Agitation or Exercise might be attended with mortal Consequences. But as soon as their Organs have attained a little more Solidity and Firmness, the more they are danced about (provided it is not done about their usual Time of Repose, which ought still to be very considerable) they are so much the better for it; and by increasing it gradually, they may be accustomed to a very quick Movement, and at length very safely to such, as may be called hard and hearty Exercise. That Sort of Motion they receive in Go-Carts, or other Vehicles, particularly contrived for their Use, is more beneficial to them, than what they have from their Nurses Arms, because they are in a better Attitude in the former; and it heats them less in Summer, which is a Circumstance of no small Importance to them; considerable Heat and Sweat disposing them to be ricketty.

§ 399. Fourthly, they should be accustomed to breathe in the free open Air as much as possible.

If Children have unhappily been lefs attended to than they ought, whence they are evidently feeble, thin, languid, obftructed, and liable to Scirrhofities (which conftitute what is termed a ricketty or confumptive State) thefe four Directions duly obferved retrieve them from that unhappy State; provided the Execution of them has not been too long delayed.

§ 400 Fifthly, If they have any natural Difcharge of a Humour by the Skin, which is very common with them, or any Eruption, fuch as Tetters, white Scurf, a Rafhe, or the like, Care muft be taken not to check or repel them, by any greafy or reftringent Applications. Not a Year paffes without Numbers of Children having been deftroyed by Imprudence in this Refpect; while others have been reduced to a deplorable and weakly Habit.

I have been a Witnefs to the moft unhappy Confequences of external Medicines applied for the Rafhe and white Scurf, which, however frightful they may appear, are never dangerous; provided nothing at all is applied to them, without the Advice and Confideration of a truly fkilful Perfon

When fuch external Diforders prove very obftinate, it is reafonable to fufpect fome Fault or Difagreement in the Milk the Child fucks; in which Cafe it fhould immediately be difcontinued, corrected, or changed. But I cannot enter here into a particular Detail of all the Treatment neceffary in fuch Cafes.

CHAPTER

Chapter XXVIII.

Directions with Respect to drowned Persons.*

Sect. 401.

WHENEVER a Person who has been drowned, has remained a Quarter of an Hour under Water, there can be no considerable Hopes of his Recovery: the Space of two or three Minutes in such a Situation being often sufficient to kill a Man irrecoverably. Nevertheless, as several Circumstances may happen to have continued Life, in such an unfortunate Situation, beyond the ordinary Term, we should always endeavour to afford them the most effectual Relief, and not give them up as irrecoverable too soon: since it has often been known, that until the Expiration of two, and sometimes even of three Hours, such Bodies have exhibited some apparent Tokens of Life.

---

* The Misfortune of a young Man drowned in bathing himself, at the Beginning of the Season, occasioned the Publication of this Chapter by itself in *June*, 1761. A few Days after, the like Misfortune happened to a labouring Man, but he was happily taken out of the Water sooner than the first (who had remained about half an Hour under it) and he was recovered by observing Part of the Advice this Chapter contains, of which Chapter several Bystanders had Copies.—This Note seems to be from the Author himself.

Water has sometimes been found in the Stomach of drowned Persons; at other times none at all. Besides, the greatest Quantity which has ever been found in it has not exceeded that, which may be drank without any Inconvenience; whence we may conclude, the meer Quantity was not mortal; neither is it very easy to conceive how drowned Persons can swallow Water. What really kills them is meer Suffocation, or the Interception of Air, of the Action of breathing; and the Water which descends into the Lungs, and which is determined there, by the Efforts they necessarily, though involuntarily make, to draw Breath, after they are under Water: for there absolutely does not any Water descend, either into the Stomach or the Lungs of Bodies plunged into Water, after they are dead; a Circumstance, which serves to establish a legal Sentence and Judgment in some criminal Cases, and Trials: This Water intimately blending itself with the Air in the Lungs, forms a viscid inactive Kind of Froth, which entirely destroys the Functions of the Lungs; whence the miserable Sufferer is not only suffocated, but the Return of the Blood from the Head being also intercepted, the Blood Vessels of the Brain are overcharged, and an Apoplexy is combined with the Suffocation. This second Cause, that is, the Descent of the Water into the Lungs, is far from being general, it having been evident from the Dissection of several drowned Bodies, that it really never had existed in them.

§ 402.

§ 402. The Intention that should be pursued, is that of unloading the Lungs and the Brain, and of reviving the extinguished Circulation. For which Purpose we should, 1, immediately strip the Sufferer of all his wet Cloaths, rub him strongly, with dry coarse Linnen; put him, as soon as possible, into a well heated Bed, and continue to rub him well a very considerable Time together.

2, A strong and healthy Person should force his own warm Breath into the Patient's Lungs; and the Smoke of Tobacco, if some was at Hand, by Means of some Pipe, Chanel, Funnel or the like, that may be introduced into the Mouth. This Air or Fume, being forcibly blown in, by stopping the Sufferer's Nostrils close at the same Time, penetrates into the Lungs, and there rarifies by its Heat that Air, which blended with the Water, composed the viscid Spume or Froth. Hence that Air becomes disengaged from the Water, recovers its Spring, dilates the Lungs, and, if there still remains within any Principle of Life, the Circulation is renewed again that Instant.

3, If a moderately expert Surgeon is at Hand, he must open the jugular Vein, or any large Vein in the Neck, and let out ten or twelve Ounces of Blood. Such a Bleeding is serviceable on many Accounts. First, merely as Bleeding, it renews the Circulation, which is the constant Effect of Bleeding in such Swoonings, as arise from an intercepted or suffocated Circulation.

Secondly, it is that particular Bleeding, which most suddenly removes, in such Cases, the Infarction or Obstruction of the Head and Lungs; and, thirdly, it is sometimes the only Vessel, whence Blood will issue under such Circumstances. The Veins of the Feet then afford none; and those of the Arms seldom; but the Jugulars almost constantly furnish it.

Fourthly, the Fume of Tobacco should be thrown up, as speedily and plentifully as possible, into the Intestines by the Fundament. There are very commodious Contrivances devised for this Purpose; but as they are not common, it may be effected by many speedy Means. One, by which a Woman's Life was preserved, consisted only in introducing the small Tube of a Tobacco Pipe well lighted up: the Head or Bowl of it was wrapped up in a Paper, in which several Holes were pricked, and through these the Breath was strongly forced. At the fifth Blast a considerable Rumbling was heard in the Woman's Belly; she threw up a little Water, and a Moment afterwards came to her Senses. Two Pipes may be thus lighted and applied, with their Bowls covered over, the Extremity of one is to be introduced into the Fundament, and the other may be blown through into the Lungs.

Any other Vapour may also be conveyed up, by introducing a *Canula*, or any other Pipe, with a Bladder firmly fixed to it. This Bladder is faltered at its other End to a large Tin Funnel, under which Tobacco is to be lighted. This Con-

Contrivance has succeeded with me upon other Occasions, in which Necessity compelled me to invent and apply it.

Fifthly, the strongest Volatiles should be applied to the Patient's Nostrils. The Powder of some strong dry Herb should be blown up his Nose, such as Sage, Rosemary, Rue, Mint, and especially Marjoram, or very well dried Tobacco; or even the Fume, the Smoke of these Herbs. But all these Means are most properly employed after Bleeding, when they are most efficacious and certain.

Sixthly, as long as the Patient shews no Signs of Life, he will be unable to swallow, and it is then useless, and even dangerous, to pour much Liquid of any kind into his Mouth, which could do nothing but keep up, or increase Suffocation. It is sufficient, in such Circumstances, to instil a few Drops of some irritating Liquor, which might also be cordial and reviving. But as soon as ever he discovers any Motion, he should take, within the Space of one Hour, five or six common Spoonfuls of Oxymel of Squills diluted with warm Water: or if that Medicine was not to be had very speedily, a strong Infusion of the blessed Thistle, or *Carduus benedictus,* of Sage, or of Chamomile Flowers sweetened with Honey, might do instead of it: and supposing nothing else to be had, some warm Water, with the Addition of a little common Salt, should be given. Some Persons are bold enough to recommend Vomits in such Cases; but they are not without their Inconvenience;

ence; and it is not as a Vomit, that I recommend the Oxymel of Squills in them.

Seventhly, Notwithstanding the Sick discover some Tokens of Life, we should not cease to continue our Assistance; since they sometimes irrecoverably expire, after these first Appearances of recovering.

And lastly, though they should be manifestly re-animated, there sometimes remains an Oppression, a Coughing and Feverishness, which effectually constitute a Disease: and then it becomes necessary sometimes to bleed them in the Arms; to give them Barley Water plentifully, or Elder-flower Tea.

§ 403. Having thus pointed out such Means as are necessary, and truly effectual, in such unfortunate Accidents, I shall very briefly mention some others, which it is the general Custom to use and apply in the first Hurry.

1, These unhappy People are sometimes wrapped up in a Sheep's, or a Calf's, or a Dog's Skin, immediately flead from the Animal: these Applications have sometimes indeed revived the Heat of the Drowned; but their Operations are more flow, and less efficacious, than the Heat of a well-warmed Bed; with the additional Vapour of burnt Sugar, and long continued Frictions with hot Flanels.

2, The Method of rolling them in an empty Hogshead is dangerous, and mispends a deal of important Time.

3, That

3, That also of hanging them up by the Feet, is attended with Danger, and ought to be wholly discontinued. The Froth or Foam, which is one of the Causes of their Death, is too thick and tough to discharge itself, in Consequence of its own Weight. Nevertheless, this is the only Effect that can be expected, from this Custom of suspending them by the Feet; which must also be hurtful, by its tending to increase the Overfulness of the Head and of the Lungs.

§ 404. It is some Years since a Girl of eighteen Years old was recovered, [though it is unknown whether she remained under Water only a little Time or some Hours] who was motionless, frozen as it were, insensible, with her Eyes closed, her Mouth wide open, a livid Colour, a swoln Visage, a Tumour or bloating of the whole Body, which was overladen as it were, or Water-soaked. This miserable Object was extended on a Kind of Bed, of hot or very warm Ashes, quickly heated in great Kettles; and by laying her quite naked on these Ashes; by covering her with others equally hot, by putting a Bonnet round her Head, with a Stocking round her Neck stuffed with the same, and heaping Coverings over all this, at the End of half an Hour her Pulse returned, she recovered her Speech, and cried out, *I freeze, I freeze*: A little Cherry-Brandy was given her, and then she remained buried, as it were, eight Hours under the Ashes; being taken out of them afterwards without any other Complaint, except that of great Lassitude or Weariness, which went entirely off the third Day. This Method was undoubtedly so effectual, that it well deserves Imitation; but it should not make us inattentive to the others. Heated Gravel or Sand mixed with Salt, or hot Salt alone, would have been equally efficacious, and they have been found so.

At the very Time of writing this, two young Ducks, who were drowned, have been revived by a dry Bath of hot Ashes. The Heat of a Dung-heap may also be beneficial; and I have just been informed, by a very creditable and sensible Spectator of it, that it effectually contributed to restore Life to a Man, who had certainly remained six Hours under Water.

§ 405. I shall conclude these Directions with an Article printed in a little Work at *Paris*, about twenty Years since, by Order of the King, to which there is not the least Doubt, but that any other Sovereign will readily accede.

" Notwithstanding the common People are
" very generally disposed to be compassionate,
" and may wish to give all Assistance to drown-
" ed Persons, it frequently happens they do not,
" only because they dare not; imagining they
" expose themselves by it to Prosecutions. It
" is therefore necessary, that they should know,
" and it cannot be too often repeated, in order
" to eradicate such a pernicious Prejudice, that
" the Magistrates have never interposed to pre-
" vent People from trying every possible Means
" to recover such unfortunate Persons, as shall
" be

" be drowned and taken out of the Water. It is
" only in those Cases, when the Persons are
" known to be absolutely and irrecoverably dead,
" that Justice renders it necessary to seize their
" Bodies."

Chapter XXIX.

Of Substances stopt between the Mouth and the Stomach.

Sect. 406.

THE Food we take in descends from the Mouth through a very strait Passage or Chanel, called the *Oesophagus*, the Gullet, which, going parallel with the Spine or Backbone, joins to, or terminates at, the Stomach.

It happens sometimes that different Bodies are stopt in this Chanel, without being able either to descend or to return up again; whether this Difficulty arises from their being too large; or whether it be owing to their having such Angles or Points, as by penetrating into, and adhering to the Sides of this membranous Canal, absolutely prevent the usual Action and Motion of it.

§ 407. Very dangerous Symptoms arise from this Stoppage, which are frequently attended with a most acute Pain in the Part; and at other Times,

Times, with a very incommodious, rather than painful, Senfation; fometimes a very ineffectual Commotion at, or rifing of, the Stomach, attended with great Anguifh; and if the Stoppage be fo circumftanced, that the *Glottis* is clofed, or the Wind-pipe compreffed, a dreadful Suffocation is the Confequence: the Patient cannot breathe, the Lungs are quite diftended; and the Blood being unable to return from the Head, the Countenance becomes red, then livid, the Neck fwells; the Oppreffion increafes, and the poor Sufferer fpeedily dies.

When the Patient's Breathing is not ftopt, nor greatly oppreffed; if the Paffage is not entirely blocked up, and he can fwallow fomething, he lives very eafily for a few Days, and then his Cafe becomes a particular Diforder of the *Oefophagus*, or Gullet But if the Paffage is abfolutely clofed, and the Obftruction cannot be removed for many Days, a terrible Death is the Confequence.

§ 408. The Danger of fuch Cafes does not depend fo much on the Nature of the obftructing Subftance, as on its Size, with Regard to that of the Paffage of the Part where it ftops, and of the Manner in which it forms the Obftruction; and frequently the very Food may occafion Death; while Subftances lefs adapted to be fwallowed are not attended with any violent Confequences, though fwallowed.

A

Of Stoppages between the Mouth and Stomach. 413

A Child of six Days old swallowed a Comfit or Sugar Plumb, which stuck in the Passage, and instantly killed it.

A grown Person perceived that a Bit of Mutton had stopt in the Passage; not to alarm any Body he arose from Table; a Moment afterwards, on looking where he might be gone, he was found dead. Another was choaked by a Bit of Cake; a third by a Piece of the Skin of a Ham; and a fourth by an Egg, which he swallowed whole in a Bravo.

A Child was killed by a Chesnut swallowed whole. Another died suddenly, choaked (which is always the Circumstance, when they die instantly after such Accidents) by a Pear which he had tossed up, and catched in his Mouth. A Woman was choaked with another Pear. A Piece of a Sinew continued eight Days in the Passage, so that it prevented the Patient from getting down any Thing else; at the Expiration of that Time it fell into the Stomach, being loosened by its Putridity: The Patient notwithstanding died soon after, being killed by the Inflammation, Gangrene and Weakness it had occasioned. Unhappily there occur but too many Instances of this Sort, of which it is unnecessary to cite more.

§ 409. Whenever any Substance is thus detained in the Gullet, there are two Ways of removing it; that is either by extracting it, or pushing it down. The safest and most certain Way is always to extract or draw it out, but this is not always the easiest: and as the Efforts made for this Purpose greatly fatigue the Patient, and are sometimes attended with grievous Consequences; and yet if the Occasion is extremely urging, it may be eligible to thrust it down, if that is easier; and if there is no Danger from the obstructing Bodies Reception into the Stomach.

The Substances which may be pushed down without Danger, are all common nourishing ones, as Bread, Meat, Cakes, Fruits, Pulse, Morsels of Tripe, and even Skin of Bacon. It is only very large Morsels of particular Aliments, that prove very difficult to digest; yet even such are rarely attended with any Fatality.

§ 410. The Substances we should endeavour to extract or draw out, though it be more painful and less easy than to push them down, are all those, whose Consequences might be highly dangerous, or even mortal, if swallowed. Such are all totally indigestible Bodies, as Cork, Linen-Rags, large Fruit Stones, Bones, Wood, Glass, Stones, Metals; and more especially if any further Danger may be superadded to that of its Indigestibility, from the Shape, whether rough, sharp, pointed, or angular, of the Substance swallowed. Wherefore we should chiefly endeavour to extract Pins, Needles, Fish-bones, other pointed Fragments of Bones, Bits of Glass, Scissars, Rings, or Buckles

Nevertheless it has happened, that every one of these Substances have at one Time or another been swallowed, and the most usual Consequences

Of Stoppages between the Mouth and Stomach. 415

quences of them are violent Pains of the Stomach, and in the Guts; Inflammations, Suppurations, Abscesses, a slow Fever, Gangrene, the *Miserere* or Iliac Passion; external Abscesses, through which the Bodies swallowed down have been discharged; and frequently, after a long Train of Maladies, a dreadful Death.

§ 411. When such Substances have not passed in too deep, we should endeavour to extract them with our Fingers, which often succeeds. If they are lower, we should make use of Nippers or a small *Forceps*; of which Surgeons are provided with different Sorts. Those which some Smoakers carry about them might be very convenient for such Purposes; and in Case of Necessity they might be made very readily out of two Bits of Wood. But this Attempt to extract rarely succeeds, if the Substance has descended far into the *Oesophagus*, and if the Substance be of a flexible Nature, which exactly applies itself to, and fills up the Cavity or Chanel of it.

§ 412. If the Fingers and the Nippers fail, or cannot be duly applied, Crotchets, a Kind of Hooks, must be employed.

These may be made at once with a pretty strong iron Wire, crooked at the End. It must be introduced in the flat Way, and for the better conducting of it, there should be another Curve or Hook at the End it is held by, to serve as a Kind of Handle to it, which has this further Use, that it may be secured by a String tied to it; a Circumstance not to be omitted in any Instrument

strument employed on such Occasions, to avoid such ill Accidents as have sometimes ensued, from these Instruments slipping out of the Operators Hold. After the Crotchet has passed beyond and below the Substance, that obstructs the Passage, it is drawn up again, and hooks up with it and extracts that Impediment to swallowing.

This Crotchet is also very convenient, whenever a Substance somewhat flexible, as a Pin or a Fishbone stick, as it were, across the Gullet: the Crotchet in such Cases seizing them about their middle Part, crooks and thus disengages them. If they are very brittle Substances, it serves to break them, and if any Fragments still stick within, some other Means must be used to extract them.

§ 413. When the obstructing Bodies are small, and only stop up Part of the Passage; and which may either easily elude the Hook, or straiten it by their Resistance, a Kind of Rings may be used, and made either solid or flexible.

The solid ones are made of iron Wire, or of a String of very fine brass Wire. For this Purpose the Wire is bent into a Circle about the middle Part of its Length, the Sides of which Circle do not touch each other, but leave a Ring, or hollow Cavity, of about an Inch Diameter. Then the long unbent Sides of the Wire are brought near each other, the circular Part or Ring is introduced into the Gullet, in order to be conducted about the obstructing Body, and so to extract it. Very flexible Rings may be made

of

of Wool, Thread, Silk, or small Packthread, which may be waxed, for their greater Strength and Consistence. Then they are to be tied fast to a Handle of Iron-Wire, of Whale-bone, or of any flexible Wood, after which the Ring is to be introduced to surround the obstructing Substance, and to draw it out.

Several of these Rings passed through one another are often made use of, the more certainly to lay hold of the obstructing Body, which may be involved by one, if another should miss it. This Sort of Rings has one Advantage, which is, that when the Substance to be extracted is once laid hold of, it may then, by turning the Handle, be retained so strongly in the Ring thus twisted, as to be moved every Way; which must be a considerable Advantage in many such Cases.

§ 414. A fourth Material employed on these unhappy Occasions is the Sponge. Its Property of swelling considerably, on being wet, is the Foundation of its Usefulness here

If any Substance is stopt in the Gullet, but without filling up the whole Passage, a Bit of Sponge is introduced, into that Part that is unstopt, and beyond the Substance. The Sponge soon dilates, and grows larger in this moist Situation, and indeed the Enlargement of it may be forwarded, by making the Patient swallow a few Drops of Water; and then drawing back the Sponge by the Handle it is fastened to, as it is now too large to return through the small Cavity, by which it was conveyed in, it draws out the obstructing Body with it, and thus unplugs, as it were, and opens the Gullet.

As dry Sponge may shrink or be contracted, this Circumstance has proved the Means of squeezing a pretty large Piece of it into a very small Space. It becomes greatly compressed by winding a String or Tape very closely about it, which Tape may be easily unwound and withdrawn, after the Sponge has been introduced. It may also be inclosed in a Piece of Whalebone, split into four Sticks at one End, and which, being endued with a considerable Spring, contracts upon the Sponge. The Whalebone is so smoothed and accommodated, as not to wound; and the Sponge is also to be safely tied to a strong Thread; that after having disengaged the Whalebone from it, the Surgeon may also draw out the Sponge at Pleasure.

Sponge is also applied on these Occasions in another Manner. When there is no Room to convey it into the Gullet, because the obstructing Substance ingrosses its whole Cavity; and supposing it not hooked into the Part, but solely detained by the Straitness of the Passage, a pretty large Bit of Sponge is to be introduced towards the Gullet, and close to the obstructing Substance. Thus applied, the Sponge swells, and thence dilates that Part of the Passage that is above this Substance. The Sponge is then withdrawn a little, and but a very little, and this Substance being less pressed upon above than below, it sometimes happens, that the greater

Straitness

Staitness and Contraction of the lower Part of the Passage, than of its upper Part, causes that Substance to ascend; and as soon as this first Loosening or Disengagement of it has happened, the total Disengagement of it easily follows.

§ 415. Finally, when all these Methods prove unavailable, there remains one more, which is to make the Patient vomit; but this can scarcely be of any Service, but when such obstructing Bodies are simply engaged in, and not hooked or stuck into the Sides of the *Oesophagus*; since under this latter Circumstance vomiting might occasion further Mischief.

If the Patient can swallow, a Vomiting may be excited with the Prescription N°. 8, or with N° 34, or 35. By this Operation a Bone was thrown out, which had stopt in the Passage four and twenty Hours.

When the Patient cannot swallow, an Attempt should be made to excite him to vomit by introducing into, and twirling about the feathery End of a Quill in, the Bottom of the Throat, which the Feather however will not effect, if the obstructing Body strongly compresses the whole Circumference of the Gullet, and then no other Resource is left, but giving a Glyster of Tobacco. A certain Person swallowed a large Morsel of Calf's Lights, which stopt in the Middle of the Gullet, and exactly filled up the Passage. A Surgeon unsuccessfully attempted various Methods to extract it, but another seeing how unavailable all of them were, and the Patient's

Visage becoming black and swelled; his Eyes ready to start, as it were, out of his Head; and falling into frequent Swoonings, attended with Convulsions too, he caused a Glyster of an Ounce of Tobacco boiled to be thrown up, the Consequence of which was a violent Vomiting, which threw up the Substance that was so very near killing him.

§ 416. A sixth Method, which I believe has never hitherto been attempted, but which may prove very useful in many Cases, when the Substances in the Passage are not too hard, and are very large, would be to fix a Worm (used for withdrawing the Charge of Guns that have been loaded) fast to a flexible Handle, with a waxed Thread fastened to the Handle, in Order to withdraw it, if the Handle slipt from the Worm; and by this Contrivance it might be very practicable, if the obstructing Substance was not too deep in the Passage of the Gullet, to extract it—It has been known that a Thorn fastened in the Throat, has been thrown out by laughing.

§ 417. In the Circumstances mentioned § 409, when it is more easy and convenient to push the obstructing Body downwards, it has been usual to make Use of Leeks, which may generally be had any where (but which indeed are very subject to break) or of a Wax-candle oiled, and but a very little heated, so as to make it flexible; or of a Piece of Whale-bone, or of Iron-Wire; one Extremity of which may be thickened and blunted

blunted in a Minute with a little melted Lead. Small Sticks of some flexible Wood may be as convenient for the same Use, such as the Birch-tree, the Hazel, the Ash, the Willow, a flexible Plummet, or a leaden Ring. All these Substances should be very smooth, that they may not give the least Irritation; for which Reason they are sometimes covered over with a thin Bit of Sheep's Gut. Sometimes a Sponge is fastened to one End of them, which, completely filling up the whole Passage, pushes down whatever Obstacle it meets with

In such Cases too, the Patient may be prompted to attempt swallowing down large Morsels of some unhurtful Substance, such as a Crust of Bread, a small Turnep, a Lettuce Stalk, or a Bullet, in Hopes of their carrying down the obstructing Cause with them. It must be acknowledged, however, that these afford but a feeble Assistance; and if they are swallowed without being well secured to a Thread, it may be apprehended they may even increase the Obstruction, by their own Stoppage.

It has sometimes very happily, though rarely, occurred, that those Substances attempted to be detruded or thrust downwards, have stuck in the Wax-Candle, or the Leek, and sprung up and out with them but this can never happen except in the Case of pointed Substances.

§ 418. Should it be impossible to extract the Bodies mentioned § 410, and all such as it must be dangerous to admit into the Stomach, we must then

then prefer the least of two Evils, and rather run the Hazard of pushing them down, than suffer the Patient to perish dreadfully in a few Moments. And we ought to scruple this Resolution the less, as a great many Instances have demonstrated, that notwithstanding several Consequences, and even a tormenting Death, have often followed the swallowing of such hurtful or indigestible Substances; yet at other times they have been attended with little or no Disorder.

§ 419. One of these four Events is always the Case, after swallowing such Things. They either, 1, go off by Stool, or, 2, they are not discharged and kill the Patient. Or else, 3, they are discharged by Urine; or, 4, are visibly extruded to the Skin. I shall give some Instances of each of these Events.

§ 420. When they are voided by Stool, they are either voided soon after they have been swallowed, and that without having occasioned scarce any troublesome Symptom; or the voiding of them has not happened till a long Time after swallowing, and is preceded with very considerable Pain. It has been seen that a Bone of the Leg of a Fowl, a Peach-stone, the Cover of a small Box of Venice Treacle, Pins, Needles, and Coins of different Sorts, have been voided within a few Days after they had slipt down into the Stomach, and that with little or no Complaint. A small Flute, or Pipe also, four Inches long, which occasioned acute Pains for three Days, has been voided happily afterwards, besides,

sides, Knives, Razors, and one Shoe-buckle. I have seen but a few Days since a Child between two and three Years old, who swallowed a Nail above an Inch long, the Head of which was more than three Tenths of an Inch broad: it stopt a few Moments about the Neck, but descended while its Friends were looking for me; and was voided with a Stool that Night, without any bad Consequence. And still more lately I have known the entire Bone of a Chicken's Wing thus swallowed, which only occasioned a slight Pain in the Stomach for three or four Days.

Sometimes such Substances are retained within for a long Time, not being voided till after several Months, and even Years, without the least ill Effect: and some of them have never either appeared, nor been complained of.

§ 421. But the Event is not always so happy; and sometimes though they are discharged through the natural Passages, the Discharges have been preceded by very acute Pains in the Stomach, and in the Bowels. A Girl swallowed down some Pins, which afflicted her with violent Pains for the Space of six Years; at the Expiration of which Term she voided them and recovered. Three Needles being swallowed brought on Cholics, Swoonings and Convulsions for a Year after: and then being voided by Stool, the Patient recovered. Another Person who swallowed two, was much happier in suffering but six Hours from them; when they were voided by Stool, and he did well.

It sometimes happens that such indigestible Substances, after having past all the Meanders, the whole Course of the Intestines, have been stopt in the Fundament, and brought on very troublesome Symptoms; but such however, as an expert Surgeon may very generally remove. If it is practicable to cut them, as it is when they happen to be thin Bones, the Jaw-bones of Fish, or Pins, they are then very easily extracted.

§ 422. The second Event is, when these fatal Substances are never voided, but cause very embarrassing Symptoms which finally kill the Patient, and of these Cases there have been but too many Examples.

A young Girl having swallowed some Pins, which she held in her Mouth, some of them were voided by Stool; but others of them pricked and pierced into her Guts, and even into the Muscles of her Belly, with the severest Pain, and killed her at the End of three Weeks.

A Man swallowed a Needle, which pierced through his Stomach, and into his Liver,* and ended in a mortal Consumption.

A Plummet

---

* I saw a very similar Instance and Event in a Lady's little favourite Bitch, whose Body she desired to be opened, from suspecting her to have been poisoned. But it appeared that a small Needle with Thread, which she had swallowed, had passed out of the Stomach into the *Duodenum* (one of the Guts) through which the Point had pierced, and pricked and corroded the con- ... Part of the Liver, which was all rough and putrid. The whole

A Plummet which flipt down, while the Throat of a Patient was fearching, killed him at the End of two Years.

It is very common for different Coins, and of different Metals, to be fwallowed without any fatal or troublefome Effects. Even a hundred Luidores * have been fwallowed, and all voided. Neverthelefs thefe fortunate Efcapes ought not to make People too fecure and incautious on fuch Occafions, fince fuch melancholy Confequences have happened, as may very juftly alarm them. One fingle Piece of Money that was fwallowed, entirely obftructed the Communication between the Stomach and the Inteftines, and killed the Patient. Whole Nuts have often been inadvertently fwallowed, but there have been fome Inftances of Perfons in whom a Heap† of them has been formed, which proved the Caufe of Death, after producing much Pain and Inquietude.

§ 423.

---

whole Carcafe was greatly bloated and extremely offenfive, very foon after the poor Animal's Death, which happened two or three Months after the Accident, and was preceded by a great Wheezing, Reftlefsnefs and Lofs of Appetite. The Needle was rufty, but the Thread entire, and very little altered. *K*

* I knew a Man of the Name of *Poole*, who being taken in the fame Ship with me, 1717 or 18, by Pirates, had fwallowed four Ginueas, and a gold Ring, all which he voided fome Days after without any Injury or Complaint, and faved them. I forget the exact Number of Days he retained them, but the Pirates ftaid with us from Saturday Night to Thurfday Noon. *K*.

† Many fatal Examples of this Kind may be feen in the *Philofophical Tranfactions*, and they fhould caution People againft fwallowing Cherry-ftones, and ftill more againft thofe of Prunes, or fuch as are pointed, though not very acutely. *K*

§ 423. The third Issue or Event is, when these Substances, thus swallowed down, have been discharged by Urine: but these Cases are very rare.

A Pin of a middling Size has been discharged by Urine, three Days after it slipt down; and a little Bone has been expelled the same Way, besides Cherry-stones, Plumb-stones, and even one Peach-stone.

§ 424. Finally, the fourth Consequence or Event is, when the indigestible Substances thus swallowed, have pierced through the Stomach or Intestines, and even to the Skin itself; and occasioning an Abscess, have made an Outlet for themselves, or have been taken out of the Abscess. A long Time is often required to effect this extraordinary Trajection and Appearance of them; sometimes the Pains they occasion are continual; in other Cases the Patient complains for a Time, after which the Pain ceases, and then returns again. The Imposthume, or Gathering, is formed in the Stomach, or in some other Part of the Belly: and sometimes these very Substances, after having pierced through the Guts, make very singular Routs, and are discharged very remotely from the Belly. One Needle that had been swallowed found its Way out, at the End of four Years, through the Leg, another at the Shoulder.

§ 425. All these Examples, and many others of cruel Deaths, from swallowing noxious Substances, demonstrate the great Necessity of an

habitual

habitual Caution in this Respect; and give in their Testimony against the horrid, I had almost said, the criminal Imprudence, of People's amusing themselves with such Tricks as may lead to such terrible Accidents, or even holding any such Substance in their Mouths, as by slipping down through Imprudence or Accident, may prove the Occasion of their Death. Is it possible that any one, without shuddering, can hold Pins or Needles in their Mouths, after reflecting on the dreadful Accidents, and cruel Deaths, that have thus been caused by them.

§ 426. It has been shewn already, that Substances obstructing the Passage of the Gullet sometimes suffocate the Patient; that at other Times they can neither be extracted nor thrust down; but that they stop in the Passage, without killing the Patient, at least not immediately and at once. This is the Case when they are so circumstanced, as not to compress the *Trachæa*, the Wind-pipe, and not totally to prevent the swallowing of Food, which last Circumstance can scarcely happen, except the Obstruction has been formed by angular or pointed Bodies. The Stoppage of such Bodies is sometimes attended, and that without much Violence, with a small Suppuration, which loosens them; and then they are either returned upwards through the Mouth, or descend into the Stomach. But at other Times an extraordinary Inflammation is produced, which kills the Patient. Or if the Contents of the Abscess attending the Inflammation

tend

tend outwardly, a Tumour is formed on the external Part of the Neck, which is to be opened, and through whose Orifice the obstructing Body is discharged. In other Instances again they take a different Course, attended with little or no Pain, and are at length discharged by a Gathering behind the Neck, on the Breast, the Shoulder, or various other Parts.

§ 427. Some Persons, astonished at the extraordinary Course and Progression of such Substances, which, from their Size, and especially from their Shape, seem to them incapable of being introduced into, and in some Sort, circulating through the human Body, without destroying it, are very desirous of having the Rout and Progression of such intruding Substances explained to them. To gratify such Inquirers, I may be indulged in a short Digression, which perhaps is the less foreign to my Plan, as in dissipating what seems marvelous, and has been thought supernatural in such Cases, I may demolish that superstitious Prejudice, which has often ascribed Effects of this Sort to Witchcraft; but which admit of an easy Explanation. This very Reason is the Motive that has determined me to give a further Extent to this Chapter.

Wherever an Incision is made through the Skin, a certain Membrane appears, which consists of two Coats or *Laminæ*, separated from each other by small Cells or Cavities, which all communicate together, and which are furnished, more or less, with Fat. There is not any Fat throughout

throughout the human Body, which is not inclosed in, or enveloped with, this Coat, which is called the adipose, fatty, or cellular Membrane.

This Membrane is not only found under the Skin, but further plying and insinuating itself in various Manners, it is extended throughout the whole Body. It distinguishes and separates all the Muscles; it constitutes a Part of the Stomach, of the Guts, of the Bladder, and of all the *Viscera* or Bowels. It is this which forms what is called the Cawl, and which also furnishes a Sheath or Envelopement to the Veins, Arteries, and Nerves. In some Parts it is very thick, and is abundantly replenished with Fat; in others it is very thin and unprovided with any; but wherever it extends, it is wholly insensible, or void of all Sensation, all Feeling.

It may be compared to a quilted Coverlet, the Cotton, or other Stuffing of which, is unequally distributed; greatly abounding in some Places, with none at all in others, so that in these the Stuff above and below touch each other. Within this Membrane, or Coverlet, as it were, such extraneous or foreign Substances are moved about; and as there is a general Communication throughout the whole Extent of the Membrane, it is no ways surprizing, that they are moved from one Part to another very distant, in a long Course and Duration of Movement. Officers and Soldiers very often experience, that Bullets which do not pass through the Parts where they have entered, are transferred to very different and remote ones.

The general Communication throughout this Membrane is daily demonstrated by Facts, which the Law prohibits; this is the Butchers inflating, or blowing up, the cellular Membrane throughout the whole Carcase of a Calf, by a small Incision in the Skin, into which they introduce a Pipe or the Nozzle of a small Bellows; and then, blowing forcibly, the Air evidently puffs up the whole Body of the Calf into this artificial Tumour or Swelling.

Some very criminal Impostors have availed themselves of this wicked Contrivance, thus to bloat up Children into a Kind of Monsters, which they afterwards expose to View for Money.

In this cellular Membrane the extravasated Waters of hydropic Patients are commonly diffused, and here they give Way to that Motion, to which their own Weight disposes them. But here I may be asked—As this Membrane is crossed and intersected in different Parts of it, by Nerves, Veins, Arteries, &c. the wounding of which unavoidably occasions grievous Symptoms, how comes it, that such do not ensue upon the Intrusion of such noxious Substances? To this I answer, 1, that such Symptoms do sometimes really ensue; and 2, that nevertheless they must happen but seldom, by Reason that all the aforesaid Parts, which traverse and intersect this Membrane, being harder than the Fat it contains; such foreign Substances must almost necessarily, whenever they rencounter those Parts, be turned aside towards the Fat which surrounds them, whose

Of Stoppages between the Mouth and Stomach. 431

whose Resistance is very considerably less, and this the more certainly so, as these Nerves, &c. are always of a cylindrical Form.——— But to return from this necessary Digression.

§ 428. To all these Methods and Expedients I have already recommended on the important Subject of this Chapter, I shall further add some general Directions

1. It is often useful, and even necessary, to take a considerable Quantity of Blood from the Arm; but especially if the Patient's Respiration, or Breathing, is extremely oppressed; or when we cannot speedily succeed in our Efforts to remove the obstructing Substance; as the Bleeding is adapted to prevent the Inflammation, which the frequent Irritations from such Substances occasion, and as by its disposing the whole Body into a State of Relaxation, it might possibly procure an immediate Discharge of the offending Substance.

2. Whenever it is manifest that all Endeavours, either to extract, or to push down the Substance stopt in the Passage, are ineffectual, they should be discontinued, because the Inflammation occasioned by persisting in them, would be as dangerous as the Obstruction itself, as there have been Instances of People's dying in Consequence of the Inflammation, notwithstanding the Body, which caused the Obstruction, had been entirely removed.

3. While the Means already advised are making Use of, the Patient should often swallow, or

if he cannot, he should frequently receive by Injection through a crooked Tube or Pipe, that may reach lower down than the *Glottis*, some very emollient Liquor, as warm Water, either alone or mixed with Milk, or a Decoction of Barley, of Mallows, or of Bran. A two-fold Advantage may arise from this; the first is, that these softening Liquors smooth and sooth the irritated Parts; and secondly, an Injection, strongly thrown in, has often been more successful in loosening the obstructing Body, than all Attempts with Instruments.

4. When after all we are obliged to leave this in the Part, the Patient must be treated as if he had an inflammatory Disease; he must be bled, ordered to a Regimen, and have his whole Neck surrounded with emollient Pultices. The like Treatment must also be used, though the obstructing Substance be removed; if there is Room to suppose any Inflammation left in the Passage.

5. A proper Degree of Agitation has sometimes loosened the inhering Body, more effectually than Instruments. It has been experienced that a Blow with the Fist on the Spine, the Middle of the Back, has often disengaged such obstructed and obstructing Bodies, and I have known two Instances of Patients who had Pins stopt in the Passage; and who getting on Horseback to ride out in Search of Relief at a neighbouring Village, found each of them the Pin disengaged after an Hour's riding: One spat it out, and the other swallowed it, without any ill Consequence.

6. When

6. When there is an immediate Apprehension of the Patient's being suffocated; when bleeding him has been of no Service; when all Hope of freeing the Passage in time is vanished, and Death seems at Hand, if Respiration be not restored; the Operation of *Bronchotomy*, or opening of the Wind-pipe, must be directly performed; an Operation neither difficult to a tolerably knowing and expert Surgeon, nor very painful to the Patient.

7. When the Substance that was stopt passes into the Stomach, the Patient must immediately be put into a very mild and smooth Regimen. He should avoid all sharp, irritating, inflaming Food; Wine, spirituous Liquors, all strong Drink, and Coffee; taking but little Nourishment at once, and no Solids, without their having been thoroughly well chewed. The best Diet would be that of farinaceous mealy Soups, made of various leguminous Grains, and of Milk and Water, which is much better than the usual Custom of swallowing different Oils.

§ 429. The Author of Nature has provided, that in eating, nothing should pass by the *Glottis* into the Wind-pipe. This Misfortune nevertheless does sometimes happen; at which very Instant there ensues an incessant and violent Cough, an acute Pain, with Suffocation; all the Blood being forced up into the Head, the Patient is in extreme Anguish, being agitated with violent and involuntary Motions, and sometimes dying on the Spot. A *Hungarian* Grenadier, by Trade a Shoemaker, was eating and working at the same time. He tumbled at once from his Seat, without uttering a single Word. His Comrades called out for Assistance; some Surgeons speedily arrived, but after all their Endeavours he discovered no Token of Life. On opening the Body, they found a Lump, or large Morsel, of Beef, weighing two Ounces, forced into the Windpipe, which it plugged up so exactly, that not the least Air could pass through it into the Lungs.

§ 430. In a Case so circumstanced, the Patient should be struck often on the Middle of the Back; some Efforts to vomit should be excited, he should be prompted to sneeze with Powder of Lilly of the Valley, Sage, or any cephalic Snuffs, which should be blown strongly up his Nose.

A Pea, pitched into the Mouth in playing, entered into the Wind-pipe, and sprung out again by vomiting the Patient with Oil. A little Bone was brought up by making another sneeze, with powdered Lilly of the Valley.

In short, if all these Means of assisting, or saving the Patient are evidently ineffectual, *Bronchotomy* must be speedily performed (See N°. 6, of the preceding Section.) By this Operation, some Bones, a Bean, and a Fish-bone have been extracted, and the Patient has been delivered from approaching Death.

§ 431. Nothing should be left untried, when the Preservation of human Life is the Object. In those Cases, when an obstructing Body can neither be disengaged from the Throat, the Passage

to

to the Stomach, nor be suffered to remain there without speedily killing the Patient, it has been proposed to make an Incision into this Passage, the *Oesophagus*, through which such a Body is to be extracted; and to employ the like Means, when a Substance which had slipt even into the Stomach itself, was of a Nature to excite such Symptoms, as must speedily destroy the Patient.

When the *Oesophagus* is so fully and strongly closed, that the Patient can receive no Food by the Mouth, he is to be nourished by Glysters of Soup, Gelly, and the like.

CHAPTER XXX.

Of external Disorders, and such as require chirurgical Application. Of Burns, Wounds, Contusions or Bruises: Of Sprains, Ulcers, frostbitten Limbs, Chilblains, Ruptures, Boils: Of Fellons, Thorns or Splinters in the Fingers or Flesh; of Warts, and of Corns.

SECT. 432.

Labouring Countrymen are exposed in the Course of their daily Work, to many outward Accidents, such as Cuts, Contusions, &c. which, however considerable in themselves, very generally end happily, and that chiefly in Consequence of the pure and simple Nature of their Blood, which is generally much less acrimonious, or sharp, in the Country, than in great Towns or Cities. Nevertheless, the very improper Treatment of such Accidents, in the Country, frequently renders them, however light in themselves, very troublesome; and indeed, I have seen so many Instances of this, that I have thought it necessary to mark out here the proper Treatment of such Accidents, as may not necessarily require the Hand or Attendance of a Surgeon. I shall also add something very briefly, concerning some external Disorders, which at the same Time result from an inward Cause.

Of Burns.

§ 433. When a Burn is very trifling and superficial, and occasions no Vesication or Blister, it is sufficient to clap a Compress of several Folds of soft Linen upon it, dipt in cold Water, and to renew it every Quarter of an Hour, till the Pain is entirely removed. But when the Burn has blistered, a Compress of very fine Linen, spread over with the Pomatum, N°. 64, should be applied over it, and changed twice a Day.

If the true Skin is burnt, and even the Muscles, the Flesh under it, be injured, the same Pomatum may be applied, but instead of a Compress, it should be spread upon a Pledget of soft Lint, to be applied very exactly over it, and over the Pledget again, a Slip of the simple Plaister N°. 65,
which

which every Body may easily prepare; or, if they should prefer it, the Plaister N°. 66.

But, independently of these external Applications, which are the most effectual ones, when they are directly to be had; whenever the Burn has been very violent, is highly inflamed, and we are apprehensive of the Progress and the Consequences of the Inflammation, the same Means and Remedies must be recurred to, which are used in violent Inflammations: the Patient should be bled, and, if it is necessary, it should be repeated more than once, and he should be put into a Regimen; drink nothing but the Ptisans N° 2 and 4, and receive daily two simple Glysters

If the Ingredients for the Ointment, called *Nutritum*, are not at Hand to make the Pomatum N°. 64, one Part of Wax should be melted in eight such Parts of Oil, to two Ounces of which Mixture the Yolk of an Egg should be added. A still more simple and sooner prepared Application, is that of one Egg, both the Yolk and the White, beat up with two common Spoonfuls of the sweetest Oil, without any Rankness. When the Pain of the Burn, and all its other Symptoms have very nearly disappeared, it is sufficient to apply the Sparadrap, or Oilcloth N°. 66.

Of Wounds.

§ 434. If a Wound has penetrated into any of the Cavities, and has wounded any Part contained in the Breast, or in the Belly: Or if, without having entered into one of the Cavities, it has opened some great Blood-vessel; or if it has wounded a considerable Nerve, which occasions Symptoms much more violent, than would otherwise have happened; if it has penetrated even to and injured the Bone. in short, if any great and severe Symptom supervenes, there is an absolute Necessity for calling in a Surgeon. But whenever the Wound is not attended with any of these Circumstances; when it affects only the Skin, the fat Membrane beneath it, the fleshy Parts and the small Vessels, it may be easily and simply dressed without such Assistance; since, in general, all that is truly necessary in such Cases is, to defend the Wound from the Impressions of the Air; and yet not so, as to give any material Obstruction to the Discharge of the Matter, that is to issue from the Wound.

§ 435 If the Blood does not particularly flow out of any considerable Vessel, but trickles almost equally from every Spot of the Wound, it may very safely be permitted to bleed, while some Lint is speedily preparing. As soon as the Lint is ready, so much of it may be introduced into the Wound as will nearly fill it, without being forced in; which is highly improper, and would be attended with the same Inconveniences as Tents and Dossils. It should be covered over with a Compress dipt in sweet Oil, or with the Cerecloth N°. 65; though I prefer the Compress for the earliest Dressings: and the whole

Dressing

Dreſſing ſhould be kept on, with a Bandage, of two Fingers Breadth, and of a Length proportioned to the Size of the Part it is to ſurround: This ſhould be rolled on tight enough to ſecure the Dreſſings, and yet ſo moderately, as to bring on no Inflammation.

This Bandage with theſe Dreſſings are to remain on twenty-four or forty-eight Hours; Wounds being healed the ſooner, for being leſs frequently dreſt. At the ſecond Dreſſing all the Lint muſt be removed, which can be done with Eaſe, and with reaſonable Speed, to the Wounded; and if any of it ſhould ſtick cloſe, in Conſequence of the clogged and dried Blood, it ſhould be left behind, adding a little freſh Lint to it; this Dreſſing in other Reſpects exactly reſembling the firſt.

When, from the Continuance of this ſimple Dreſſing, the Wound is become very ſuperficial, it is ſufficient to apply the Cerecloth, or Plaiſter, without any Lint.

Such as have conceived an extraordinary Opinion of any medical Oils, impregnated with the Virtues of particular Plants, may, if that will increaſe their Satisfaction, make uſe of the common Oil of Yarrow, of Trefoil, of Lilies, of Chamomile, of Balſamines, or of red Roſes; only being very careful, that ſuch Oils are not become ſtale and rank.

§ 436. When the Wound is conſiderable, it muſt be expected to inflame before Suppuration (which, in ſuch a Caſe, advances more ſlowly) can enſue; which Inflammation will neceſſarily be attended with Pain, with a Fever, and ſometimes with a Raving, or Wandering, too. In ſuch a Situation, a Pultice of Bread and Milk, with the Addition of a little Oil, that it may not ſtick too cloſe, muſt be applied inſtead of the Compreſs or the Plaiſter: which Pultice is to be changed, but without uncovering the Wound, thrice and even four times every Day.

§ 437. Should ſome pretty conſiderable Blood-veſſel be opened by the Wound, there muſt be applied over it, a Piece of Agaric of the Oak, N° 67, with which no Country Place ought to be unprovided. It is to be kept on, by applying a good deal of Lint over it; covering the whole with a thick Compreſs, and then with a Bandage a little tighter than uſual. If this ſhould not be ſufficient to prevent the Bleeding from the large Veſſel, and the Wound be in the Leg or Arm, a ſtrong Ligature muſt be made above the Wound with a *Turniquet*, which is made in a Moment with a Skain of Thread, or of Hemp, that is paſſed round the Arm circularly, into the Middle of which is inſerted a Piece of Wood or Stick of an Inch Thickneſs, and four or five Inches long; ſo that by turning round this Piece of Wood, any Tightneſs or Compreſſion may be effected at Pleaſure; exactly as a Country-man ſecures a Hogſhead, or a Piece of Timber on his Cart, with a Chain and Ring. But Care muſt be taken, 1, to diſpoſe the Skain in ſuch a Manner, that it muſt always be two Inches wider than

than the Part it surrounds: and, 2, not to strain it so tight as to bring on an Inflammation, which might terminate in a Gangrene.

§ 438. All the boasted Virtues of a Multitude of Ointments are downright Nonsense or Quackery. Art, strictly considered, does not in the least contribute to the healing of Wounds; the utmost we can do amounting only to our removing those Accidents, which are so many Obstacles to their Re-union. On this Account, if there is any extraneous Body in the Wound, such as Iron, Lead, Wood, Glass, Bits of Cloth or Linen, they must be extracted, if that can be very easily done; but if not, Application must be made to a good Surgeon, who considers what Measures are to be taken, and then dresses the Wound, as I have already advised.

Very far from being useful, there are many Ointments that are pernicious on these Occasions; and the only Cases in which they should be used, are those in which the Wounds are distinguished with some particular Appearances, which ought to be removed by particular Applications: But a simple recent Wound, in a healthy Man, requires no other Treatment but what I have already directed, besides that of the general Regimen.

Spirituous Applications are commonly hurtful, and can be suitable and proper but in a few Cases, which Physicians and Surgeons only can distinguish.

When Wounds occur in the Head, instead of the Compress dipt in Oil, or of the Cerecloth, the Wound should be covered with a Betony Plaister; or, when none is to be had in time, with a Compress squeezed out of hot Wine.

§ 439. As the following Symptoms, of which we should be most apprehensive, are such as attend on Inflammations, the Means we ought to have Recourse to are those which are most likely to prevent them; such as Bleeding, the usual Regimen, moderate Coolers and Glysters.

Should the Wound be very inconsiderable in its Degree, and in its Situation, it may be sufficient to avoid taking any Thing heating; and above all Things to retrench the Use of any strong Drink, and of Flesh-meat.

But when it is considerable, and an Inflammation must be expected, there is a Necessity for Bleeding; the Patient should be kept in the most quiet and easy Situation, he should be ordered immediately to a Regimen; and sometimes the Bleeding also must be repeated. Now all these Means are the more indispensably necessary, when the Wound has penetrated to some internal Part, in which Situation, no Remedy is more certain than that of an extremely light Diet. Such wounded Persons as have been supposed incapable of living many Hours, after Wounds in the Breast, in the Belly, or in the Kidnies, have been completely recovered, by living for the Course of several Weeks, on nothing but a Barley, or other farinaceous mealy, Ptisans, without

out Salt, without Soup, without any Medicine; and especially without the Use of any Ointments.

§ 440. In the same Proportion that Bleeding, moderately and judiciously employed, is serviceable, in that very same an Excess of it becomes pernicious. Great Wounds are generally attended with a considerable Loss of Blood, which has already exhausted the wounded Person; and the Fever is often a Consequence of this copious Loss of Blood. Now if under such a Circumstance, Bleeding should be ordered and performed, the Patient's Strength is totally sunk; the Humours stagnate and corrupt; a Gangrene supervenes, and he dies miserably, at the End of two or three Days, of a *Series* of repeated Bleedings, but not of the Wound. Notwithstanding the Certainty of this, the Surgeon frequently boasts of his ten, twelve, or even his fifteen Bleedings, assuring his Hearers of the insuperable Mortality of the Wound, since the letting out such a Quantity of Blood could not recover the Patient, when it really was that excessive artificial Profusion of it, that downright dispatched him. —— The Pleasures of Love are very mortal ones to the Wounded.

§ 441. The Balsams and vulnerary Plants, which have often been so highly celebrated for the Cure of Wounds, are very noxious, when taken inwardly; because the Introduction of them gives or heightens the Fever, which ought to have been abated.

Of Contusions, or Bruises.

§ 442. A Contusion, which is commonly called a Bruise, is the Effect of the forcible Impression or Stroke of a Substance not sharp or cutting, on the Body of a Man, or any Animal; whether such an Impression be violently made on the Man, as when he is struck by a Stick, or by a Stone thrown at him; or whether the Man be involuntarily forced against a Post, a Stone, or any hard Substance by a Fall; or whether, in short, he is squeezed and oppressed betwixt two hard Bodies, as when his Finger is squeezed betwixt the Door and the Door-Post, or the whole Body jammed in betwixt any Carriage and the Wall. These Bruises, however, are still more frequent in the Country than Wounds, and commonly more dangerous too; and indeed the more so, as we cannot judge so exactly, and so soon, of the whole Injury that has been incurred; and because all that is immediately visible of it is often but a small Part of the real Damage attending it: since it frequently happens that no Hurt appears for a few successive Days, nor does it become manifest, until it is too late to admit of an effectual Cure.

§ 443. It is but a few Weeks since a Cooper came to ask my Advice. His Manner of breathing, his Aspect, the Quickness, Smallness, and Irregularity of his Pulse, made me apprehensive at once, that some Matter was formed within his Breast.

Nevertheless he still kept up, and went about, working also at some Part of his Trade. He had fallen in removing some Casks or Hogsheads; and the whole Weight of his Body had been violently impressed upon the right Side of his Breast. Notwithstanding this, he was sensible of no Hurt at first; but some Days afterwards he began to feel a dull heavy Pain in that Part, which continued and brought on a Difficulty of Breathing, Weakness, broken Sleep and Loss of Appetite. I ordered him immediately to Stilness and Repose, and I advised him to drink a Ptisan of Barley sweetened with Honey, in a plentiful Quantity. He regularly obeyed only the latter Part of my Directions: yet on meeting him a few Days after, he told me he was better. The very same Week, however, I was informed he had been found dead in his Bed. The Imposthume had undoubtedly broke, and suffocated him

§ 444. A young Man, run away with by his Horse, was forced with Violence against a Stable-Door, without being sensible of any Damage at the Time. But at the Expiration of twelve Days, he found himself attacked by some such Complaints, as generally occur at the Beginning of a Fever. This Fever was mistaken for a putrid one, and he was very improperly treated, for the Fever it really was, above a Month. In short, it was agreed at a Consultation, that Matter was collected in the Breast. In Consequence of this, he was more properly attended, and at length

length happily cured by the Operation for an *Empyema*, after languishing a whole Year. I have published these two Instances, to demonstrate the great Danger of neglecting violent Strokes or Bruises; since the first of these Patients might have escaped Death; and the second a tedious and afflicting Disorder, if they had taken, immediately after each Accident, the necessary Precautions against its Consequences.

§ 445. Whenever any Part is bruised, one of two Things always ensues, and commonly both happen together; especially if the Contusion is pretty considerable: Either the small Blood-vessels of the contused Part are broken, and the Blood they contained is spread about in the adjoining Parts; or else, without such an Effusion of it, these Vessels have lost their Tone, their active Force, and no longer contributing to the Circulation, their Contents stagnate. In each of these Cases, if Nature, either without or with the Assistance of Art, does not remove the Impediment, an Inflammation comes on, attended with an imperfect, unkindly Suppuration, with Putrefaction and a Gangrene; without mentioning the Symptoms that arise from the Contusion of some particular Substance, as a Nerve, a large Vessel, a Bone, &c. Hence we may also conceive the Danger of a Contusion happening to any inward Part, from which the Blood is either internally effused, or the Circulation wholly obstructed in some vital Organ. This is the Cause of the sudden Death of Persons after a violent Fall,

Fall; or of those who have received the violent Force of heavy descending Bodies on their Heads; or of some violent Strokes, without any evident external Hurt or Mark.

There have been many Instances of sudden Deaths after one Blow on the Pit of the Stomach, which has occasioned a Rupture of the Spleen.

It is in Consequence of Falls occasioning a general slight Contusion, as well internal as external, that they are sometimes attended with such grievous Consequences, especially in old Men, where Nature, already enfeebled, is less able to redress such Disorders. And thus in Fact has it been, that many such, who had before enjoyed a firm State of Health, have immediately lost it after a Fall (which seemed at first to have affected them little or not at all) and languished soon after to the Moment of their Death, which such Accidents very generally accelerate.

§ 446. Different external and internal Remedies are applicable in Contusions. When the Accident has occurred in a slight Degree, and there has been no great nor general Shock, which might produce an internal Soreness or Contusion, external Applications may be sufficient. They should consist of such Things as are adapted, first, to attenuate and resolve the effused and stagnant Blood, which shews itself so apparently; and which, from its manifest Blackness very soon after the Contusion, becomes successively brown, yellow, and greyish, in Proportion as the Magnitude of the Suffusion or Settling decreases,

till

till at last it disappears entirely; and the Skin recovers its Colour, without the Blood's having been discharged through the external Surface, as it has been insensibly and gradually dissolved, and been taken in again by the Vessels: And secondly, the Medicines should be such as are qualified to restore the Tone, and to recover the Strength of the affected Vessels.

The best Application is Vinegar, diluted, if very sharp, with twice as much warm Water; in which Mixture Folds of Linnen are to be dipt, within which the contused Parts are to be involved; and these Folds are to be remoistened and re-applied every two Hours on the first Day.

Parsley, Chervil, and Houseleek Leaves, lightly pounded, have also been successfully employed; and these Applications are preferable to Vinegar, when a Wound is joined to the Bruise. The Pultices, N°. 68, may also be used with Advantage.

§ 447. It has been a common Practice immediately to apply spirituous Liquors, such as Brandy, Arquebussade and * Alibour Water, and the like; but a long Abuse ought not to be established by Prescription. These Liquids which coagulate the Blood, instead of resolving it, are truly pernicious; notwithstanding they are sometimes employed

---

* This Dr Tissot informs me is a Solution of white Vitriol and in the other Drugs in Spirit of Wine, and is never used in regular Practice now. It has its Name from the Author of the Second. A.

ployed without any visible Disadvantage, on very slight Occasions. Frequently by determining the settled Blood towards the Insterstices of the Muscles, the fleshy Parts; or sometimes even by preventing the Effusion, or visible Settling of the Blood, and fixing it, as it were, within the bruised Vessels, they seem to be well; though this only arises from their concentring and concealing the Evil, which, at the End of a few Months, breaks forth again in a very troublesome Shape. Of this I have seen some miserable Examples, whence it has been abundantly evinced, that Applications of this Sort should never be admitted; and that Vinegar should be used, instead of them. At the utmost it should only be allowed, (after there is Reason to suppose all the stagnant Blood resolved and resorbed into the Circulation) to add a third Part of Arquebusade Water to the Vinegar; with an Intention to restore some Strength to the relaxed and weakened Parts.

§ 448. It is still a more pernicious Practice to apply, in Bruises, Plaisters composed of greasy Substances, Rosins, Gums, Earths, &c. The most boasted of these is always hurtful, and there have been many Instances of very slight Contusions being aggravated into Gangrenes by such Plaisters ignorantly applied, which Bruises would have been entirely subdued by the Oeconomy of Nature, if left to herself, in the Space of four Days.

Those Sacs or Suffusions of coagulated Blood, which are visible under the Skin, should never be be opened, except for some urgent Reason; since however large they may be, they insensibly disappear and dissipate; instead of which Termination, by opening them, they sometimes terminate in a dangerous Ulceration.

§ 449. The internal Treatment of Contusions is exactly the same with that of Wounds; only that in these Cases the best Drink is the Prescription, N°. 1, to each Pot of which a Drachm of Nitre must be added.

When any Person has got a violent Fall; has lost his Senses, or is become very stupid, when the Blood starts out of his Nostrils, or his Ears; when he is greatly oppressed, or his Belly feels very tight and tense, which import an Effusion of Blood either into the Head, the Breast or the Belly, he must, first of all, be bled upon the Spot, and all the Means must be recurred to, which have been mentioned § 439, giving the wretched Patient the least possible Disturbance or Motion; and by all means avoiding to jog or shake him, with a Design to bring him to his Senses; which would be directly and effectually killing him, by causing a further Effusion of Blood. Instead of this the whole Body should be fomented, with some one of the Decoctions already mentioned: and when the Violence has been chiefly impressed on the Head, Wine and Water should be prefered to Vinegar.

Falls attended with Wounds, and even a Fracture of the Skull, and with the most alarming Symptoms, have been cured by these internal Remedies,

Of external Disorders.

Remedies, and without any other external Assistance, except the Use of the aromatic Fomentation, N°. 68.

A Man from *Pully-petit* came to consult me some Months ago, concerning his Father, who had a high Fall out of a Tree. He had been twenty-four Hours without Feeling or Sense, and without any other Motion than frequent Efforts to vomit, and Blood had issued both from his Nose and Ears. He had no visible outward Hurt neither on his Head, nor any other Part; and, very fortunately for him, they had not as yet exerted the least Effort to relieve him. I immediately directed a plentiful Bleeding in the Arm; and a large Quantity of Whey sweetened with Honey to be drank, and to be also injected by Way of Glyster. This Advice was very punctually observed; and fifteen Days after the Father came to *Lausanne*, which is four Leagues from *Pully-petit*, and told me he was very well. It is proper, in all considerable Bruises, to open the Patient's Belly with a mild cooling Purge, such as N°. 11, 23, 32, 49. The Prescription N°. 24, and the honyed Whey are excellent Remedies, from the same Reason.

§ 450. In these Circumstances, Wine, distilled Spirits, and whatever has been supposed to revive and to rouse, is mortal. For this Reason People should not be too impatient, because the Patients remain some Time without Sense or Feeling. The giving of Turpentine is more likely to do Mischief than Good; and if it has been sometimes serviceable, it must have been in Consequence of its purging the Patient, who probably then needed to be purged. The Fat of a Whale, *(Sperma cæti)* Dragons Blood, Crabs-Eyes, and Ointments of whatsoever Sort are at least useless and dangerous Medicines, if the Case be very hazardous; either by the Mischief they do, or the Good they prevent from being done. The proper Indication is to dilute the Blood, to render it more fluid and disposed to circulate; and the Medicines just mentioned produce a very contrary Effect.

§ 451. When an aged Person gets a Fall, which is the more dangerous in Proportion to his Age and Grossness; notwithstanding he should not seem in the least incommoded by it, if he is sanguine and still somewhat vigorous, he should part with three or four Ounces of Blood. He should take immediately a few successive Cups of a lightly aromatic Drink, which should be given him hot; such, for Instance, as an Infusion of Tea sweetened with Honey, and he should be advised to move gently about. He must retrench a little from the usual Quantity of his Food, and accustom himself to very gentle, but very frequent, Exercise.

§ 452. Sprains or Wrenches, which very often happen, produce a Kind of Contusion, in the Parts adjoining to the sprained Joint. This Contusion is caused by the violent Friction of the Bone against the neighbouring Parts; and as soon as the Bones are immediately returned into their

proper

proper Situation, the Disorder should be treated as a Contusion. Indeed if the Bones should not of themselves return into their proper natural Position, Recourse must be had to the Hand of a Surgeon.

The best Remedy in this Case is absolute Rest and Repose, after applying a Compress moistened in Vinegar and Water, which is to be renewed and continued, till the Marks of the Contusion entirely disappear; and there remains not the smallest Apprehension of an Inflammation. Then indeed, and not before, a little Brandy or Arquebusade Water may be added to the Vinegar; and the Part (which is almost constantly the Foot) should be strengthened and secured for a considerable Time with a Bandage, as it might, otherwise be liable to fresh Sprains, which would daily more and more enfeeble it: and if this Evil is overlooked too much in its Infancy, the Part never recovers its full Strength; and a small Swelling often remains to the End of the Patient's Life.

If the Sprain is very slight and moderate, a Plunging of the Part into cold Water is excellent, but if this is not done at once immediately after the Sprain, or if the Contusion is violent, it is even hurtful.

The Custom of rolling the naked Foot upon some round Body is insufficient, when the Bones are not perfectly replaced; and hurtful, when the Sprain is accompanied with a Contusion.

It happens continually almost that Country People, who encounter such Accidents, apply themselves either to ignorant or knavish Impostors, who find, or are determined to find, a Disorder or Dislocation of the Bones, where there is none; and who, by their violent Manner of handling the Parts, or by the Plaisters they surround them with, bring on a dangerous Inflammation, and change the Patient's Dread of a small Disorder, into a very grievous Malady.

These are the very Persons who have created, or indeed rather imagined, some impossible Diseases, such as the Opening, the Splitting of the Stomach, and of the Kidnies. But these big Words terrify the poor Country People, and dispose them to be more easily and effectually duped.

Of Ulcers

§ 453 Whenever Ulcers arise from a general Fault of the Blood, it is impossible to cure them, without destroying the Cause and Fuel of them. It is in Fact imprudent to attempt to heal them up by outward Remedies; and a real Misfortune to the Patient, if his Assistant effectually heals and closes them.

But, for the greater Part, Ulcers in the Country are the Consequence of some Wound, Bruise, or Tumour improperly treated; and especially of such as have been dressed with too sharp, or too spirituous Applications. Rancid Oils are also one

one of the Causes, which change the most simple Wounds into obstinate Ulcers, for which Reason they should be avoided; and Apothecaries should be careful, when they compound greasy Ointments, to make but little at a Time, and the oftner, as a very considerable Quantity of any of them becomes rank before it is all sold; notwithstanding sweet fresh Oil may have been employed in preparing them.

§ 454. What serves to distinguish Ulcers from Wounds, is the Dryness and Hardness of the Sides or Borders of Ulcers, and the Quality of the Humour discharged from them; which, instead of being ripe consistent Matter, is a Liquid more thin, less white, sometimes yielding a disagreeable Scent, and so very sharp, that if it touch the adjoining Skin, it produces Redness, Inflammation, or Pustules there; sometimes a serpiginous, or Ring-worm like Eruption, and even a further Ulceration.

§ 455 Such Ulcers as are of a long Duration, which spread wide, and discharge much, prey upon the Patient, and throw him into a slow Fever, which melts and consumes him. Besides, when an Ulcer is of a long Standing, it is dangerous to dry it up, and indeed this never should be done, but by substituting in the Place of one Discharge that is become almost natural, some other Evacuation, such as Purging from Time to Time.

We may daily see sudden Deaths, or very tormenting Diseases, ensue the sudden drying up such Humours and Drains as have been of a long Continuance. and whenever any Quack (and as many as promise the speedy Cure of such, deserve that Title) assures the Patient of his curing an inveterate Ulcer in a few Days, he demonstrates himself to be a very dangerous and ignorant Intermeddler, who must kill the Patient, if he keeps his Word. Some of these impudent Impostors make use of the most corrrosive Applications, and even arsenical ones; notwithstanding the most violent Death is generally the Consequence of them.

§ 456. The utmost that Art can effect, with Regard to Ulcers, which do not arise from any Fault in the Humours, is to change them into Wounds. To this End, the Hardness and Dryness of the Edges of the Ulcer, and indeed of the whole Ulcer, must be diminished, and its Inflammation removed. But sometimes the Hardness is so obstinate, that this cannot be mollified any other Way, than by scarifying the Edges with a Lancet. But when it may be effected by other Means, let a Pledget spread with the Ointment, N°. 69, be applied all over the Ulcer, and this Pledget be covered again with a Compress of several Folds, moistened in the Liquid, N°. 70, which should be renewed three times daily; though it is sufficient to apply a fresh Pledget only twice.

As I have already affirmed that Ulcers were often the Consequence of sharp and spirituous Dressings, it is evident such should be abstained from,

with-

Of external Disorders.

without which Abstinence they will prove incurable.

To forward the Cure, salted Food, Spices, and strong Drink should be avoided; the Quantity of Flesh-meat should be lessened, and the Body be kept open by a Regimen of Pulse, of Vegetables, and by the habitual Use of Whey sweetened with Honey.

If the Ulcers are in the Legs, a very common Situation of them, it is of great Importance, as well as in Wounds of the same Parts, that the Patient should walk about but little; and yet never stand up without walking. This indeed is one of these Cases, in which those, who have some Credit and Influence in the Estimation of the People, should omit nothing to make them thoroughly comprehend the Necessity of confining themselves, some Days, to undisturbed Tranquillity and Rest, and they should also convince them, that this Term of Rest is so far from being lost Time, that it is likely to prove their most profitable Time of Life. Negligence, in this material Point, changes the slightest Wounds into Ulcers, and the most trifling Ulcers into obstinate and incurable ones: insomuch that there is scarcely any Man, who may not observe some Family in his Neighbourhood, reduced to the Hospital,* from their having been too inattentive

---

* This seems just the same as *coming on the Parish*, or being received into an Alms house here, in Consequence of such an incurable Disability happening to the poor working Father of a Family K

tive to the due Care of some Complaint of this Sort.

I conclude this Article on Ulcers with repeating, that those which are owing to some internal Cause, or even such as happen from an external one, in Persons of a bad Habit of Body, frequently require a more particular Treatment.

Of Frozen Limbs.

§ 457. It is but too common, in very rigorous Winters, for some Persons to be pierced with so violent a Degree of Cold, that their Hands or Feet, or sometimes both together are frozen at once, just like a Piece of Flesh-meat exposed to the Air

If a Person thus pierced with the Cold, dispose himself to walk about, which seems so natural and obvious a Means to get warm, and especially, if he attempts to * warm the Parts that have been frozen, his Case proves irrecoverable. Intolerable Pains are the Consequence, which Pains are speedily attended with an incurable Gangrene, and there is no Means left to save the

---

* The Reason of the Fatality of Heat, in these Cases, and of the Success of an opposite Application, (See § 459) seems strictly and even beautifully analogous to what *Hippocrates* has observed of the Danger, and even Fatality, of all great and sudden Changes in the human Body, whether from the Weather or otherwise. Whence this truly great Founder of Physick, when he observes elsewhere that Diseases are to be cured by something contrary to their Causes, very consistently advises, not a direct and violent Contrariety, but a gradual and regulated one, a *Sub-contrariety* K.

the Patient's Life, but by cutting off the gangrened Limbs.

There was a very late and terrible Example of this, in the Case of an Inhabitant at *Cossonay*, who had both his Hands frozen. Some greasy Ointments were app'ied hot to them, the Consequence of which was, the Necessity of cutting off six of his Fingers.

§ 458. In short, there is but one certain Remedy in such Cases, and this is to convey the Person affected into some Place where it does not freeze, but where, however, it is but very moderately hot, and there continually to apply, to the frozen Parts, Snow, if it be at hand, and if not, to keep washing them incessantly, but very gently (since all Friction would at this Juncture prove dangerous) in Ice-water, as the Ice thaws in the Chamber. By this Application, the Patients will be sensible of their Feeling's returning very gradually to the Part, and that they begin to recover their Motion. In this State they may safely be moved into a Place a little warmer, and drink some Cups of the Potion N°. 13, or of another of the like Quality.

§ 459. Every Person may be a competent Judge of the manifest Danger of attempting to relieve such Parts by heating them, and of the Use of Ice-water, by a common, a daily Experience. Frozen Pears, Apples, and Radishes, being put into Water just about to freeze, recover their former State, and prove quickly eatable. But if they are put into warm Water, or into a

hot

hot Place,—Rottenness, which is one Sort of Gangrene, is the immediate Effect. The following Case will make this right Method of treating them still more intelligible, and demonstrate its Efficacy.

A Man was travelling to the Distance of six Leagues in very cold Weather; the Road being covered with Snow and Ice. His Shoes, not being very good, failed him on his March, so that he walked the three last Leagues bare-footed; and felt, immediately after the first Half League, sharp Pains in his Legs and Feet, which increased as he proceeded. He arrived at his Journey's End in a Manner nearly deprived of his lower Extremities. They set him before a great Fire, heated a Bed well, and put him into it. His Pains immediately became intolerable: he was incessantly in the most violent Agitations, and cried out in the most piercing and affecting Manner. A Physician, being sent for in the Night, found his Toes of a blackish Colour, and beginning to lose their Feeling. His Legs and the upper Part of his Feet, which were excessively swelled, of a purplish Red, and varied with Spots of a violet Colour, were still sensible of the most excruciating Pains. The Physician ordered in a Pail of Water from the adjoining River, adding more to it, and some Ice withal. In this he obliged the Patient to plunge his Legs, they were kept in near an Hour, and within that Time, the Pains became less violent. After another Hour he ordered a second cold Bath, from which the Patient perceiving still further Relief, prolonged it to the Extent of two Hours. During that Time, some Water was taken out of the Pail, and some Ice and Snow were put into it. Now his Toes, which had been black, grew red, the violet Spots in his Legs disappeared; the Swelling abated; the Pains became moderate, and intermitted. The Bath was nevertheless repeated six times; after which there remained no other Complaint, but that of a great Tenderness or extraordinary Sensibility in the Soles of his Feet, which hindered him from walking. The Parts were afterwards bathed with some aromatic Fomentations; and he drank a Ptisan of Sarsaparilla [one of Elder Flowers would have answered the same Purpose, and have been less expensive.] On the eighth Day from his Seizure he was perfectly recovered, and returned home on Foot on the fifteenth.

§ 460. When cold Weather is extremely severe, and a Person is exposed to it for a long Time at once, it proves mortal, in Consequence of its congealing the Blood, and because it forces too great a Proportion of Blood up to the Brain; so that the Patient dies of a Kind of Apoplexy, which is preceded by a Sleepiness. In this Circumstance the Traveller, who finds himself drowsy, should redouble his Efforts to extricate himself from the eminent Danger he is exposed to. This Sleep, which he might consider as some Alleviation of his Sufferings, if indulged, would prove his last.

§ 461.

§ 461. The Remedies in such Cases are the same with those directed in frozen Limbs. The Patient must be conducted to an Apartment rather cold than hot, and be rubbed with Snow or with Ice-water. There have been many well attested Instances of this Method; and as such Cases are still more frequent in more northern Climates, a Bath of the very coldest Water has been found the surest Remedy.

Since it is known that many People have been revived, who had remained in the Snow, or had been exposed to the freezing Air during five, or even six successive Days, and who had discovered no one Mark of Life for several Hours, the utmost Endeavours should be used for the Recovery of Persons in the like Circumstances and Situation.

Of Kibes, or Chilblains.

§ 462. These troublesome and smarting Complaints attack the Hands, Feet, Heels, Ears, Nose and Lips, those of Children especially, and mostly in Winter; when these Extremities are exposed to the sudden Changes from hot to cold, and from cold to hot Weather. They begin with an Inflation or kind of Swelling, which, at first, occasions but little Heat, Pain or Itching. Sometimes they do not exceed this first State, and go off spontaneously without any Application: But at other Times (which may be termed the second Degree of the Disorder, whether it happens from

their

their being neglected, or improperly treated) their Heat, Redness, Itching and Pain increase confiderably; fo that the Patient is often deprived of the free Ufe of his Fingers by the Pain, Swelling and Numbnefs: in which Cafe the Malady is ftill aggravated, if effectual Means are not ufed.

Whenever the Inflammation mounts to a ftill higher Degree, fmall Vefications or Blifters are formed, which are not long without burfting; when they leave a flight Excoriation, or Rawnefs, as it were, which fpeedily ulcerates, and frequently proves a very deep and obftinate Ulcer, difcharging a fharp and ill-conditioned Matter.

The laft and moft virulent Degree of Chilblains, which is not infrequent in the very coldeft Countries, though very rare in the temperate ones, is, when the Inflammation degenerates into a Gangrene.

§ 463. Thefe Tumours are owing to a Fulnefs and Obftruction of the Veffels of the Skin, which occurs from this Circumftance, that the Veins, which are more fuperficial than the Arteries, being proportionably more affected and ftraitened by the Cold, do not carry off all the Blood communicated to them by the Arteries; and perhaps alfo the Particles or Atoms of Cold, which are admitted through the Pores of the Skin, may act upon our Fluids, as it does upon Water, and occafion a Congelation of them, or a confiderable Approach towards it.

If

If these Complaints are chiefly felt, which in Fact is the Case, rather on the extreme Parts, than on others, it arises from two Causes, the principal one being, that the Circulation's being weaker at the Extremities than elsewhere, the Effect of those Causes, that may impair it, must be more considerably felt there. The second Reason is, because these Parts are more exposed to the Impressions from without than the others.

They occur most frequently to Children, from their Weakness and the greater Tenderness and Sensibility of their Organs, which necessarily increases the Effect of external Impressions. It is the frequent and strong Alteration from Heat to Cold, that seems to contribute the most powerfully to the Production of Chilblains, and this Effect of it is most considerable, when the Heat of the Air is at the same Time blended with Moisture; whence the extreme and superficial Parts pass suddenly as it were, out of a hot, into a cold, Bath. A Man sixty Years of Age, who never before was troubled with Kibes, having worn, for some Hours on a Journey, a Pair of furred Gloves, in which his Hands sweated, felt them very tender, and found them swelled up with Blood: as the common Effect of the warm Bath is to soften and relax, and to draw Blood abundantly to the bathed Parts, whence it renders them more sensible.

This Man, I say, thus circumstanced, was at that Age first attacked with Chilblains, which proved extremely troublesome, and he was every ry succeeding Winter as certainly infested with them, within Half an Hour after he left off his Gloves, and was exposed to a very cold Air.

It is for this Reason, that several Persons are never infested with Chilblains, but when they use themselves to Muffs, which are scarcely known in hot Countries; nor are they very common among the more northern ones, in which the extraordinary Changes from Cold to Heat are very rare and unusual.

Some People are subject to this troublesome Complaint in the Fall; while others have it only in the Spring. The Child of a labouring Peasant, who has a hard Skin, and one inured to all the Impressions of the Seasons and of the Elements, is, and indeed necessarily must be, less liable to Kibes, than the Child of a rich Citizen, whose Skin is often cherished, at the Expence of his Constitution. But even among Children of the same Rank in Life and Circumstances, who seem pretty much of the same Complexion, and live much in the same Manner; whence they might of Course be supposed equally liable to the same Impressions, and to the like Effects of them, there is, nevertheless, a very great Difference with Respect to their constitutional Propensity to contract Chilblains. Some are very cruelly tormented with them, from the setting in of Autumn, to the very End of the Spring. others have either none at all, or have them but very slightly, and for a very short Time. This Difference undoubtedly arises from

the

the different Quality of their Humours, and the Texture of their whole Surface, but particularly from that of the Skin of their Hands, though we readily confess it is by no Means easy to determine, with Certainty and Precision, in what this Difference essentially consists.

Children of a sanguine Complexion and delicate Skin are pretty generally subject to this Disorder, which is often regarded much too slightly, though it is really severe enough to engage our Attention more, since, even abstracted from the sharp Pains which smart these unhappy Children for several Months; it sometimes gives them a Fever, hinders them from sleeping, and yet confines them to their Bed, which is very prejudicial to their Constitution. It also breaks in upon the Order of their different Duties and Employments; it interrupts their innocent salutary Pleasures; and sometimes, when they are obliged to earn their daily Bread by doing some Work or other, it sinks them down to Misery. I knew a young Man, who from being rendered incapable by Chilblains, of serving out his Apprenticeship to a Watch-maker, is become a lazy Beggar

Chilblains which attack the Nose, often leave a Mark that alters the Physiognomy, the Aspect of the Patient, for the Remainder of his Life. and the Hands of such as have suffered from very obstinate ones, are commonly ever sensible of their Consequences.

§ 464. With Respect, therefore, to these afflicting Tumours and Ulcerations, we should, in the first Place, do our utmost to prevent them, and next exert our best Endeavours to cure such as we could not prevent.

§ 465. Since they manifestly depend on the Sensibility of the Skin, the Nature of the Humours, and the Changes of the Weather from Heat to Cold, in Order to prevent them, in the first Place, the Skin must be rendered firmer or less tender. 2, That vicious Quality of the Temperament, which contributes to their Existence, must be corrected; and, 3, the Persons so liable must guard themselves as well as possible, against these Changes of the Weather.

Now the Skin of the Hands, as well as that of the whole Body, may be strengthened by that Habit of washing or bathing in cold Water, which I have described at large, § 384, and in Fact I have never seen Children, who had been early accustomed and inured to this Habit, as much afflicted with Chilblains as others. But still a more particular Regard should be had to fortify the Skin of the Hands, which are more obnoxious to this Disorder than the Feet, by making Children dip them in cold Water, and keep them for some Moments together in it every Morning, and every Evening too before Supper, from the very Beginning of the Fall. It will give the Children no Sort of Pain, during that Season, to contract this Habit, and when it is once contracted, it will give them no Trouble to continue it throughout the Winter, even when the Water is ready to freeze every where.

They may also be habituated to plunge their Feet into cold Water twice or thrice a Week: and this Method, which might be less adapted for grown Persons, who had not been accustomed to it, must be without Objection with Respect to such Children, as have been accustomed to it; to whom all its Consequences must be useful and salutary.

At the same Time Care must be taken not to defeat or lessen the Effect of the cold bathing, by suffering the Bather or Washer, to grow too warm between two Baths or Dippings; which is also avoiding the too speedy Successions of Heat and Cold. For this Purpose, 1, the Children must be taught never to warm their Hands before the Fire at such Times, and still less before the Stoves, which very probably are one of the principal Causes of Chilblains, that are less usual in Countries which use no such Stoves, and among those Individuals who make the least Use of them, where they are. Above all, the Use of *Cavettes* (that is, of Seats or little Stairs, as it were, contrived between the Stove and the Wall) is prejudicial to Children, and even to grown People, upon several Accounts. 2, They should never accustom themselves to wear Muffs. 3, It would be also proper they should never use Gloves, unless some particular Circumstances require it, and I recommend this Abstinence from Gloves, especially to young Boys. but if any should be allowed them, let the Gloves be thin and smooth

§ 466

§ 466. When Chilblains seem to be nourished by some Fault in the Temperament or Humours, the Consideration of a Physician becomes necessary, to direct a proper Method of removing or altering it. I have seen Children from the Age of three, to that of twelve or thirteen Years, in whom their Chilblains, raw and flead, as it were, for eight Months of the Year, seemed to be a particular Kind of Issue, by which Nature freed herself of an inconvenient Superfluity of Humours, when the Perspiration was diminished by the Abatement of the violent Heats. In such Cases I have been obliged to carry them through a pretty long Course of Regimen and Remedies; which, however, being necessarily various from a Variety of Circumstances, cannot be detailed here. The milder Preparations of Antimony are often necessary in such Cases; and some Purges conduce in particular ones to allay and to abridge the Disorder.

§ 467 The first Degree of this Complaint goes off, as I have already said, without the Aid of Medicine, or should it prove somewhat more obstinate, it may easily be dissipated by some of the following Remedies But when they rise to the second Degree, they must be treated like other Complaints from Congelation, or Frost-biting (of which they are the first Degree) with cold Water, Ice-water and Snow.

No other Method of Medicine is nearly as efficacious as very cold Water, so as to be ready to freeze, in which the Hands are to be dipt and retained for some Minutes together, and several Times daily. In short it is the only Remedy which ought to be applied, when the Hands are the Parts affected; when the Patient has the Courage to bear this Degree of Cold; and when he is under no Circumstance which may render it prejudicial. It is the only Application I have used for myself, after having been attacked with Chilblains for some Years past, from having accustomed myself to too warm a Muff.

There ensues a slight Degree of Pain for some Moments after plunging the Hand into Water, but it diminishes gradually. On taking the Hand out, the Fingers are numbed with the Cold, but they presently grow warm again; and within a Quarter of an Hour, it is entirely over.

The Hands, on being taken out of the Water, are to be well dried, and put into Skin Gloves; after bathing three or four Times, their Swelling subsides, so that the Skin wrinkles: but by continuing the cold Bathing, it grows tight and smooth again, the Cure is compleated after using it three or four Days; and, in general, the Disorder never returns again the same Winter.

The most troublesome raging Itching is certainly assuaged by plunging the Hands into cold Water.

The Effect of Snow is, perhaps, still more speedy the Hands are to be gently and often rubbed with it for a considerable Time, they grow hot, and are of a very high Red for
some

some Moments, but entire Ease very quickly succeeds

Nevertheless, a very small Number of Persons, who must have extremely delicate and sensible Skins, do not experience the Efficacy of this Application. It seems too active for them, it affects the Skin much like a common blistering Plaister, and by bringing on a large flow of Humours there, it increases, instead of lessening the Complaint.

§ 468. When this last Reason indeed, or some other Circumstance exists; such as the Child's Want of Courage, or its Affliction; the monthly Discharges in a Woman; a violent Cough; habitual Colics; and some other Maladies, which have been observed to be renewed or aggravated by the Influence of Cold at the Extremities, do really forbid this very cold Application, some others must be substituted.

One of the best is to wear Day and Night, without ever putting it off, a Glove made of some smooth Skin, such as that of a Dog; which seldom fails to extinguish the Disorder in some Days time.

When the Feet are affected with Chilblains, Socks of the same Skin should be worn, and the Patient keep close to his Bed for some Days.

§ 469 When the Disorder is violent, the Use of cold Water prohibited, and the Gloves just recommended have but a slow Effect, the diseased Parts should be gently fomented or moistened several times a Day, with some Decoction,

rather

rather more than warm, which at the same time should be dissolving and emollient. Such is that celebrated Decoction of the Scrapings, the Peel of Radishes, whose Efficacy is still further increased, by adding one sixth Part of Vinegar to the Decoction.

Another Decoction, of whose great Efficacy I have been a Witness, but which dies the Hands yellow for a few Days, is the Prescription N°. 71. Many others may be made, of nearly the same Virtues, with all the vulnerary Herbs, and even with the *Faltranc*.

Urine, which some boast of in these Cases, from their having used it with Success, and the Mixture of Urine and Lime-water have the like Virtues with the former Decoctions.*

As soon as the Hands affected are taken out of these Decoctions, they must be defended from the Air by Gloves.

§ 470. Vapours or Steams are often more efficacious than Decoctions; whence instead of dipping the Hands into these already mentioned, we may expose them to their Vapours, with still more Success. That of hot Vinegar is one of the most powerful Remedies; those of †*Asphalt*,

or

---

* Chilblains may also be advantageously washed with Water and Flower of Mustard, which will concur, in a certain and easy Manner, both to cleanse and to cure them. *L L*

† This so should be, the same with the *Bitumen Judaicum*, formerly kept in the Shops, but which is never directed, except in that strange Medley the *Venice* Treacle, according to the old Prescription. The best is found in *Egypt*, and on the *Red Sea*: but a different Sort from *Germany*, *France*, and *Switzerland*, is now generally substituted here. *K*

or of Turpentine have frequently succeeded too. It may be needless to add that the affected Parts must be defended from the Air, as well after the Steams as the Decoctions; since it is from this Cause of keeping off the Air, that the Cerecloths are of Service; and hence also the Application of Suet has sometimes answered.

When the Distemper is subdued by the Use of Bathings or Steams, which make the Skin supple and soft, then it should be strengthened by washing the Parts with a little camphorated Brandy, diluted with an equal Quantity of Water.

§ 471. When the Nose is affected with a Chilblain, the Steam of Vinegar, and an artificial Nose, or Covering for it, made of Dog-skin, are the most effectual Applications. The same Treatment is equally proper for the Ears and the Chin, when infested with them. Frequently washing these Parts in cold Water is a good Preservative from their being attacked.

§ 472. Whenever the Inflammation rises very high, and brings on some Degree of a Fever, the Patient's usual Quantity of strong Drink and of Flesh-meat must be lessened, his Body should be kept open by a few Glysters, he should take every Evening a Dose of Nitre as prescribed, N°. 20; and if the Fever proved strong, he should lose some Blood too.

As many as are troubled with obstinate Chilblains, should always be denied the Use of strong Liquor and Flesh.

§ 473.

§ 473. When this Diftemper prevails in its third Degree, and the Parts are ulcerated; befides keeping the Patients ftrictly to the Regimen of Perfons in a Way of Recovery, and giving them a Purge of Manna, the fwelled Parts fhould be expofed to the Steams of Vinegar, the Ulcerations fhould be covered with a Diapalma Plaifter; and the whole Part fhould be enveloped in a fmooth foft Skin, or in thin Cerecloths.

§ 474 The fourth Degree of this Difeafe, in which the Parts become gangrenous, muft be prevented by the Method and Medicines which remove an Inflammation, but if unhappily a Gangrene has already appeared, the Affiftance of a Surgeon proves indifpenfably neceffary.

Of Ruptures.

§ 475. *Hernias* or Ruptures, which Country-People term *being burften*, are a Diforder which fometimes occurs at the very Birth, though more frequently they are the Effects of violent crying, of a ftrong forcing Cough, or of repeated Efforts to vomit, in the firft Months of Infancy.

They may happen afterwards indifcriminately at every Age, either as Confequences of particular Maladies, or Accidents, or from Peoples' violent Exertions of their Strength. They happen much oftner to Men than Women; and the moft common Sort, indeed the only one of which I propofe to treat, and that but briefly, is that which confifts in the Defcent of a Part of the

Of external Diforders. 475

the Guts, or of the Cawl, into the Bag or Cod-piece.

It is not difficult to diftinguifh this Rupture. When it occurs in little Children, it is almoft ever cured by making them conftantly wear a Bandage which fhould be made only of Fuftian, with a little Pillow or Pincufhion, ftuffed with Linen Rags, Hair or Bran. There fhould be at leaft two of thefe Bandages, to change them alternately, nor fhould it ever be applied, but when the Child is laid down on its Back, and after being well affured that the Gut or Cawl, which had fallen down, has been fafely returned into the Cavity of the Belly, fince without this Precaution it might occafion the worft Confequences.

The good Effect of the Bandage may be ftill further promoted, by applying upon the Skin, and within the Plait or Fold of the Groin (under which Place the Rings, or Paffage out of the Belly into the Bag lie) fome pretty aftringent or ftrengthening Plaifter, fuch as that commonly ufed for Fractures, or that I have already mentioned, § 144 Here we may obferve by the Way, that ruptured Children fhould never be fet on a Horfe, nor be carried by any Perfon on Horfeback, before the Rupture is perfectly cured.

§ 476. In a more advanced Age, a Bandage only of Fuftian is not fufficient, one muft be procured with a Plate of Steel, even fo as to conftrain and incommode the Wearer a little at firft:

first: nevertheless it soon becomes habitual, and is then no longer inconvenient to them.

§ 477. Ruptures sometimes attain a monstrous Size; and a great Part of the Guts fall down into the *Scrotum* or Bag, without any Symptom of an actual Disease. This Circumstance, nevertheless, is accompanied with very great Inconvenience, which disables Persons affected with it to work; and whenever the Malady is so considerable, and of a long Standing too, there are commonly some Obstacles that prevent a compleat Return of the Guts into the Belly. In this State indeed, the Application of the Bandage or Truss is impracticable, and the miserable Patients are condemned to carry their grievous Burthen for the Remainder of their Lives, which may however, be palliated a little by the Use of a Suspensory and Bag, adapted to the Size of the Rupture. This Dread of its increasing Magnitude is a strong Motive for checking the Progress of it, when it first appears. But there is another still stronger, which is, that Ruptures expose the Patient to a Symptom frequently mortal. This occurs when that Part of the Intestines fallen into the *Scrotum* inflames; when still increasing in its Bulk, and being extremely compressed, acute Pains come on: for now from the Increase of the Rupture's Extent, the Passage which gave Way to its Descent, cannot admit of its Return or Ascent; the Blood-vessels themselves being oppressed, the Inflammation increases every Moment, the Communication between the Stomach and

Of external Disorders.

and the Fundament is often entirely cut off; so that nothing passes through, but incessant Vomitings come on [this being the Kind of *Miserere*, or Iliac Passion I have mentioned, § 320] which are succeeded by the Hickup, Raving, Swooning, cold Sweats, and Death.

§ 478. This Symptom supervenes in Ruptures, when the Excrements become hard in that Part of the Guts fallen into the *Scrotum*; when the Patient is overheated with Wine, Drams, an inflammatory Diet, &c. or when he has received a Stroke on the ailing Part, or had a Fall.

§ 479. The best Means and Remedies are, 1, as soon as ever this Symptom or Accident is manifest, to bleed the Patient very plentifully, as he lies down in his Bed and upon his Back, with his Head a little raised, and his Legs somewhat bent, so that his Knees may be erect. This is the Attitude or Posture they should always preserve as much as possible When the Malady is not too far advanced, the first Bleeding often makes a compleat Cure; and the Guts return up as soon as it is over. At other Times this Bleeding is less successful, and leaves a Necessity for its Repetition.

2, A Glyster must be thrown up consisting of a strong Decoction of the large white Beet Leaves, with a small Spoonful or Pinch of common Salt, and a Bit of fresh Butter of the Size of an Egg.

3, Folds of Linen dipt in Ice-water must be applied all over the Tumour, and constantly renewed

newed every Quarter of an Hour. This Remedy, when immediately applied, has produced the moſt happy Effects; but if the Symptom has endured violently more than ten or twelve Hours, it is often too late to apply it; and then it is better to make Uſe of Flanels dipt in a warm Decoction of Mallow and Elder Flowers, ſhifting them frequently. It has been known however, that Ice-water, or Ice itſelf has ſucceeded as late as the third Day.*

4, When theſe Endeavours are inſufficient, Glyſters of Tobacco Smoke muſt be tried, which has often redreſſed and returned Ruptures, when every Thing elſe had failed.

5, And laſtly, if all theſe Attempts are fruitleſs, the Operation muſt be reſolved on, without loſing a Moment's Time; as this local Diſeaſe proves ſometimes mortal in the Space of two Days; but for this Operation an excellent Surgeon is indiſpenſably neceſſary. The happy Conſequence with which I have ordered it, in a moſt deſperate Caſe ſince the firſt Edition of this Work, on the ſixth Day after a Labour, has convinced me, ſtill more than any former Obſervation I had

---

* Pieces of Ice applied between two Pieces of Linen, directly upon the Rupture, as ſoon as poſſible after its firſt Appearance, is one of thoſe extraordinary Remedies, which we ſhould never heſitate to make immediate Uſe of. We may be certain by this Application, if the Rupture is ſimple, and not complicated from ſome aggravating Cauſe, to remove ſpeedily, and with very little Pain, a Diſorder, that might be attended with the moſt dreadful Conſequences. But the Continuance of this Application muſt be proportioned to the Strength of the Perſon ruptured, which may be efficaciouſly eſtimated by his Pulſe. L L

had made, that the Trial of it ought never to be omitted, when other Attempts have been unavailing. It cannot even haften the Patient's Death, which muſt be inevitable without it, but it rather renders that more gentle, where it might fail to prevent it. When it is performed as Mr. LEVADE effected it, in the Caſe I have juſt referred to, the Pain attending it is very tolerable and ſoon over.

I ſhall not attempt to deſcribe the Operation, as I could not explain myſelf ſufficiently to inſtruct an ignorant Surgeon in it, and an excellent and experienced one muſt be ſufficiently apprized of all I could ſay concerning it.

A certain Woman in this Place, but now dead, had the great and impudent Temerity to attempt this Operation, and killed her Patients after the moſt excruciating Torments, and an Extirpation, or cutting away of the Teſticle, which Quacks and ignorant Surgeons always do, but which a good Surgeon never does in this Operation. This is often the Cuſtom too (in Country Places) of thoſe Caitiffs, who perform this Operation without the leaſt Neceſſity; and mercileſsly emaſculate a Multitude of Infants; whom Nature, if left to her own Conduct, or aſſiſted only by a ſimple Bandage, would have perfectly cured, inſtead of which, they abſolutely kill a great many, and deprive thoſe of their Virility, who ſurvive their Robbery and Violence. It were religiouſly to be wiſhed ſuch Caitiffs were to be duly, that is, ſeverely puniſhed, and it cannot

cannot be too much inculcated into the People, that this Operation (termed the *Bubonocele*) in the Manner it is performed by the best Surgeons, is not necessary, except in the Symptoms and Circumstances I have mentioned, and that the cutting off the Testicle never is so.

Of Phlegmons or Boils.

§ 480. Every Person knows what Boils are at Sight, which are considerably painful when large, highly inflamed, or so situated as to incommode the Motions, or different Positions of the Body. Whenever their Inflammation is very considerable, when there are a great many of them at once, and they prevent the Patients from sleeping, it becomes necessary to enter them into a cooling Regimen, to throw up some opening Glysters; and to make them drink plentifully of the Ptisan, N°. 2. Sometimes it is also necessary to bleed the Patient.

Should the Inflammation be very high indeed, a Pultice of Bread and Milk, or of Sorrel a little boiled and bruised, must be applied to it. But if the Inflammation is only moderate, a Mucilage Plaister, or one of the simple Diachylon, may be sufficient. Diachylon with the Gums is more active and efficacious, but it so greatly augments the Pain of some Persons afflicted with Boils, that they cannot bear it.

Boils, which often return, signify some Fault in the Temperament, and frequently one so considerable,

siderable, that might dispose a Physician to be so far apprehensive of its Consequences, as to enquire into the Cause, and to attempt the Extinction of it. But the Detail of this is no Part nor Purpose of the present Work.

§ 481. The Phlegmon, or Boil, commonly terminates in Suppuration, but a Suppuration of a singular Kind. It breaks open at first on its Top, or the most pointed Part, when some Drops of a *Pus* like that of an Abscess comes out, after which the Germ, or what is called the Core of it may be discerned. This is a purulent Matter or Substance, but so thick and tenacious, that it appears like a solid Body; which may be drawn out entirely in the Shape of a small Cylinder, like the Pith of Elder, to the Length of some Lines of an Inch; sometimes to the Length of a full Inch, and even more. The Emission of this Core is commonly followed by the Discharge of a certain Quantity, according to the Size of the Tumour, of liquid Matter, spread throughout the Bottom of it. As soon as ever this Discharge is made, the Pain goes entirely off; and the Swelling disappears at the End of a few Days, by continuing to apply the simple Diachylon, or the Ointment N°. 66

Of Fellons or Whitlows.

§ 482. The Danger of these small Tumours is much greater than is generally supposed. It is an Inflammation at the Extremity or End of a Finger,

Finger, which is often the Effect of a small Quantity of Humour extravasated, or stagnant, in that Part; whether this has happened in Consequence of a Bruise, a Sting, or a Bite. At other times it is evident that it has resulted from no external Cause, but is the Effect of some inward one.

It is distinguished into many Kinds, according to the Place in which the Inflammation begins; but the essential Nature of the Malady is always the same, and requires the same Sort of Remedies. Hence such as are neither Physicians nor Surgeons, may spare themselves the Trouble of enquiring into the Divisions of this Distemper; which, though they vary the Danger of it, and diversify the Manner of the Surgeons Operation, yet have no Relation to the general Treatment of it; the Power and Activity of which must be regulated by the Violence of the Symptoms.

§ 483. This Disorder begins with a slow heavy Pain, attended by a slight Pulsation, without Swelling, without Redness, and without Heat; but in a little Time the Pain, Heat, and Pulsation or Throbbing becomes intolerable The Part grows very large and red; the adjoining Fingers and the whole Hand swelling up. In some Cases a Kind of red and inflated Fuse or Streak may be observed, which, beginning at the affected Part, is continued almost to the Elbow; neither is it unusual for the Patients to complain of a very sharp Pain under the Shoulder; and sometimes the whole Arm is excessively inflamed and swelled.

led. The Sick have not a Wink of Sleep, the Fever and other Symptoms quickly increasing. If the Distemper rises to a violent Degree indeed, a *Delirium* and Convulsions supervene.

This Inflammation of the Finger determines, either in Suppuration, or in a Gangrene. When the last of these occurs, the Patient is in very great Danger, if he is not very speedily relieved; and it has proved necessary more than once to cut off the Arm, for the Preservation of his Life. When Suppuration is effected, if the Matter lies very deep and sharp, or if the Assistance of a Surgeon has arrived too late, the Bone of the last *Phalanx*, or Row of Bones of the Finger, is generally carious and lost. But how gentle soever the Complaint has been, the Nail is very generally separated and falls off.

§ 484. The internal Treatment in Whitlows, is the same with that in other inflammatory Distempers. The Patient must enter upon a Regimen more or less strict, in Proportion to the Degree of the Fever; and if this runs very high, and the Inflammation be very considerable, there may be a Necessity for several Bleedings.

The external Treatment consists in allaying the Inflammation; in softening the Skin; and in procuring a Discharge of the Matter, as soon as it is formed. For this Purpose,

1, The Finger affected is to be plunged, as soon as the Disorder is manifest, in Water a little more than warm: the Steam of boiling Water may also be admitted into it, and by doing these

Things almoſt conſtantly for the firſt Day, a total Diſſipation of the Malady has often been obtained. But unhappily it has been generally ſuppoſed, that ſuch ſlight Attacks could have but very ſlight Conſequences, whence they have been neglected until the Diſorder has greatly advanced; in which State Suppuration becomes abſolutely neceſſary.

2, This Suppuration therefore may be forwarded, by continually involving the Finger, as it were, in a Decoction of Mallow Flowers boiled in Milk, or with a Cataplaſm of Bread and Milk. This may be rendered ſtill more active and ripening, by adding a few white Lilly Roots, or a little Honey. But this laſt muſt not be applied before the Inflammation is ſomewhat abated, and Suppuration begins; before which Term, all ſharp Applications are very dangerous. At this Time, Yeaſt or Leaven may be advantagiouſly uſed, which powerfully promotes Suppuration. The Sorrel Pultice, mentioned § 480, is alſo a very efficacious one.

§ 485. A ſpeedy Diſcharge of the ripe Matter is of conſiderable Importance, but this particularly requires the Attention of the Surgeon, as it is not proper to wait till the Tumour breaks and diſcharges of itſelf; and this the rather, as from the Skin's proving ſometimes extremely hard, the Matter might be inwardly effuſed between the Muſcles, and upon their Membranes, before it could penetrate through the Skin. For this Reaſon, as ſoon as Matter is ſuſpected to be formed,

formed, a Surgeon should be called in, to determine exactly on the Time, when an Opening should be made; which had better be performed a little too soon than too late; and a little too deep, than not deep enough.

When the Orifice has been made, and the Discharge is effected, it is to be dressed up with the Plaister N°. 66, spread upon Linen, or with the Cerecloth; and these Dressings are to be repeated daily.

§ 486. When the Whitlow is caused by a Humour extravasated very near the Nail, an expert Surgeon speedily checks it Progress, and cures it effectually by an Incision which lets out the Humour. Yet, notwithstanding this Operation is in no wise difficult, all Surgeons are not qualified to perform it, and but too many have no Idea at all of it.

§ 487. Fungous, or, as it is commonly called, proud Flesh sometimes appears during the incarning or healing of the Incision. Such may be kept down with sprinkling a little *Minium* (red Lead) or burnt Alum over it.

§ 488. If a *Caries*, a Rottenness of the Bone, should be a Consequence, there is a Necessity for a Surgeon's Attendance, as much as if there was a Gangrene, for which Reason, I shall add nothing with Respect to either of these Symptoms, only observing, there are three very essential Remedies against the last; viz. the Bark, N°. 14, a Drachm of which must be taken every two Hours, Scarifications throughout the whole gangrened Part; and Fomentations with a Decoction of the Bark; and the Addition of Spirit of Sulphur. This Medicine is certainly no cheap one; but a Decoction of other bitter Plants, with the Addition of Spirit of Salt, may sometimes do instead of it. And here I take leave to insist again upon it, that in most Cases of gangrened Limbs, it is judicious not to proceed to an Amputation of the mortified Part, till the Gangrene stops, which may be known by a very perceivable Circle, (and easily distinguished by the most ignorant Persons) that marks the Bounds of the Gangrene, and separates the living from the mortified Parts.

Of Thorns, Splinters, or other pointed Substances piercing into the Skin, or Flesh.

§ 489 It is very common for the Hands, Feet or Legs, to be pierced by the forcible Intrusion of small pointed Substances, such as Thorns or Prickles, whether of Roses, Thistles or Chestnuts, or little Splinters of Wood, Bone, &c.

If such Substances are immediately and entirely extracted, the Accident is generally attended with no bad Consequences, though more certainly to obviate any such, Compresses of Linen dipt in warm Water may be applied to the Part, or it may be kept a little while in a warm Bath. But if any such pointed penetrating Body cannot be directly extracted, or a Part of it be left within, it causes an Inflammation, which, in its Progress,

Progress, soon produces the same Symptoms as a Whitlow: or if it happens in the Leg, it inflames and forms a confiderable Abscefs there.

§ 490. To prevent fuch Confequences, if the penetrating Subftance is ftill near the Surface, and an expert Surgeon is at Hand, he muft immediately make a fmall Incifion, and thence extract it. But if the Inflammation were already formed, this would be ufelefs, and even dangerous.

When the Incifion, therefore, is improper; theie fhould be applied to the affected Parts, (after conveying the Steam of fome hot Water into it) either fome very emollient Pultices of the Crumb of Bread, Milk and Oil, or fome very emollient unctuous Matter alone, the Fat of a * Hare being generally employed in fuch Cafes, and being indeed very effectual to relax and fupple the Skin, and, by thus diminifhing its Refiftance, to afford the offenfive penetrating Body an Opportunity of fpringing forth. Nothing however, but the groffeft Prejudice, could make any one imagine, that this Fat attracted the Splinter, Thorn, or any other intruded Subftance by any fympathetic Virtue; no other Sympathy in Nature being clearly demonftrated, except that very common one between wrong Heads, and abfurd extravagant Opinions.

It is abfolutely neceffary that the injured Part should

---

* Thefe Creatures perhaps are fatter in *Swifferland*, than we often fee them here. *K.*

should be kept in the easiest Posture, and as immoveable as possible.

If Suppuration has not been prevented by an immediate Extraction of the offending Substance, the Abscess should be opened as soon as ever Matter is formed. I have known very troublesome Events from its being too long delayed.

§ 491. Sometimes the Thorn, after having very painfully penetrated through the Teguments, the Skin, enters directly into the Fat; upon which the Pain ceases, and the Patient begins to conclude no sharp prickling Substance had ever been introduced into the Part; and of Course supposes none can remain there. Nevertheless some Days after, or, in other Instances, some Weeks, fresh Pains are excited, to which an Inflammation and Abscess succeed, which are to be treated as usual, with Emollients, and seasonably opened.

A Patient has been reduced to lose his Hand, in Consequence of a sharp Thorn's piercing into his Finger; from its having been neglected at first, and improperly treated afterwards.

Of Warts.

§ 492. Warts are sometimes the Effects of a particular Fault in the Blood, which feeds and extrudes a surprizing Quantity of them. This happens to some Children, from four to ten Years old, and especially to those who feed most plentifully on Milk or Milk-meats. They may be removed

Of external Disorders.

removed by a moderate Change of their Diet, and the Pills prescribed N°. 18.

But they are more frequently an accidental Disorder of the Skin, arising from some external Cause.

In this last Case, if they are very troublesome in Consequence of their great Size, their Situation or their long Standing, they may be destroyed, 1, by tying them closely with a Silk Thread, or with a strong flaxen one waxed. 2, By cutting them off with a sharp Scissars or a Bistory, and applying a Plaister of Diachylon, with the Gums, over the cut Wart, which brings on a small Suppuration that may destroy or dissolve the Root of the Wart: and, 3, By drying, or, as it were, withering them up by some moderately corroding Application, such as that of the milky Juice of † Purslain, of Fig-leaves, of *Chelidonium* (Swallow-wort) or of Spurge. But besides these corroding vegetable Milks being procurable only in Summer, People who have very delicate thin Skins should not make Use of them, as they may occasion a considerable and painful Swelling. Strong

---

† Our Garden Purslain, though a very juicy Herb, cannot strictly be termed milky. In the hotter Climates where it is wild, and grows very rankly, they sometimes boil the Leaves and Stalks (besides eating them as a cooling Salad) and find the whole an insipid mucilaginous Pot-herb. But Dr Tissot observes to me, that its Juice will inflame the Skin; and that some Writers on Diet, who disapprove it internally, affirm they have known it productive of bad Effects. Yet none such have ever happened to myself, nor to many others, who have frequently eaten of it. Its Seeds have sometimes been directed in cooling Emulsions. The Wart Spurge is a very milky and common Herb, which flowers in Summer here. *K.*

Strong Vinegar, charged with as much common Salt as it will dissolve, is a very proper Application to them. A Plaister may also be composed from Sal Ammoniac and some Galbanum, which being kneaded up well together and applied, seldom fails of destroying them.

The most powerful Corrosives should never be used, without the Direction of a Surgeon; and even then it is full as prudent not to meddle with them, any more than with actual Cauteries. I have lately seen some very tedious and troublesome Disorders and Ulcerations of the Kidnies, ensue the Application of a corrosive Water, by the Advice of a Quack. Cutting them away is a more certain, a less painful, and a less dangerous Way of removing them.

Wens, if of a pretty considerable Size, and Duration, are incurable by any other Remedy, except Amputation.

Of Corns.

§ 493. The very general or only Causes of Corns, are Shoes either too hard and stiff, or too small.

The whole Cure consists in softening the Corns by repeated Washings and Soakings of the Feet in pretty hot Water, then in cutting them, when softened, with a Penknife or Scissars, without wounding the sound Parts (which are the more sensible, in Proportion as they are more extended than usual) and next in applying a Leaf of House-

House-leek, of Ground-ivy, or of Purſlain dipt in Vinegar, upon the Part. Inſtead of theſe Leaves, if any Perſon will give himſelf the little Trouble of dreſſing them every Day, he may apply a Plaiſter of ſimple Diachylon, or of Gum Ammoniacum ſoftened in Vinegar.

The Increaſe or Return of Corns can only be prevented, by avoiding the Cauſes that produce them.

Chapter XXXI.

Of ſome Caſes which require immediate Aſſiſtance; ſuch as Swoonings; Hæmorrhages, or involuntary Loſs of Blood; Convulſion Fitts, and Suffocations, the ſudden Effects of great Fear; of Diſorders cauſed by noxious Vapours, of Poiſons, and of acute Pains.

Of Swoonings.

Sect. 494.

THERE are many Degrees of Swooning, or fainting away: the ſlighteſt is that in which the Patient conſtantly perceives and underſtands, yet without the Power of ſpeaking. This is called a Fainting, which happens very often to vapouriſh Perſons,

sons, and without any remarkable Alteration of the Pulse.

If the Patient entirely loses Sensation, or Feeling, and Understanding, with a very considerable Sinking of the Pulse, this is called a *Syncopè*, and is the second Degree of Swooning.

But if this *Syncopè* is so violent, that the Pulse seems totally extinguished; without any discernible Breathing, with a manifest Coldness of the whole Body; and a wanly livid Countenance, it constitutes a third and last Degree, which is the true Image of Death, that in Effect sometimes attends it, and it is called an *Asphixy*, which may signify a total Resolution.

Swoonings result from many different Causes, of which I shall only enumerate the principal; and these are, 1, Too large a Quantity of Blood. 2, A Defect or insufficient Proportion of it, and a general Weakness. 3, A Load at and violent Disorders of the Stomach 4, Nervous Maladies. 5, The Passions, and, 6, some Kinds of Diseases.

Of Swoonings occasioned by Excess of Blood.

§ 495. An excessive Quantity of Blood is frequently a Cause of Swooning, and it may be inferred that it is owing to this Cause, when it attacks sanguine, hearty and robust Persons; and more especially when it attacks them, after being combined with any additional or supervening Cause, that suddenly increased the Motion of the Blood;

Blood; such as heating Meats or Drinks, Wine, spirituous Liquors: smaller Drinks, if taken very hot and plentifully, such as Coffee, Indian Tea, Bawm Tea and the like; a long Exposure to the hot Sun, or being detained in a very hot Place; much and violent Exercise; an over intense and assiduous Study or Application, or some excessive Passion.

In such Cases, first of all the Patient should be made to smell to, or even to snuff up, some Vinegar; and his Forehead, his Temples and his Wrists should be bathed with it; adding an equal Quantity of warm Water, if at Hand. Bathing them with distilled or spirituous Liquids would be prejudicial in this Kind of Swooning.

2, The Patient should be made, if possible, to swallow two or three Spoonfuls of Vinegar, with four or five Times as much Water.

3, The Patient's Garters should be tied very tightly above his Knees; as by this Means a greater Quantity of Blood is retained in the Legs, whence the Heart may be less overladen with it

4, If the Fainting proves obstinate, that is, if it continues longer than a Quarter of an Hour, or degenerates into a *Syncope*, an Abolition of Feeling and Understanding, he must be bled in the Arm, which quickly revives him.

5, After the Bleeding, the Injection of a Glyster will be highly proper; and then the Patient should be kept still and calm, only letting him drink, every half Hour, some Cups of Elder

Flower

Flower Tea, with the Addition of a little Sugar and Vinegar.

When Swoonings which refult from this Caufe occur frequently in the fame Perfon, he fhould, in Order to efcape them, purfue the Directions I fhall hereafter mention, § 544, when treating of Perfons who fuperabound with Blood.

The very fame Caufe, or Caufes, which occafion thefe Swoonings, alfo frequently produce violent Palpitations, under the fame Circumftances; the Palpitation often preceding or following the *Deliquium*, or Swooning.

Of Swoonings occafioned by Weaknefs.

§ 496. If too great a Quantity of Blood, which may be confidered as fome Excefs of Health, is fometimes the Caufe of Swooning, this laft is oftener the Effect of a very contrary Caufe, that is, of a Want of Blood, or an Exhauftion of too much.

This Sort of Swooning happens after great Hæmorrhages, or Difcharges of Blood; after fudden or exceffive Evacuations, fuch as one of fome Hours Continuance in a *Cholera Morbus* (§ 321) or fuch as are more flow, but of longer Duration, as for Inftance, after an inveterate *Diarrhæa*, or Purging, exceffive Sweats; a Flood of Urine, fuch Exceffes as tend to exhauft Nature; obftinate Wakefulnefs; a long Inappetency, which, by depriving the Body of its neceffary

Of Cases which require immediate Assistance. 495

cessary Sustenance, is attended with the same Consequence as profuse Evacuations.

These different Causes of Swooning should be opposed by the Means and Remedies adapted to each of them. A Detail of all these would be improper here, but the Assistances that are necessary at the Time of Swooning, are nearly the same for all Cases of this Class; excepting for that attending a great Loss of Blood, of which I shall treat hereafter: first of all, the Patients should be laid down on a Bed, and being covered, should have their Legs and Thighs, their Arms, and their whole Bodies rubbed pretty strongly with hot Flanels and no Ligature should remain on any Part of them.

2, They should have very spirituous Things to smell or snuff up, such as the Carmelite Water, Hungary Water, the *English Salt, Spirit of Sal Ammoniac, strong swelling Herbs, such as Rue, Sage, Rosemary, Mint, Wormwood, and the like.

3, These should be conveyed into their Mouths; and they should be forced, if possible, to swallow some Drops of Carmelite Water, or of Brandy, or of some other potable Liquor,
mixed

---

* Dr. TISSOT informs me, that in *Swisserland*, they call a volatile Salt of Vipers, or the volatile Salt of raw Silk, *Sel d'Angleterre*, of which one *Goddard* made a Secret, and which he brought into Vogue the latter End of the last Century. But he justly observes at the same Time, that on the present Occasion every other volatile Alkali will equally answer the Purpose; and indeed the Smell of some of them, as the Spirit of Sal Ammoniac with Quicklime, *Eau de Luce*, &c. seem more penetrating. K.

mixed with a little Water; while some hot Wine mixed with Sugar and Cinnamon, which makes one of the best Cordials, is getting ready.

4, A Compress of Flanel, or of some other woollen Stuff, dipt in hot Wine, in which some aromatic Herb has been steeped, must be applied to the Pit of the Stomach.

5, If the Swooning seems likely to continue, the Patient must be put into a well heated Bed, which has before been perfumed with burning Sugar and Cinnamon; the Frictions of the whole Body with hot Flanels being still continued.

6, As soon as the Patient can swallow, he should take some Soup or Broth, with the Yolk of an Egg; or a little Bread or Biscuit, soaked in the hot spiced Wine.

7, Lastly, during the whole Time that all other Precautions are taken to oppose the Cause of the Swooning, Care must be had for some Days to prevent any *Deliquium* or Fainting, by giving them often, and but little at a time, some light yet strengthening Nourishment, such as Panada made with Soup instead of Water, new laid Eggs very lightly poached, light roast Meats with sweet Sauce, Chocolate, Soups of the most nourishing Meats, Jellies, Milk, &c.

§ 497. Those Swoonings, which are the Effect of Bleeding, or of the violent Operation of some Purge, are to be ranged in this Class.

Such as happen after artificial Bleeding, are generally very moderate, commonly terminating as soon as the Patient is laid upon the Bed; and

Persons subject to this Kind, should be bled lying down, in Order to prevent it. But should the Fainting continue longer than usual, some Vinegar smelt to, and a little swallowed with some Water, is a very good Remedy.

The Treatment of such Faintings or Swoonings, as are the Consequences of too violent Vomits or Purges, may be seen hereafter § 552.

Of Faintings occasioned by a Load, or Uneasiness at Stomach.

§ 498. It has been already observed, § 308, that Indigestions were sometimes attended with Swoonings, and indeed such vehement ones, as required speedy and very active Succour too, such as that of a Vomit. The Indigestion is sometimes less the Effect of the Quantity, than of the Quality, or the Corruption of the Food, contained in the Stomach. Thus we see there are some Persons, who are disordered by eating Eggs, Fish, Craw Fish, or any fat Meat; being thrown by them into inexpressible Anguish attended with Swooning too. It may be supposed to depend on this Cause, when these very Aliments have been lately eaten; and when it evidently neither depends on the other Causes I have mentioned; nor on such as I shall soon proceed to enumerate.

We should in Cases of this Sort, excite and revive the Patients as in the former, by making them receive some very strong Smell, of whatever

Kind is at hand; but the most essential Point is to make them swallow down a large Quantity of light warm Fluid; which may serve to drown, as it were, the indigested Matter; which may soften its Acrimony; and either effect the Discharge of it by vomiting, or force it down into the Chanel of the Intestines.

A light Infusion of Chamomile Flowers, of Tea, of Sage, of Elder Flowers, or of *Carduus Benedictus*, operate with much the same Efficacy; though the Chamomile and Carduus promote the Operation of vomiting rather more powerfully; which warm Water alone will sometimes sufficiently do.

The Swooning ceases, or at least, considerably abates in these Cases, as soon as ever the Vomiting commences. It frequently happens too, that, during the Swooning, Nature herself brings on certain *Nausea*, a Wambling and sickish Commotion of the Stomach, that revives or rouses the Patient for a Moment; but yet not being sufficient to excite an actual Vomiting, lets him soon sink down again into this temporary Dissolution, which often continues a pretty confiderable Time; leaving behind it a Sickness at Stomach, Vertigos, and a Depression and Anxiety, which do not occur in the former Species of this Malady.

Whenever these Swoonings from this Cause are entirely terminated, the Patient must be kept for some Days to a very light Diet, and take, at the same Time, every Morning fasting, a Dose of of the Powder, N°. 38, which relieves and exonerates the Stomach of whatever noxious Contents might remain in it; and then restores its natural Strength and Functions.

§ 499. There is another Kind of Swooning, which also results from a Cause in the Stomach; but which is, nevertheless, very different from this we have just been treating of; and which requires a very different Kind of Assistance. It arises from an extraordinary Sensibility of this important Organ, and from a general Weakness of the Patient.

Those subject to this Malady are valetudinary weakly Persons, who are disordered from many slight Causes, and whose Stomachs are at once very feeble and extremely sensible. They have almost continually a little Uneasiness after a Meal, though they should indulge but a little more than usual; or if they eat of any Food not quite so easy of Digestion, they have some Qualm or Commotion after it: Nay, should the Weather only be unfavourable, and sometimes without any perceivable assignable Cause, their Uneasiness terminates in a Swoon.

Patients swooning, from these Causes, have a greater Necessity for great Tranquillity and Repose, than for any other Remedy; and it might be sufficient to lay them down on the Bed: But as the Bystanders in such Cases find it difficult to remain inactive Spectators of Persons in a Swoon, some spirituous Liquid may be held to their Nose, while their Temples and Wrists are rubbed with it; and at the same Time a little Wine should be given them. Frictions are also useful in these Cases.

This Species of Swooning is oftener attended with a little Feverishness than the others.

Of those Swoonings, which arise from nervous Disorders.

§ 500. This Species of Swooning is almost wholely unknown to those Persons, for whom this Treatise is chiefly intended. Yet as there are some Citizens who pass a Part of their Lives in the Country; and some Country People who are unhappily afflicted with the Ailments of the Inhabitants of large Towns and Cities, it seemed necessary to treat briefly of them

By Disorders of the Nerves, I understand in this Place, only that Fault or Defect in them, which is the Cause of their exciting in the Body, either irregular Motions, that is, Motions without any external Cause, at least any perceivable one; and without our Will's consenting to the Production of them · or such Motions, as are greatly more considerable than they should be, if they had been proportioned to the Force of the Impression from without. This is very exactly that State, or Affection termed the *Vapours*; and by the common People, the *Mother*. And as there is no Organ unprovided with Nerves, and none, or hardly any Function, in which the Nerves have not their Influence, it may be easily ly comprehended, that the Vapours being a State or Condition, which arises from the Nerves exerting irregular involuntary Motions, without any evident Cause, and all the Functions of the Body depending partly on the Nerves; there is no one Symptom of other Diseases which the Vapours may not produce or imitate; and that these Symptoms, for the same Reason, must vary infinitely, according to those Branches of the Nerves which are disordered. It may also hence be conceived, why the Vapours of one Person have frequently no Resemblance to those of another: and why the Vapours of the very same Person, in one Day, are so very different from those in the next. It is also very conceivable that the Vapours are a certain, a real Malady; and that Oddity of the Symptoms, which cannot be accounted for, by People unacquainted with the animal Oeconomy, has been the Cause of their being considered rather as the Effect of a depraved Imagination, than as a real Disease. It is very conceiveable, I say, that this surprizing Oddity of the Symptoms is a necessary Effect of the Cause of the Vapours; and that no Person can any more prevent his being invaded by the Vapours, than he can prevent the Attack of a Fever, or of the Tooth-ach.

§ 501. A few plain Instances will furnish out a more compleat Notion of the Mechanism, or Nature, of Vapours. An Emetic, a vomiting Medicine, excites the Act, or rather the Passion, the Convulsion of Vomiting, chiefly by the Irritation

tation it gives to the Nerves of the Stomach; which Irritation produces a Spasm, a Contraction of this Organ. Now if in Consequence of this morbid or defective Texture of the Nerves, which constitutes the Vapours, those of the Stomach are excited to act with the same Violence, as in Consequence of taking a Vomit, the Patient will be agitated and worked by violent Efforts to vomit, as much as if he had really taken one.

If an involuntary unusual Motion in the Nerves, that are distributed through the Lungs, should constrain and straiten the very little Vesicles, or Bladders, as it were, which admit the fresh Air at every Respiration, the Patient will feel a Degree of Suffocation; just as if that Straitening or Contraction of the Vesicles were occasioned by some noxious Steam or Vapour.

Should the Nerves which are distributed throughout the whole Skin, by a Succession of these irregular morbid Motions, contract themselves, as they may from external Cold, or by some stimulating Application, Perspiration by the Pores will be prevented or checked; whence the Humours, which should be evacuated through the Pores of the Skin, will be thrown upon the Kidnies, and the Patient will make a great Quantity of thin clear Urine, a Symptom very common to vapourish People, or it may be diverted to the Glands of the Intestines, the Guts, and terminate in a watery *Diarrhæa*, or Looseness, which frequently proves a very obstinate one.

§ 502.

§ 502. Neither are Swoonings the least usual Symptoms attending the Vapours: and we may be certain they spring from this Source, when they happen to a Person subject to the Vapours; and none of the other Causes producing them are evident, or have lately preceded them.

Such Swoonings, however, are indeed very rarely dangerous, and scarcely require any medical Assistance. The Patient should be laid upon a Bed; the fresh Air should be very freely admitted to him; and he should be made to smell rather to some disagreeable and fetid, than to any fragrant, Substance. It is in such Faintings as these that the Smell of burnt Leather, of Feathers, or of Paper, have often proved of great Service.

§ 503. Patients also frequently faint away, in Consequence of fasting too long, or from having eat a little too much; from being confined in too hot a Chamber; from having seen too much Company; from smelling too over-powering a Scent; from being too costive; from being too forcibly affected with some Discourse or Sentiments; and, in a Word, from a great Variety of Causes, which might not make the least Impression on Persons in perfect Health; but which violently operate upon those vapourish People, because, as I have said, the Fault of their Nerves consists in their being too vividly, too acutely affected; the Force of their Sensation being nowise proportioned to the external Cause of it.

As soon as that particular Cause is distinguished from all the rest, which has occasioned the present Swooning; it is manifest that this Swooning is to be remedied by removing that particular Cause of it.

Of Swoonings occasioned by the Passions

§ 504. There have been some Instances of Persons dying within a Moment, through excessive Joy. But such Instances are so very rare and sudden, that Assistance has seldom been sought for on this Occasion. The Case is otherwise with Respect to those produced from Rage, Vexation, and Dread or Horror. I shall treat in a separate Article of those resulting from great Fear; and shall briefly consider here such as ensue from Rage, and vehement Grief or Disappointment.

§ 505. Excessive Rage and violent Affliction are sometimes fatal in the Twinkling of an Eye, though they oftener terminate in fainting only. Excessive Grief or Chagrine is especially accompanied with this Consequence; and it is very common to see Persons thus affected, sink into successive Faintings for several Hours. It is plainly obvious that very little Assistance can be given in such Cases: it is proper, however, they should smell to strong Vinegar, and frequently take a few Cups of some hot and temperately cordial Drink, such as Bawm Tea, or Lemonade with a little Orange or Lemon-peel

The calming assuaging Cordial, that has seemed

ed the most efficacious to me, is one small Coffee-Spoonful of a Mixture of three Parts of the Mineral Anodyne Liquor of HOFFMAN,* and one Part of the spirituous Tincture of Amber, which should be swallowed in a Spoonful of Water, taking after it a few Cups of such Drinks as I shall presently direct.

It is not to be supposed that Swoonings or Faintings, from excessive Passions, can be cured by Nourishment. The physical State or Condition, into which vehement Grief throws the Body, is that, of all others, in which Nourishment would be most injurious to it: and as long as the Vehemence of the Affliction endures, the Sufferer should take nothing but some Spoonfuls of Soup or Broth, or a few Morsels of some light Meat roasted.

§ 506. When Wrath or Rage has risen to so high a Pitch, that the human Machine, the Body, entirely exhausted, as it were, by that violent Effort, sinks down at once into excessive Relaxation, a Fainting sometimes succeeds, and even the most perilous Degree of it, a *Syncopè*.

It is sufficient, or rather the most that can be done here, to let the Patient be perfectly still a while in this State, only making him smell to some Vinegar. But when he is come to himself, he should drink plentifully of hot Lemonade, and take one or more of the Glysters N°. 5.

Sometimes there remain in these Cases Sicknesses at Stomach, Reachings to vomit, a Bitterness

* Our sweet Spirit of Vitriol is a similar, and as effectual a Medicine. K.

ness in the Mouth, and some vertiginous Symptoms which seem to require a Vomit. But such a Medicine must be very carefully avoided, since it may be attended with the most fatal Consequence; and Lemonade with Glysters generally and gradually remove these Swoonings. If the *Nausea* and Sickness at Stomach continue, the utmost Medicine we should allow besides, would be that of N°. 23, or a few Doses of N°. 24.

Of symptomatical Swoonings, or such as happen in the Progress of other Diseases.

§ 507. Swoonings, which supervene in the Course of other Diseases, never afford a favourable Prognostic, as they denote Weakness, and Weakness is an Obstacle to Recovery.

In the Beginning of putrid Diseases, they also denote an Oppression at Stomach, or a Mass of corrupt Humours, and they cease as soon as an Evacution supervenes, whether by Vomit or Stool.

When they occur at the Beginning of malignant Fevers, they declare the high Degree of their Malignancy, and the great Diminution of the Patient's natural Strength.

In each of these Cases Vinegar, used externally and internally, is the best Remedy during the Exacerbation or Height of the Paroxysm; and Plenty of Lemon Juice and Water after it.

§ 508 Swoonings which supervene in Diseases, accompanied with great Evacuations, are cured

cured like those which are owing to Weakness; and Endeavours should be used to restrain or moderate the Evacuations.

§ 509. Those who have any inward Abscess or Imposthume are apt to swoon frequently. They may sometimes be revived a little by Vinegar, but they prove too frequently mortal.

§ 510. Many Persons have a slighter or a deeper Swooning, at the End of a violent Fit of an intermitting Fever, or at that of each Exacerbation of a continual Fever; this constantly shews the Fever has run very high, the Swooning having been the Consequence of that great Relaxation, which has succeeded to a very high Tension. A Spoonful or two of light white Wine, with an equal Quantity of Water, affords all the Succour proper in such a Case.

§ 511. Persons subject to frequent Swoonings, should neglect nothing that may enable them to remove them when known; since the Consequences of them are always detrimental, except in some Fevers, in which they seem to mark the *Crisis*.

Every swooning Fit leaves the Patient in Dejection and Weakness; the Secretions from the Blood are suspended, the Humours disposed to Stagnation, Grumosities, or Coagulations, and Obstructions are formed; and if the Motion of the Blood is totally intercepted, or considerably checked, *Polypus's*, and these often incurable, are formed in the Heart, or in the larger Vessels, the Consequences of which are dreadful, and sometimes give Rise to internal Aneurisms, which

which always prove mortal, after long Anxiety and Oppression.

Swoonings which attack old People, without any manifest Cause, always afford an unfavourable Prognostic.

Of Hæmorrhages, or an involuntary Loss of Blood.

§ 512. Hæmorrhages of the Nose, supervening in inflammatory Fevers, commonly prove a favourable *Crysis*; which Bleeding we should carefully avoid stopping; except it becomes excessive, and seems to threaten the Patient's Life.

As they scarcely ever happen in very healthy Subjects, but from a superfluous Abundance of Blood, it is very improper to check them too soon, lest some internal Stuffings and Obstructions should prove the Consequence.

A Swooning sometimes ensues after the Loss of only a moderate Quantity of Blood. This Swooning stops the Hæmorrhage, and goes off without any further Assistance, except the smelling to Vinegar. But in other Cases there is a Succession of fainting Fits, without the Blood's stopping; while at the same time slight convulsive Motions and Twitchings ensue, attended with a Raving, when it becomes really necessary to stop the Bleeding and indeed, without waiting till these violent Symptoms appear, the following Signs will sufficiently direct us, when it is right to stop the Flux of Blood, or to permit its Continuance — As long as the Pulse is still pretty

pretty full; while the Heat of the Body is equally extended to the very Extremities; and the Countenance and Lips preserve their natural Redness, no ill Consequence is to be apprehended from the Hæmorrhage, though it has been very copious, and even somewhat profuse.

But whenever the Pulse begins to faulter and tremble; when the Countenance and the Lips grow pale, and the Patient complains of a Sickness at Stomach, it is absolutely necessary to stop the Discharge of Blood. And considering that the Operation of Remedies does not immediately follow the Exhibition or Application of them, it is safer to begin a little too early with them, than to delay them, though ever so little too long.

§ 513. First of all then, tight Bandages, or Ligatures, should be applied round both Arms, on the Part they are applied over in order to Bleeding; and round the lower Part of both Thighs, on the gaitering Place; and all these are to be drawn very tight, with an Intention to detain and accumulate the Blood in the Extremities.

2, In Order to increase this Effect, the Legs are to be plunged in warm Water up to the Knees; for by relaxing the Blood-vessels of the Legs and Feet, they are dilated at the same time, and thence receive, and, in Consequence of the Ligatures above the Knees, retain the more Blood. If the Water were cold, it would repel the Blood to the Head, if hot, it would increase
the

the Motion of it; and, by giving a greater Quickness to the Pulse, would even contribute to increase the Hæmorrhage.

As soon however, as the Hæmorrhage is stopt, these Ligatures [on the Thighs] may be relaxed a little, or one of them be entirely removed; allowing the others to continue on an Hour or two longer without touching them: but great Precaution should be taken not to slacken them entirely, nor all at once.

3, Seven or eight Grains of Nitre, and a Spoonful of Vinegar, in half a Glass of cool Water, should be given the Patient every half Hour

4, One Drachm of white Vitriol must be dissolved in two common Spoonfuls of Spring Water, and a Tent of Lint, or Bits of soft fine Linen dipt in this Solution, are to be introduced into the Nostrils, horizontally at first, but afterwards to be intruded upwards, and as high as may be, by the Assistance of a flexible Bit of Wood or Whale-bone. But should this Application be ineffectual, the Mineral Anodyne Liquor of HOFFMAN is certain to succeed: and in the Country, where it often happens that neither of these Applications are to be had speedily, Brandy, and even Spirit of Wine, mixt with a third Part Vinegar, have answered entirely well, of which I have been a Witness

The Prescription N° 67, which I have already referred to, on the Article of Wounds, may also be serviceable on this Occasion. It must be reduced

reduced to Powder, and conveyed up the Nostrils as high as may be, on the Point or Extremity of a Tent of Lint, which may easily be covered with it. Or a Quill, well charged with the Powder, may be introduced high into the Nostrils, and its Countents be strongly blown up from its other Extremity: though after all the former Method is preferable.

5, When the Flux of Blood is totally stopt, the Patient is to be kept as still and quiet as possible; taking great Care not to extract the Tent which remains in the Nose; not to remove the Clots of coagulated Blood which fill up the Passage. The loosening and removing of these should be effected very gradually and cautiously; and frequently the Tent does not spring out spontaneously, till after many Days.

§ 514. I have not, hitherto, said any thing of artificial Bleeding in these Cases, as I think it at best unserviceable; since, though it may sometimes have stopt the morbid Loss of Blood, it has at other times increased it. Neither have I mentioned Anodynes here, whose constant Effect is to determine a larger Quantity of Blood to the Head.

Applications of cold Water to the Nape of the Neck ought to be wholly disused, having sometimes been attended with the most embarrassing Consequences.

In all Hæmorrhages, all Fluxes of Blood, great Tranquillity, Ligatures, and the Use of the Drinks N°. 2 or 4, are very useful.

§ 515.

§ 515. People who are very liable to frequent Hæmorrhages, ought to manage themselves conformably to the Directions contained in the next Chapter, § 544. They should take very little Supper; avoid all sharp and spirituous Liquors; Apartments that are over hot, and cover their Heads but very lightly.

When a Patient has for a long time been subject to Hæmorrhages, if they cease, he should retrench from his usual Quantity of Food, accustom himself to artificial Bleedings at proper Intervals, and take some gentle opening Purges, especially that of N°. 24, and frequently a little Nitre in an Evening.

Of Convulsion Fits.

§ 516. Convulsions are, in general, more terrifying than dangerous; they result from many and various Causes; and on the Removal or Extirpation of these, their Cure depends.

In the very Fit itself very little is to be done or attempted.

As nothing does shorten the Duration, nor even lessen the Violence, of an epileptic Fit, so nothing at all should be attempted in it, and the rather, because Means and Medicines often aggravate the Disease. We should confine our Endeavours solely to the Security of the Patient, by preventing him from giving himself any violent Strokes; by getting something, if possible, between his Teeth, such as a small Roller of Linen to pre-

prevent his Tongue from being hurt, or very dangerously squeezed and bruised, in a strong Convulsion.

The only Case which requires immediate Assistance in the Fit, is, when it is so extremely violent, the Neck so swelled, and the Face so very red, that there is Room to be apprehensive of an Apoplexy, which we should endeavour to obviate, by drawing eight or ten Ounces of Blood from the Arm

As this terrible Disease is common in the Country, it is doing a real Service to the unfortunate Victims of it, to inform them how very dangerous it is to give themselves blindly up to take all the Medicines, which are cried up to them in such Cases. If there be any one Disease, which requires a more attentive, delicate, and exquisite Kind of Treatment, it is this very Disease. Some Species of it are wholly incurable: and such as may be susceptible of a Cure, require the utmost Care and Consideration of the most enlightned and most experienced Physicians: while those who pretend to cure all epileptic Patients, with one invariable Medicine, are either Ignorants, or Impostors, and sometimes both in one.

§ 517 Simple Convulsion Fits, which are not epileptic, are frequently of a long Continuance, persevering, with very few and short Intervals, for Days and even for Weeks.

The true genuine Cause should be investigated as strictly as possible, though nothing should be attempted in the Fit. The Nerves are, during that Term, in so high a Degree of Tension and Sensibility, that the very Medicines, supposed to be strongly indicated, often redouble the Storm they were intended to appease.

Thin watery Liquors, moderately imbued with Aromatics, are the least hurtful, the most innocent Things that can be given, such as Bawm, Lime-tree, and Elder Flower Tea. A Ptisan of Liquorice Root only has sometimes answered better than any other.

Of suffocating, or strangling Fits.

§ 518. These Fits (by whatever other Name they may be called) whenever they very suddenly attack a Person, whose Breathing was easy and natural just before, depend almost constantly on a Spasm or Contraction of the Nerves, in the Vesicles of the Lungs; or upon an Infarction, a Stuffing of the same Parts, produced by viscid clammy Humours.

That Suffocation which arises from a Spasm is not dangerous, it goes off of itself, or it may be treated like Swoonings owing to the same Cause. See § 502.

§ 519. That Suffocation, which is the Effect of a sanguineous Fulness and Obstruction, may be distinguished by its attacking strong, vigorous, sanguine Persons, who are great Eaters, using much juicy nutritious Food, and strong Wine and Liquors, and who frequently eat and inflame themselves; and when the Fit has come on
after

after any inflaming Cause; when the Pulse is full and strong, and the Countenance red.

Such are cured, 1, by a very plentiful Discharge of Blood from the Arm, which is to be repeated, if necessary.

2, By the Use of Glysters.

3, By drinking plentifully of the Ptisan N°. 1; to each Pot of which, a Drachm of Nitre is to be added, and,

4, By the Vapour of hot Vinegar, continually received by Respiration or Breathing. See § 55

§ 520. There is Reason to think that one of these Fits is owing to a Quantity of tough viscid Humours in the Lungs, when it attacks Persons, whose Temperament, and whose Manner of living are opposite to those I have just described; such as valetudinary, weakly, phlegmatic, pituitous, inactive, and squeamish Persons, who feed badly, or on fat, viscid, and insipid Diet, and who drink much hot Water, either alone, or in Tea-like Infusions And these Signs of Suffocation, resulting from such Causes, are still more probable, if the Fit came on in rainy Weather, and during a southerly Wind; and when the Pulse is soft and small, the Visage pale and hollow.

The most efficacious Treatment we can advise, is, 1, To give every half Hour half a Cup of the Potion, N° 8, if it can be readily had. 2, To make the Patient drink very plentifully of the

Drink N°. 12; and, 3, to apply two strong Blisters to the fleshy Parts of his Legs.

If he was strong and hearty before the Fit, and the Pulse still continues vigorous, and feels somewhat full withall, the Loss of seven or eight Ounces of Blood is sometimes indispensably necessary. A Glyster has also frequently been attended with extraordinary good Effects.

Those afflicted with this oppressing Malady are commonly relieved, as soon as they expectorate, and sometimes even by vomiting a little.

The Medicine N°. 25, a Dose of which may be taken every two Hours, with a Cup of the Ptisan N°. 12, often succeeds very well.

But if neither this Medicine, nor the Prescription of N°. 8 are at Hand, which may be the Case in Country Places; an Onion of a moderate Size should be pounded in an Iron or Marble Mortar; upon this, a Glass of Vinegar is to be poured, and then strongly squeezed out again through a Piece of Linen. An equal Quantity of Honey is then to be added to it. A Spoonful of this Mixture, whose remarkable Efficacy I have been a Witness of, is to be given every half Hour.

Of the violent Effects of Fear.

§ 521 Here I shall insert some Directions to prevent the ill Consequences of great Fear or Terror, which are very prejudicial at every Term of Life, but chiefly during Infancy.

The

The general Effects of Terror, are a great Straitening or Contraction of all the small Vessels, and a Repulsion of the Blood into the large and internal ones. Hence follows the Suppression of Perspiration, the general Seizure or Oppression, the Trembling, the Palpitations and Anguish, from the Heart and the Lungs being overcharged with Blood; and sometimes attended with Swoonings, irremediable Disorders of the Heart, and Death itself. A heavy Drowsiness, Raving, and a Kind of furious or raging *Delirium* happen in other Cases, which I have frequently observed in Children, when the Blood-vessels of the Neck were swelled and stuffed up; and Convulsions, and even the Epilepsy have come on, all which have proved the horrible Consequence of a most senseless and wicked Foolery or Sporting. One half of those Epilepsies which do not depend on such Causes, as might exist before the Child's Birth, are owing to this detestable Custom, and it cannot be too much inculcated into Children, never to frighten one another; a Point which Persons intrusted with their Education, ought to have the strictest Regard to.

When the Humours that should have passed off by Perspiration, are repelled to the Intestines, a tedious and very obstinate Looseness is the frequent Consequence.

§ 522. Our Endeavours should be directed, to re-establish the disordered Circulation, to restore the obstructed Perspiration; and to allay the Agitation of the Nerves.

The popular Custom in these Cases has been to give the terrified Patient some cold Water directly; but when the Fright has been considerable, this is a very pernicious custom, and I have seen some terrible Consequences from it.

They should, on the contrary, be conveyed into some very quiet Situation, leaving there but very few Persons, and such only as they are thoroughly familiar with. They should take a few Cups of pretty warm Drink, particularly of an Infusion of Lime-tree Flowers and Bawm. Their Legs should be put into warm Water, and remain there an Hour, if they will patiently permit it, rubbing them gently now and then, and giving them every half-quarter of an Hour, a small Cup of the said Drink. When their Composure and Tranquillity are returned a little, and their Skin seems to have recovered its wonted and general Warmth, Care should be taken to dispose them to sleep, and to perspire plentifully. For this Purpose they may be allowed a few Spoonfuls of Wine, on putting them into Bed, with one Cup of the former Infusion, or, which is more certain and effectual, a few Drops of SYDENHAM's Liquid Laudanum, N°. 44, but should that not be near at Hand, a small Dose of *Venice* Treacle.

§ 523. It sometimes happens that Children do not seem at first extremely terrified; but the Fright is renewed while they sleep, and with no small Violence. The Directions I have just given

Of Cases which require immediate Assistance. 519

given must then be observed, for some successive Evenings, before they are put to Bed.

Their Fright frequently returns about the latter End of the Night, and agitates them violently every Day. The same Treatment should be continued in such Cases; and we should endeavour to dispose them to be a-sleep at the usual Hour of its Return.

By this very Method, I have dissipated the dismal Consequences of Fear of Women in Child-bed, which is so commonly, and often speedily, mortal.

If a Suffocation from this Cause is violent, there is sometimes a Necessity for opening a Vein in the Arm.

These Patients should gradually be inured to an almost continual, but gentle, Kind of Exercise.

All violent Medicines render those Diseases, which are the Consequences of great Fear, incurable. A pretty common one is, that of an Obstruction of the Liver, which has been productive of a Jaundice.*

Of Accidents or Symptoms produced by the Vapours of Coal, and of Wine.

§ 524 Not a single Year passes over here, without the Destruction of many People by the

---

* I have seen this actually verified by great and disagreeable Surprize, attended indeed with much Concern, in a Person of exquisite Sensations. *K.*

Vapour of Charcoal, or of small Coal, and by the Steam or Vapour of Wine.

The Symptoms by Coal occur, when * small Coal, and especially when † Charcoal is burnt in a Chamber close shut, which is direct Poison to a Person shut up in it. The sulphureous Oil, which is set at Liberty and diffused by the Action of Fire, expands itself through the Chamber; while those who are in it perceive a Disorder and Confusion in their Heads; contract Vertigos, Sickness at Stomach, a Weakness, and very unusual Kind of Numbness; become raving, convulsed and trembling; and if they fail of Presence of Mind, or of Strength, to get out of the Chamber, they die within a short Time.

I have seen a Woman who had vertiginous Commotions in her Head for two Days, and almost continual Vomitings, from her having been confined less than six Minutes in a Chamber (and that notwithstanding, both one Window and one Door were open) in which there was a Chafing-dish with some burning Coals. Had the Room been quite close, she must have perished by it.

This Vapour is narcotic or stupefying, and proves mortal in Consequence of its producing a

sleepy

---

* *La Braise.*

† *Ccarbon.* Dr Tissot informs me, their Difference consists in this, that the Charcoal is prepared from Wood burnt in a close or stifled Fire, and that the small Coal is made of Wood (and of smaller Wood) burnt in an open Fire, and extinguished before it is reduced to the State of a Cinder. He says the latter is smaller, softer, less durable in the Fire, and the Vapour of it less dangerous than that of Charcoal.

sleepy or apoplectic Disorder, though blended, at the same time, with something convulsive; which sufficiently appears from the Closure of the Mouth, and the strict Contraction or Locking of the Jaws.

The Condition of the Brain, in the dissected Bodies of Persons thus destroyed, proves that they die of an Apoplexy: notwithstanding it is very probable that Suffocation is also partly the Cause of their Deaths; as the Lungs have been found stuffed up with Blood and livid.

It has also been observed in some other such Bodies, that Patients killed by the Vapour of burning Coals, have commonly their whole Body swelled out to one third more than their Magnitude, when living. The Face, Neck, and Arms are swelled out, as if they had been blown up; and the whole human Machine appears in such a State, as the dead Body of a Person would, who had been violently strangled; and who had made all possible Resistance for a long time, before he was overpowered.

§ 525. Such as are sensible of the great Danger they are in, and retreat seasonably from it, are generally relieved as soon as they get into the open Air; or if they have any remaining Uneasiness, a little Water and Vinegar, or Lemonade, drank hot, affords them speedy Relief. But when they are so far poisoned, as to have lost their Feeling and Understanding, if there be any Means of reviving them, such Means consist,

1, In

1, In exposing them to a very pure, fresh and open Air.

2, In making them smell to some very penetrating Odour, which is somewhat stimulating and reviving, such as the volatile Spirit of Sal Ammoniac, the †*English* Salt; and afterwards to surround them, as it were, with the Steam of Vinegar.

3, In taking some Blood from their Arm.

4, In putting their Legs into warm or hot Water, and chafing them well.

5, In making them swallow, if practicable, much Lemonade, or Water and Vinegar, with the Addition of Nitre: and,

6, In throwing up some sharp Glysters.

As it is manifest there is something spasmodic in these Cases, it were proper to be provided with some antispasmodic Remedies, such as the Mineral Anodyne Liquid of HOFFMAN. Even Opium has sometimes been successfully given here, but it should be allowed to Physicians only to direct it in such Cases.

A Vomit would be hurtful; and the Reachings to vomit arise only from the Oppression on the Brain.

It is a common but erroneous Opinion, that if the Coal be suffered to burn for a Minute or so in the open Air, or in a Chimney, it is sufficient to prevent any Danger from the Vapour of it.

Hence it amounts even to a criminal Degree of Imprudence, to sleep in a Chamber while Charcoal

---

† See Note * Page 495.

Charcoal or small Coal is burning in it; and the Number of such imprudent Persons, as have never awaked after it, is so considerable, and so generally known too, that the Continuance of this unhappy Custom is astonishing.

§ 526. The Bakers, who make Use of much small Coal, often keep great Quantities of it in their Cellars, which frequently abound so much with the Vapour of it, that it seizes them violently the Moment they enter into the Cellar. They sink down at once deprived of all Sensation, and die if they are not drawn out of it soon enough to be assisted, according to the Directions I have just given.

One certain Means of preventing such fatal Accidents is, upon going into the Cellar to throw some flaming Paper or Straw into it, and if these continue to flame out and consume, there is no Reason for dreading the Vapour: but if they should be extinguished, no Person should venture in. But after opening the Vent-hole, a Bundle of flaming Straw must be set at the Door, which serves to attract the external Air strongly. Soon after the Experiment of the flaming Paper must be repeated, and if it goes out, more Straw is to be set on Fire before the Cellar Door.

§ 527. Small Coal, burnt in an open Fire, is not near so dangerous as *Charcoal*, properly so called, the Danger of which arises from this, that in extinguishing it by the usual Methods, all those sulphureous Particles of it, in which its Danger consists, are concentred. Nevertheless, small
Coal

Coal is not entirely deprived of all its noxious Quality, without some of which it could not strictly be Coal.

The common Method of throwing some Salt on live Coals, before they are conveyed into a Chamber; or of casting a Piece of Iron among them to imbibe some Part of their deadly narcotic Sulphur, is not without its Utility; though by no means sufficient to prevent all Danger from them.

§ 528. When the most dangerous Symptoms from this Cause disappear, and there remains only some Degree of Weakness, of Numbness, and a little Inappetency, or Loathing at Stomach, nothing is better than Lemonade with one fourth Part Wine, half a Cup of which should frequently be taken, with a small Crust of Bread.

§ 529. The Vapour which exhales from Wine, and in general from all fermenting Liquors, such as Beer, Cyder, &c. contains something poisonous, which kills in the like Manner with the Vapour of Coal, and there is always some Danger in going into a Cellar, where there is much Wine in the State of Fermentation; if it has been shut up close for several Hours. There have been many Examples of Persons struck dead on entering one, and of others who have escaped out of it with Difficulty.

When such unhappy Accidents occur, Men should not be successively exposed, one after another, to perish, by endeavouring to fetch out the first who sunk down upon his Entrance; but the

the Air should immediately be purified by the Method already directed, or by discharging some Guns into the Cellar; after which People may venture in with Precaution. And when the Persons unfortunately affected are brought out, they are to be treated like those, who were affected with the Coal-Vapour.

I saw a Man, about eight Years since, who was not sensible of the Application of Spirit of Sal Ammoniac, till about an Hour after he was struck down, and who was entirely freed at last by a plentiful Bleeding; though he had been so insensible, that it was several Hours before he discovered a very great Wound he had, which extended from the Middle of his Arm to his Armpit, and which was made by a Hook intended to be used, in Case of a House catching Fire, to assist Persons in escaping from the Flames.

§ 530. When subterraneous Caves that have been very long shut are opened; or when deep Wells are cleaned, that have not been emptied for several Years, the Vapours arising from them produce the same Symptoms I have mentioned, and require the same Assistance. They are to be cleansed and purified by burning Sulphur and Salt Petre in them, or Gunpowder, as compounded of both.

§ 531 The offensive Stink of Lamps and of Candles, especially when their Flames are extinguished, operate like other Vapours, though with less Violence, and less suddenly. Nevertheless there have been Instances of People killed by the Fumes of Lamps fed with Nut Oil, which had been extinguished in a close Room. These last Smells or Fumes prove noxious also, in Consequence of their Greasiness, which being conveyed, together with the Air, into the Lungs, prevent their Respiration: And hence we may observe, that Persons of weak delicate Breasts find themselves quickly oppressed in Chambers or Apartments, illuminated with many Candles.

The proper Remedies have been already directed, § 525. The Steam of Vinegar is very serviceable in such Cases.

Of Poisons.

§ 532. There are a great Number of Poisons, whose Manner of acting is not alike; and whose ill Effects are to be opposed by different Remedies: But Arsenic, or Ratsbane, and some particular Plants are the Poisons which are the most frequently productive of Mischief, in Country Places

§ 533. It is in Consequence of its excessive Acrimony, or violent Heat and Sharpness, which corrodes or gnaws, that Arsenic destroys by an excessive Inflammation, with a burning Fire as it were, most torturing Pains in the Mouth, Throat, Stomach, Guts, with rending and often bloody Vomitings, and Stools, Convulsions, Faintings, &c.

The

The best Remedy of all is pouring down whole Torrents of Milk, or, where there is not Milk, of warm Water. Nothing but a prodigious Quantity of such weak Liquids can avail such a miserable Patient. If the Cause of the Disorder is immediately known, after having very speedily taken down a large Quantity of warm Water, Vomiting may be excited with Oil, or with melted Butter, and by tickling the Inside of the Throat with a Feather. But when the Poison has already inflamed the Stomach and the Guts, we must not expect to discharge it by vomiting. Whatever is healing or emollient, Decoctions of mealy Pulse, of Barley, of Oatmeal, of Marshmallows, and Butter and Oil are the most suitable.

As soon as ever the tormenting Pains are felt in the Belly, and the Intestines seem attacked, Glysters of Milk must be very frequently thrown up.

If at the very Beginning of the Attack, the Patient has a strong Pulse, a very large Bleeding may be considerably serviceable by its delaying the Progress, and diminishing the Degree of Inflammation.

And even though it should happen that a Patient overcomes the first Violence of this dreadful Accident, it is too common for him to continue in a languid State for a long Time, and sometimes for all the Remainder of his Life. The most certain Method of preventing this Misery, is to live for some Months solely upon Milk, and

and some very new laid Eggs, just received from the Hen, and dissolved or blended in the Milk, without boiling them.

§ 534. The Plants which chiefly produce these unhappy Accidents are some Kinds of Hemlock, whether it be the Leaf or the Root; the Berries of the *Bella Donna*, or deadly Nightshade, which Children eat by mistake for Cherries; some Kind of Mushrooms, the Seed of the *Datura*, or the stinking Thorn-Apple.

All the Poisons of this Class prove mortal rather from a narcotic, or stupefying, than from an acrid, or very sharp Quality. Vertigos, Faintings, Reachings to vomit, and actual Vomitings are the first Symptoms produced by them.

The Patient should immediately swallow down a large Quantity of Water, moderately seasoned with Salt or with Sugar, and then a Vomiting should be excited as soon as possible by the Prescription Nº. 34 or 35: or, if neither of these is very readily procurable, with Radish-seed pounded, to the Quantity of a Coffee Spoonful, swallowed in warm Water, soon after forcing a Feather or a Finger into the Patient's Throat, to expedite the Vomiting.

After the Operation of the Vomit, he must continue to take a large Quantity of Water, sweetened with Honey or Sugar, together with a considerable Quantity of Vinegar, which is the true Specific, or Antidote, as it were, against those Poisons: the Intestines must also be emptied by a few Glysters.

Thirty

Thirty-seven Soldiers having unhappily eaten, instead of Carrots, of the Roots of the *Oenanthe*, or Water-hemlock, became all extremely sick; when the Emetic, N° 34, with the Assistance of Glysters, and very plentiful drinking of warm Water, saved all but one of them, who died before he could be assisted.

§ 535. If a Person has taken too much Opium; or any Medicine into which it enters, as *Venice* Treacle, Mithridate, Diascordium, &c. whether by Imprudence, Mistake, Ignorance, or through any bad Design, he must be bled upon the Spot, and treated as if he had a sanguine Apoplexy, (See § 147) by Reason that Opium in Effect produces such a one. He should snuff up and inhale the Vapour of Vinegar plentifully, adding it also liberally to the Water he is to drink.

Of acute Pains.

§ 536. It is not my Intention to treat here of those Pains, that accompany any evident known Disease, and which should be conducted as relating to such Diseases; nor of such Pains as infirm valetudinary Persons are habitually subject to; since Experience has informed such of the most effectual Relief for them: But when a Person sound and hale, finds himself suddenly attacked with some excessive Pain, in whatever Part it occurs, without knowing either the Nature, or the Cause of it, they may, till proper Advice can be procured,

1, Part with some Blood, which, by abating the Fulness and Tension, almost constantly assuages the Pains, at least for some Time: and it may even be repeated, if, without weakening the Patient much, it has lessened the Violence of the Pain.

2, The Patient should drink abundantly of some very mild temperate Drink, such as the Ptisan N° 2, the Almond Emulsion N°. 4, or warm Water with a fourth or fifth Part Milk.

3, Several emollient Glysters should be given.

4, The whole Part that is affected, and the adjoining Parts should be covered with Cataplasms, or soothed with the emollient Fomentation, N°. 9.

5, The warm Bath may also be advantagiously used.

6, If notwithstanding all these Assistances, the Pain should still continue violent, and the Pulse is neither full nor hard, the grown Patient may take an Ounce of Syrup of Diacodium, or sixteen Drops of liquid Laudanum, and when neither of these are to be had,* an *English* Pint of boiling Water must be poured upon three or four Poppy-heads with their Seeds, but without the Leaves, and this Decoction is to be drank like Tea.

§ 537. Persons very subject to frequent Pains, and especially to violent Head-achs, should abstain

from

---

* *Une Quartelle.*

from all strong Drink; such Abstinence being often the only Means of curing them: And People are very often mistaken in supposing Wine necessary for as many as seem to have a weak Stomach.

Chapter XXXII.

Of Medicines taken by Way of Precaution, or Prevention.

Sect. 538.

I Have pointed out, in some Parts of this Work, the Means of preventing the bad Effects of several Causes of Diseases; and of prohibiting the Return of some habitual Disorders. In the present Chapter I shall adjoin some Observations, on the Use of the principal Remedies, which are employed as general Preservatives; pretty regularly too at certain stated Times, and almost always from meer Custom only, without knowing, and often with very little Consideration, whether they are right or wrong

Nevertheless, the Use, the Habit of taking Medicines, is certainly no indifferent Matter: it is ridiculous, dangerous, and even criminal to omit them, when they are necessary, but not less so to take them when they are not wanted. A good Medicine taken seasonably, when there is some Disorder, some *Disarrangement* in the Body, which would in a short time occasion a Distemper, has often prevented it. But yet the very same Medicine, if given to a Person in perfect Health, if it does not directly make him sick, leaves him at the best in a greater Propensity to the Impressions of Diseases; and there are but too many Examples of People, who having very unhappily contracted a Habit, a Disposition to take Physick, have really injured their Health, and impaired their Constitution, however naturally strong, by an Abuse of those Materials which Providence has given for the Recovery and Re-establishment of it, an Abuse which, though it should not injure the Health of the Person, would occasion those Remedies, when he should be really sick, to be less efficacious and serviceable to him, from their having been familiar to his Constitution; and thus he becomes deprived of the Assistance he would have received from them, if taken only in those Times and Circumstances, in which they were necessary for him.

Of Bleeding

§ 539. Bleeding is necessary only in these four Cases. 1, When there is too great a Quantity of Blood in the Body. 2, When there is any Inflammation, or an inflammatory Disease. 3, When some Cause supervenes, or is about to super-

supervene, in the Constitution, which would speedily produce an Inflammation, or some other dangerous Symptom, if the Vessels were not relaxed by Bleeding. It is upon this Principle that Patients are bled after Wounds, and after Bruises, that Bleeding is directed for a pregnant Woman, if she has a violent Cough, and that Bleeding is performed, by Way of Precaution, in several other Cases. 4, We also advise Bleeding sometimes to assuage an excessive Pain, though such Pain is not owing to Excess of Blood, nor arrives from an inflamed Blood; but in Order to appease and moderate the Pain by Bleeding; and thereby to obtain Time for destroying the Cause of it by other Remedies. But as these two last Reasons are in Effect involved or implied in the two first; it may be very generally concluded, that an Excess of Blood, and an inflamed State of it, are the only two necessary Motives for Bleeding.

§ 540 An Inflammation of the Blood is known by the Symptoms accompanying those Diseases, which that Cause produces. Of these I have already spoken, and I have at the same time regulated the Practice of Bleeding in such Cases. Here I shall point out those Symptoms and Circumstances, which manifest an Excess of Blood.

The first, then, is the general Course and Manner of the Patient's living, while in Health. If he is a great Eater, and indulges in juicy nutritious Food, and especially on much Flesh-meat,

meat; if he drinks rich and nourishing Wine, or other strong Drink, and at the same time enjoys a good Digestion; if he takes but little Exercise, sleeps much, and has not been subject to any very considerable Evacuation, he may well be supposed to abound in Blood. It is very obvious that all these Causes rarely occur in Country People; if we except only the Abatement of their Exercise, during some Weeks in Winter, which indeed may contribute to their generating more Blood than they commonly do.

The labouring Country-man, for much the greater Part of his Time, lives only on Bread, Water and Vegetables; Materials but very moderately nourishing, as one Pound of Bread probably does not make, in the same Body, more Blood than one Ounce of Flesh; though a general Prejudice seems to have established a contrary Opinion. 2, The total Stopping or long Interruption of some involuntary Bleeding or Hæmorrhage, to which he had been accustomed. 3, A full and strong Pulse, and Veins visibly filled with Blood, in a Body that is not lean and thin, and when he is not heated. 4, A florid lively Ruddiness. 5, A considerable and unusual Numbness; Sleep more profound, of more Duration, and yet less tranquil and calm, than at other times; a greater Propensity than ordinary to be fatigued after moderate Exercise or Work, and a little Oppression and Heaviness from walking. 6, Palpitations, accompanied sometimes with very great Dejection, and even with a slight fainting Fit; especially on

being

being in any hot Place, or after moving about confiderably. 7, Vertigos, or Swimmings of the Head, especially on bowing down and raising it up at once, and after sleeping. 8, Frequent Pains of the Head, to which the Person was not formerly subject; and which seem not to arise from any Defect in the Digestions. 9, An evident Sensation of Heat, pretty generally diffused over the whole Body. 10, A smarting Sort of Itching all over, from a very little more Heat than usual. And lastly, frequent Hæmorrhages, and these attended with manifest Relief, and more Vivacity.

People should, notwithstanding, be cautious of supposing an unhealthy Excess of Blood, from any one of these Symptoms only. Many of them must concur; and they should endeavour to be certain that even such a Concurrence of them does not result from a very different Cause, and wholly opposite in Effect to that of an Excess of Blood.

But when it is certain, from the whole Appearance, that such an Excess doth really exist, then a single, or even a second Bleeding is attended with very good Effects. Nor is it material, in such Cases, from what Part the Blood is taken.

§ 541. On the other Hand, when these Circumstances do not exist, Bleeding is in no wise necessary: nor should it ever be practised in these following Conditions and Circumstances; except for some particular and very strong Reasons; of the due Force of which none but Physicians can judge.

First, when the Person is in a very advanced Age, or in very early Infancy. 2, When he is either naturally of a weakly Constitution, or it has been rendered such by Sickness, or by some other Accident. 3, When the Pulse is small, soft, feeble, and intermits, and the Skin is manifestly pale. 4, When the Limbs, the Extremities of the Body, are often cold, puffed up and soft. 5, When their Appetite has been very small for a long time, their Food but little nourishing, and their Perspiration too plentiful, from great Exercise. 6, When the Stomach has long been disordered, and the Digestion bad, whence very little Blood could be generated. 7, When the Patient has been considerably emptied, whether by Hæmorrhages, a Looseness, profuse Urine or Sweat: or when the *Crisis* of some Distemper has been effected by any one of these Evacuations. 8, When the Patient has long been afflicted with some depressing Disease, and troubled with many such Obstructions as prevent the Formation of Blood. 9, Whenever a Person is exhausted, from whatever Cause. 10, When the Blood is in a thin, pale, and dissolved State

§ 542, In all these Cases, and in some others less frequent, a single Bleeding often precipitates the Patient into an absolutely incurable State, an irreparable Train of Evils. Many dismal Examples of it are but too obvious.

What-

Whatever, therefore, be the Situation of the Patient, and however naturally robuſt, that Bleeding, which is unneceſſary, is noxious. Repeated, re-iterated Bleedings, weaken and enervate, haſten old Age, diminiſh the Force of the Circulation, thence fatten and puff up the Body, and next by weakening, and laſtly by deſtroying, the Digeſtions, they lead to a fatal Dropſy. They diſorder the Perſpiration by the Skin, and leave the Patient liable to Colds and Defluxions. They weaken the nervous Syſtem, and render them ſubject to Vapours, to the hypochondriac Diſorders, and to all nervous Maladies.

The ill Conſequence of a ſingle, though erroneous Bleeding is not immediately diſcernible: on the contrary, when it was not performed in ſuch a Quantity, as to weaken the Patient perceivably, it appears to have been rather beneficial. Yet I ſtill here inſiſt upon it, that it is not the leſs true that, when unneceſſary, it is prejudicial; and that People ſhould never bleed, as ſometimes has been done, for meer Whim, or, as it were, for Diverſion It avails nothing to affirm, that within a few Days after it, they have got more Blood than they had before it, that is, that they weigh more than at firſt, whence they infer the Loſs of Blood very ſpeedily repaired. The Fact of their augmented Weight is admitted; but this very Fact teſtifies againſt the real Benefit of that Bleeding; ſince it is a Proof, that the natural Evacuations of the Body are leſs com-

compleatly made; and that Humours, which ought to be expelled, are retained in it. There remains the same Quantity of Blood, and perhaps a little more; but it is not a Blood so well made, so perfectly elaborated; and this is so very true, that if the thing were otherwise; if some Days after the Bleeding they had a greater Quantity of the same Kind of Blood, it would amount to a Demonstration, that more re-iterated Bleedings must necessarily have brought on an inflammatory Disease, in a Man of a robust Habit of Body.

§ 543. The Quantity of Blood, which a grown Man may Part with, by Way of Precaution, is about ten Ounces.

§ 544. Persons so constituted as to breed much Blood, should carefully avoid all those Causes which tend to augment it, (See § 540, N°. 1) and when they are sensible of the Quantity augmented, they should confine themselves to a light frugal Diet, on Pulse, Fruits, Bread and Water, they should often bathe their Feet in warm Water, taking Night and Morning the Powder N° 20; drink of the Ptisan N°. 1; sleep but very moderately, and take much Exercise. By using these Precautions they may either prevent any Occasion for Bleeding, or should they really be obliged to admit of it, they would increase and prolong its good Effects. These are also the very Means, which may remove all the Danger that might ensue from a Person's omitting to bleed, at the usual Season or Interval, when

when the Habit, the Fashion of Bleeding had been inveterately established in him.

§ 545. We learn with Horror and Astonishment, that some have been bled eighteen, twenty and even twenty-four times in two Days; and some others, some * hundred times, in the Course of some Months. Such Instances irrefragably demonstrate the continual Ignorance of their Physician or Surgeon, and should the Patient escape, we ought to admire the inexhaustible Resources of Nature, that survived so many murderous Incisions.

§ 546. The People entertain a common Notion, which is, that the first Time of bleeding certainly saves the Life of the Patient; but to convince them of the Falsity of this silly Notion, they need only open their Eyes, and see the very contrary Fact to this occur but too unhappily every Day; many People dying soon after their first Bleeding. Were their Opinion right, it would be impossible that any Person should die of the first Disease that seized him, which yet daily happens. Now the Extirpation of this absurd Opinion is really become important, as the

Con-

---

* How shocking is this! and yet how true in some Countries! I have been most certainly assured, that Bleeding has been inflicted and repeated in the last sinking and totally relaxing Stage of a Sea-Scurvy, whose fatal Termination it doubtless accelerated. This did not happen in our own Fleet, yet we are not as yet wholly exempt on Shore, from some Abuse of Bleeding, which a few raw unthinking Operators are apt to consider as a meer Matter of Course. I have in some other Place stigmatized the Madness of Bleeding in Convulsions, from manifest Exhaustion and Emptiness, with the Abhorrence it deserves K

Continuance of it is attended with some unhappy Consequences: their Faith in, their great Dependance on, the extraordinary Virtue of this first Bleeding makes them willing to omit it, that is, to treasure it up against a Distemper, from which they shall be in the greatest Danger, and thus it is deferred as long as the Patient is not extremely bad, in Hopes that if they can do without it then, they shall keep it for another and more pressing Occasion. Their present Disease in the mean time rises to a violent Height, and then they bleed, but when it is too late, and I have seen Instances of many Patients, who were permitted to die, that the first Bleeding might be reserved for a more important Occasion. The only Difference between the first Bleeding, and any subsequent one is, that the first commonly gives the Patient an Emotion, that is rather hurtful than salutary.

Of Purges

§ 547 The Stomach and Bowels are emptied either by Vomiting, or by Stools, the latter Discharge being much more natural than the first, which is not effected without a violent Motion, and one indeed to which Nature is repugnant. Nevertheless, there are some Cases, which really require this artificial Vomiting; but these excepted (some of which I have already pointed out) we should rather prefer those Remedies, which empty the Belly by Stool.

§ 548.

§ 548. The Signs, which indicate a Neceffity for Purging, are, 1, a difagreeable Taft or Savour of the Mouth in a Morning, and especially a bitter Taft; a foul, furred Tongue and Teeth, difagreable Eructations or Belchings, Windinefs and Diftenfion.

2, A Want of Appetite which increafes very gradually, without any Fever, which degenerates into a Difguft or total Averfion to Food; and fometimes communicates a bad Taft to the very little fuch Perfons do eat.

3, Reachings to vomit in a Morning fafting, and fometimes throughout the Day, fuppofing fuch not to depend on a Woman's Pregnancy, or fome other Diforder, in which Purges would be either ufelefs or hurtful.

4, A vomiting up of bitter, or corrupted, Humours.

5, A manifeft Senfation of a Weight, or Heavinefs in the Stomach, the Loins, or the Knees.

6, A Want of Strength fometimes attended with Reftleffnefs, ill Humour, or Peevifhnefs, and Melancholy.

7, Pains of the Stomach, frequent Pains of the Head, or Vertigos; fometimes a Drowfinefs, which increafes after Meals.

8, Some Species of Cholics, irregular Stools which are fometimes very great in Quantity, and too liquid for many Days together, after which an obftinate Coftivenefs enfues.

9, A

9, A Pulse less regular, and less strong, than what is natural to the Patient, and which sometimes intermits.

§ 549. When these Symptoms, or some of them, ascertain the Necessity of purging a Person, not then attacked by any manifest Disease (for I am not speaking here of Purges in such Cases) a proper purging Medicine may be given him. The bad Tast in his Mouth; the continual Belchings, the frequent Reachings to vomit, the actual Vomitings and Melancholy discover, that the Cause of his Disorder resides in the Stomach, and shew that a Vomit will be of Service to him. But when such Signs or Symptoms are not evident, the Patient should take such purging or opening Remedies, as are particularly indicated by the Pains, whether of the Loins, from the Cholic; or by a Sensation of Weight or Heaviness in the Knees.

§ 550. But we should abstain from either vomiting or purging, 1, Whenever the Complaints of the Patient are founded in their Weakness, and their being already exhausted 2, When there is a general Dryness of the Habit, a very considerable Degree of Heat, some Inflammation, or a strong Fever. 3, Whenever Nature is exerting herself in some other salutary Evacuation; whence purging must never be attempted in critical Sweats, during the monthly Discharges, nor during a Fit of the Gout. 4, Nor in such inveterate Obstructions as Purges cannot remove, and really do augment. 5, Neither when

when the nervous System is considerably weakened.

§ 551. There are other Cases again, in which it may be proper to purge, but not to give a Vomit. These Cases are, 1, When the Patient abounds too much with Blood, (See § 540) since the Efforts which attend vomiting, greatly augment the Force of the Circulation; whence the Blood-vessels of the Head and of the Breast, being extremely distended with Blood, might burst, which must prove fatal on the Spot, and has repeatedly proved so. 2, For the same Reason they should not be given to Persons, who are subject to frequent Bleeding from the Nose, or to coughing up or vomiting of Blood; to Women who are subject to excessive or unseasonable Discharges of Blood, &c. from the *Vagina*, the Neck of the Womb; nor to those who are with Child. 3, Vomits are improper for ruptured Persons.

§ 552. When any Person has taken too acrid, too sharp, a Vomit, or a Purge, which operates with excessive Violence; whether this consists in the most vehement Efforts and Agitations, the Pains, Convulsions, or Swoonings, which are their frequent Consequences, or whether that prodigious Evacuation and Emptiness their Operation causes, (which is commonly termed a *Super-purgation*) and which may hurry the Patient off. Instances of which are but too common among the lower Class of the People, who much too frequently confide themselves to the Conduct
of

of ignorant Men-flayers: In all such unhappy Accidents, I say, we should treat these unfortunate Persons, as if they had been actually poisoned, by violent corroding Poisons, (See § 533) that is, we should fill them, as it were, with Draughts of warm Water, Milk, Oil, Barley-water, Almond Milk, emollient Glysters with Milk, and the Yolks of Eggs; and also bleed them plentifully, if their Pains are excessive, and their Pulses strong and feverish.

The Super-purgation, the excessive Discharge, is to be stopt, after having plied the Patient plentifully with diluting Drinks, by giving the calming Anodyne Medicines directed in the Removal of acute Pains, § 536, N°. 6.

Flanels dipt in hot Water, in which some *Venice* Treacle is dissolved, are very serviceable: and should the Evacuations by Stool be excessive, and the Patient has not a high Fever, and a parching Kind of Heat, a Morsel of the same Treacle, as large as a Nutmeg, may be dissolved in his Glyster.

But should the Vomiting solely be excessive, without any Purging, the Number of the emollient Glysters with Oil and the Yolk of an Egg must be increased; and the Patient should be placed in a warm Bath.

§ 553. Purges frequently repeated, without just and necessary Indications, are attended with much the same ill Effects as frequent Bleedings. They destroy the Digestions; the Stomach no longer, or very languidly, exerts its Functions; the

the Intestines prove inactive, the Patient becomes liable to very severe Cholics; the Plight of the Body, deprived of its salutary Nutrition, falls off; Perspiration is disordered; Defluxions ensue; nervous Maladies come on, with a general Languor; and the Patient proves old, long before the Number of his Years have made him so.

Much irreparable Mischief has been done to the Health of Children, by Purges injudiciously given and repeated. They prevent them from attaining their utmost natural Strength, and frequently contract their due Growth. They ruin their Teeth, dispose young Girls to future Obstructions; and when they have been already affected by them, they render them still more obstinate.

It is a Prejudice too generally received, that Persons who have little or no Appetite need purging; since this is often very false, and most of those Causes, which lessen or destroy the Appetite, cannot be removed by purging; though many of them may be increased by it.

Persons whose Stomachs contain much glairy viscid Matter suppose, they may be cured by Purges, which seem indeed at first to relieve them: but this proves a very slight and deceitful Relief. These Humours are owing to that Weakness and Laxity of the Stomach, which Purges augment, since notwithstanding they carry off Part of these viscid Humours generated in it, at the Expiration of a few Days there is a greater Accumulation of them than before; and thus, by a Re-iteration of purging Medicines, the Malady soon becomes incurable, and Health irrecoverably-lost. The real Cure of such Cases is effected by directly opposite Medicines. Those referred to, or mentioned, § 272, are highly conducive to it.

§ 554 The Custom of taking stomachic Medicines infused in Brandy, Spirit of Wine, Cherry Water, &c. is always dangerous; for notwithstanding the present immediate Relief such Infusions afford in some Disorders of the Stomach, they really by slow Degrees impair and ruin that Organ; and it may be observed, that as many as accustom themselves to Drams, go off, just like excessive Drinkers, in Consequence of their having no Digestion; whence they sink into a State of Depression and Languor, and die dropsical.

§ 555. Either Vomits or Purges may be often beneficially omitted, even when they have some Appearance of seeming necessary, by abating one Meal a Day for some time; by abstaining from the most nourishing Sorts of Food, and especially from those which are fat, by drinking freely of cool Water, and taking extraordinary Exercise. The same Regimen also serves to subdue, without the Use of Purges, the various Complaints which often invade those, who omit taking purging Medicines, at those Seasons and Intervals, in which they have made it a Custom to take them.

§ 556

§ 556. The Medicines, N°. 34 and 35, are the moſt certain Vomits. The Powder, N° 21, is a good Purge, when the Patient is in no wiſe feveriſh.

The Doſes recommended in the Table of Remedies are thoſe, which are proper for a grown Man, of a vigorous Conſtitution. Neverthelefs there are ſome few, for whom they may be too weak: in ſuch Circumſtances they may be increaſed by the Addition of a third or fourth Part of the Doſe preſcribed. But ſhould they not operate in that Quantity, we muſt be careful not to double the Doſe, much leſs to give a three-fold Quantity, which has ſometimes been done; and that even without its Operation, and at the Riſque of killing the Patient, which has not ſeldom been the Conſequence. In Caſe of ſuch purging not enſuing, we ſhould rather give large Draughts of Whey ſweetened with Honey, or of warm Water, in a Pot of which an Ounce, or an Ounce and a half of common Salt muſt be diſſolved; and this Quantity is to be taken from time to time in ſmall Cups, moving about with it.

The Fibres of Country People who inhabit the Mountains, and live almoſt ſolely on Milk, are ſo little ſuſceptible of Senſation, that they muſt take ſuch large Doſes to purge them, as would kill all the Peaſantry in the Vallies. In the Mountains of *Valais* there are Men who take twenty, and even twenty-four Grains of Glafs of

Antimony for a single Dose, a Grain or two of which were sufficient to poison ordinary Men.

§ 557. Notwithstanding our Cautions on this important Head, whenever an urgent Necessity commands it, Purging must be recurred to at all Times and Seasons. but when the Season may be safely selected, it were right to decline Purging in the Extremities of either Heat or Cold, and to take the Purge early in the Morning, that the Medicines may find less Obstruction or Embarrassment from the Contents of the Stomach. Every other Consideration, with Relation to the Stars and the Moon, is ridiculous, and void of any Foundation. The People are particularly averse to purging in the Dog-days; and if this were only on Account of the great Heat, it would be very pardonable. but it is from an astrological Prejudice, which is so much the more absurd, as the real Dog-days are at thirty-six Days Distance from those commonly reckoned such; and it is a melancholy Reflection, that the Ignorance of the People should be so gross, in this Respect, in our enlightened Age; and that they should still imagine the Virtue and Efficacy of Medicines to depend on what Sign of the Zodiac the Sun is in, or in any particular Quarter of the Moon. Yet it is certain in this Point, they are so inveterately attached to this Prejudice, that it is but too common to see Country-People die, in waiting for the Sign or Quarter most favourable to the Operation and Effect of a Medicine, which was truly necessary five or six Days before either of them

Some

Sometimes too that particular Medicine is given, to which a certain Day is supposed to be auspicious and favourable, in Preference to that which is most prevalent against the Disease. And thus it is, than an ignorant Almanack Maker determines on the Lives of the human Race, and contracts the Duration of them with Impunity.

§ 558 When a Vomit or a Purge is to be taken, the Patient's Body should be prepared for the Reception of it twenty-four Hours beforehand, by taking very little Food, and drinking some Glasses of warm Water, or of a light Tea of some Herbs.

He should not drink after a Vomit, until it begins to work; but then he should drink very plentifully of warm Water, or a light Infusion of Chamomile Flowers, which is preferable.

It is usual, after Purges, to take some thin Broth or Soup during their Operation; but warm Water sweetened with Sugar or Honey, or an Infusion of Succory Flowers, would sometimes be more suitable.

§ 559 As the Stomach suffers, in some Degree, as often as either a Vomit, or a Purge, is taken, the Patient should be careful how he lives and orders himself for some Days after taking them, as well in Regard to the Quantity as Quality of his Food.

§ 560. I shall say nothing of other Articles taken by Way of Precaution, such as Soups, Whey, Waters, &c. which are but little used among the People, but confine myself to this general Remark, that when they take any of these precautionary Things, they should enter on a Regimen or Way of living, that may co-operate with them, and contribute to the same Purpose. Whey is commonly taken to refresh and cool the Body, and while they drink it, they deny themselves Pulse, Fruits, and Sallads. They eat nothing then, but the best and heartiest Flesh-meats they can come at, such Vegetables as are used in good Soups, Eggs, and good Wine, notwithstanding this is to destroy, by high and heating Aliments, all the attemperating cooling Effects expected from the Whey.

Some Persons propose to cool and attemperate their Blood by Soups and a thin Diet, into which they cram Craw-fish, that heat considerably, or *Nasturtium*, Cresses which also heat, and thus defeat their own Purpose. Happily, in such a Case, the Error in one Respect often cures that in the other; and these Kinds of Soup, which are in no wise cooling, prove very serviceable, in Consequence of the Cause of the Symptoms, which they were intended to remove, not requiring any Coolers at all.

The general physical Practice of the Community, which unhappily is but too much in Fashion, abounds with similar Errors. I will just cite one, because I have seen its dismal Effects. Many People suppose Pepper cooling, though their Smell, Taste, and common Sense concur to inform them of the contrary. It is the very hottest of Spices.

§ 561.

§ 561. The most certain Preservative, and the most attainable too by every Man, is to avoid all Excess, and especially Excess in eating and in drinking. People generally eat more than thoroughly consists with Health, or permits them to attain the utmost Vigour, of which their natural Constitutions are capable. The Custom is established, and it is difficult to eradicate it: notwithstanding we should at least resolve not to eat, but through Hunger, and always under a Subjection to Reason, because, except in a very few Cases, Reason constantly suggests to us not to eat, when the Stomach has an Aversion to Food. A sober moderate Person is capable of Labour, I may say, even of excessive Labour of some Kinds, of which greater Eaters are absolutely incapable. Sobriety of itself cures such Maladies as are otherwise incurable, and may recover the most shattered and unhealthy Persons.

CHAPTER XXXIII.

Of Mountebanks, Quacks, and Conjurers.

SECT. 562.

ONE dreadful Scourge still remains to be treated of, which occasions a greater Mortality, than all the Distempers I have hitherto described, and which, as long as it continues, will defeat our most Precaution cautions to preserve the Healths and Lives of the common People. This, or rather, these Scourges, for they are very numerous, are Quacks; of which there are two Species: The Mountebanks or travelling Quacks, and those pretended Physicians in Villages and Country-Places, both male and female, known in *Swifferland* by the Name of Conjurers, and who very effectually unpeople it.

The first of these, the Mountebanks, without visiting the Sick, or thinking of their Distempers, sell different Medicines, some of which are for external Use, and these often do little or no Mischief; but their internal ones are much oftener pernicious. I have been a Witness of their dreadful Effects, and we are not visited by one of these wandering Caitiffs, whose Admission into our Country is not mortally fatal to some of its Inhabitants. They are injurious also in another Respect, as they carry off great Sums of Money with them, and levy annually some thousands of Livres, amongst that Order of the People, who have the least to spare. I have seen, and with a very painful Concern, the poor Labourer and the Artisan, who have scarcely possessed the common Necessaries of Life, borrow wherewithal to purchase, and at a dear Price, the Poison that was to compleat their Misery, by increasing their Maladies; and which, where they escaped with their Lives, has left them in such a languid and inactive State, as has reduced their whole Family to Beggary.

§ 563

§ 563. An ignorant, knavish, lying and impudent Fellow will always seduce the gross and credulous Mass of People, incapable to judge of and estimate any thing rightly; and adapted to be the eternal Dupes of such, as are base enough to endeavour to dazzle their weak Understandings; by which Method these vile Quacks will certainly defraud them, as long as they are tolerated. But ought not the Magistrates, the Guardians, the Protectors, the political Fathers of the People interpose, and defend them from this Danger, by severely prohibiting the Entrance of such pernicious Fellows into a Country, where Mens' Lives are very estimable, and where Money is scarce; since they extinguish the first, and carry off the last, without the least Possibility of their being in anywise useful to it. Can such forcible Motives as these suffer our Magistrates to delay *their* Expulsion any longer, *whom* there never was the least Reason for admitting?

§ 564. It is acknowledged the Conjurers, the residing Conjurers, do not carry out the current Money of the Country, like the itinerant Quacks; but the Havock they make among their Fellow Subjects is without Intermission, whence it must be very great, as every Day in the Year is marked with many of their Victims. Without the least Knowledge or Experience, and offensively armed with three or four Medicines, whose Nature they are as thoroughly ignorant of, as of their unhappy Patients Diseases, and which Medicines, being almost all violent ones, are very certainly

tainly so many Swords in the Hands of raging Madmen. Thus armed and qualified, I say, they aggravate the slightest Disorders, and make those that are a little more considerable, mortal; but from which the Patients would have recovered, if left solely to the Conduct of Nature; and, for a still stronger Reason, if they had confided to the Guidance of her experienced Observers and Assistants.

§ 565. The Robber who assassinates on the High-way, leaves the Traveller the Resource of defending himself, and the Chance of being aided by the Arrival of other Travellers: But the Poisoner, who forces himself into the Confidence of a sick Person, is a hundred times more dangerous, and as just an Object of Punishment.

The Bands of Highwaymen, and their Individuals, that enter into any Country or District, are described as particularly as possible to the Publick. It were equally to be wished, we had also a List of these physical Impostors and Ignorants male and female; and that a most exact Description of them, with the Number, and a brief summary of their murderous Exploits, were faithfully published. By this Means the Populace might probably be inspired with such a wholesome Dread of them, that they would no longer expose their Lives to the Mercy of such Executioners.

§ 566. But their Blindness, with Respect to these two Sorts of maleficent Beings, is inconceivable. That indeed in Favour of the Mountebank

tebank is somewhat less gross, because as they are not personally acquainted with him, they may the more easily credit him with some Part of the Talents and the Knowledge he arrogates. I shall therefore inform them, and it cannot be repeated too often, that whatever ostentatious Dress and Figure some of these Impostors make, they are constantly vile Wretches, who, incapable of earning a Livelyhood in any honest Way, have laid the Foundation of their Subsistence on their own amazing Stock of Impudence, and that of the weak Credulity of the People; that they have no scientific Knowledge; that their Titles and Patents are so many Impositions, and inauthentic; since by a shameful Abuse, such Patents and Titles are become Articles of Commerce, which are to be obtained at very low Prices; just like the second-hand laced Cloaks which they purchase at the Brokers. That their Certificates of Cures are so many Chimeras or Forgeries, and that in short, if among the prodigious Multitudes of People who take their Medicines, some of them should recover, which it is almost physically impossible must not sometimes be the Case, yet it would not be the less certain, that they are a pernicious destructive Set of Men. A Thrust of a Rapier into the Breast has saved a Man's Life by seasonably opening an Imposthume in it, which might otherwise have killed him: and yet internal penetrating Wounds, with a small Sword, are not the less mortal for one such extraordinary Consequence. Nor is it even surprizing that these

these Mountebanks, which is equally applicable to Conjurers, who kill thousands of People, whom Nature alone, or assisted by a Physician, would have saved, should now and then cure a Patient, who had been treated before by the ablest Physicians Frequently Patients of that Class, who apply to these Mountebanks and Conjurers (whether it has been, that they would not submit to the Treatment proper for their Distempers, or whether the real Physician tired of the intractable Creatures has discontinued his Advice and Attendance) look out for such Doctors, as assure them of a speedy Cure, and venture to give them such Medicines as kill many, and cure one (who has had Constitution enough to overcome them) a little sooner than a justly reputable Physician would have done. It is but too easy to procure, in every Parish, such Lists of their Patients, and of their Feats, as would clearly evince the Truth of whatever has been said here relating to them.

§ 567. The Credit of this Market, this Fair-hunting Doctor, surrounded by five or six hundred Peasants, staring and gaping at him, and counting themselves happy in his condescending to cheat them of their very scarce and necessary Cash, by selling them, for twenty times more than its real Worth, a Medicine whose best Quality were to be only a useless one, the Credit, I say, of this vile yet tolerated Cheat, would quickly vanish, could each of his Auditors be persuaded, of what is strictly true, that except a

little

little more Tenderness and Agility of Hand, he knows full as much as his Doctor; and that if he could assume as much Impudence, he would immediately have as much Ability, would equally deserve the same Reputation, and to have the same Confidence reposed in him.

§ 568. Were the Populace capable of reasoning, it were easy to disabuse them in these Respects, but as it is, their Guardians and Conductors should reason for them. I have already proved the Absurdity of reposing any Confidence in Mountebanks, properly so called; and that Reliance some have on the Conjurers is still more stupid and ridiculous.

The very meanest Trade requires some Instruction. A Man does not commence even a Cobler, a Botcher of old Leather, without serving an Apprenticeship to it; and yet no Time has been served, no Instruction has been attended to, by these Pretenders to the most necessary, useful and elegant Profession. We do not confide the mending, the cleaning of a Watch to any, who have not spent several Years in considering how a Watch is made, what are the Requisites and Causes of its going right; and the Defects or Impediments that make it go wrong: and yet the preserving and rectifying the Movements of the most complex, the most delicate and exquisite, and the most estimable Machine upon Earth, is entrusted to People who have not the least Notion of its Structure, of the Causes of its Motions; nor of the Instruments proper to rectify their Deviations.

Let a Soldier discarded from his Regiment for his roguish Tricks, or who is a Deserter from it, a Bankrupt, a disreputable Ecclesiastic, a drunken Barber, or a Multitude of such other worthless People, advertize that they mount, set and fit up all Kinds of Jewels and Trinkets in Perfection; if any of these are not known; if no Person in the Place has ever seen any of their Work; or if they cannot produce authentic Testimonials of their Honesty, and their Ability in their Business, not a single Individual will trust them with two Pennyworth of false Stones to work upon; in short they must be famished. But if instead of professing themselves Jewellers, they post themselves up as Physicians, the Croud purchase, at a high Rate, the Pleasure of trusting them with the Care of their Lives, the remaining Part of which they rarely fail to empoison.

§ 569. The most genuine and excellent Physicians, these extraordinary Men, who, born with the happiest Talents, have began to inform their Understandings from their earliest Youth; who have afterwards carefully qualified themselves by cultivating every Branch of Physic; who have sacrificed the best and most pleasurable Days of their Lives, to a regular and assiduous Investigation of the human Body, of its various Functions, of the Causes that may impair or embarrass them, and informed themselves of the Qualities and Virtues of every simple and com-

Of Mountebanks, Quacks, and Conjurers.

compound Medicine; who have surmounted the Difficulty and Loathsomness of living in Hospitals among thousands of Patients; and who have added the medical Observations of all Ages and Places to their own; these few and extraordinary Men, I say, still consider themselves as short of that perfect Ability and consummate Knowledge, which they contemplate and wish for, as necessary to guarding the precious *Depositum* of human Life and Health, confided to their Charge. Nevertheless we see the same inestimable Treasures, intrusted to gross and stupid Men, born without Talents; brought up without Education or Culture; who frequently can scarcely read; who are as profoundly ignorant of every Subject that has any Relation to Physic, as the Savages of *Asia*; who awake only to drink away; who often exercise their horrid Trade merely to find themselves in strong Liquor, and execute it chiefly when they are drunk who, in short, became Physicians, only from their Incapacity to arrive at any Trade or Attainment! Certainly such a Conduct in Creatures of the human Species must appear very astonishing, and even melancholy, to every sensible thinking Man; and constitute the highest Degree of Absurdity and Extravagance.

Should any Person duly qualified enter into an Examination of the Medicines they use, and compare them with the Situation and Symptoms of the Patients to whom they give them, he must be struck with Horror; and heartily deplore the

Fate

Fate of that unfortunate Part of the human Race, whose Lives, so important to the Community, are committed to the Charge of the most murderous Set of Beings.

§ 570. Some of these Caitiffs however, apprehending the Force and Danger of that Objection, founded on their Want of Study and Education, have endeavoured to elude it, by infusing and spreading a false, and indeed, an impudent impious Prejudice among the People, which prevails too much at present; and this is, that their Talents for Physic are a supernatural Gift, and, of Course, greatly superior to all human Knowledge It were going out of my Province to expatiate on the Indecency, the Sin, and the Irreligion of such Knavery, and incroaching upon the Rights and perhaps the Duty of the Clergy, but I intreat the Liberty of observing to this respectable Order of Men, that this Superstition, which is attended with dreadful Consequences, seems to call for their utmost Attention. and in general the Expulsion of Superstition is the more to be wished, as a Mind, imbued with false Prejudices, is less adapted to imbibe a true and valuable Doctrine There are some very callous hardened Villians among this murdering Band, who, with a View to establish their Influence and Revenue as well upon Fear as upon Hope, have horridly ventured so far as to incline the Populace to doubt, whether they received their boasted Gift and Power from Heaven or from Hell' And yet these are the Men who

who are trusted with the Health and the Lives of many others.

§ 571. One Fact which I have already mentioned, and which it seems impossible to account for is, that great Earnestness of the Peasant to procure the best Assistance he can for his sick Cattle. At whatever Distance the Farrier lives, or some Person who is supposed qualified to be one (for unfortunately there is not one in *Swisserland*) if he has considerable Reputation in this Way, the Country-man goes to consult him, or purchases his Visit at any Price. However expensive the Medicines are, which the Horse-doctor directs, if they are accounted the best, he procures them for his poor Beast. But if himself, his Wife or Children fall sick, he either calls in no Assistance nor Medicines; or contents himself with such as are next at Hand, however pernicious they may be, though nothing the cheaper on that account: for certainly the Money, extorted by some of these physical Conjurers from their Patients, but oftner from their Heirs, is a very shameful Injustice, and calls loudly for Reformation.

§ 572. In an excellent Memoir or Tract, which will shortly be published, on the Population of *Swisserland*, we shall find an important and very affecting Remark, which strictly demonstrates the Havock made by these immedical Magicians or Conjurers, and which is this: That in the common Course of Years, the Proportion between the Numbers and Deaths of the Inhabitants of any one Place, is not extremely different in City and Country: but when the very same epidemical Disease attacks the City and the Villages, the Difference is enormous; and the Number of Deaths of the former compared with that of the Inhabitants of the Villages, where the Conjurer exercises his bloody Dominion, is infinitely more than the Deaths in the City.

I find in the second Volume of the Memoirs of the oeconomical Society of *Berne*, for the Year 1762, another Fact equally interesting, which is related by one of the most intelligent and sagacious Observers, concerned in that Work. " Pleurifies and Peripneumonies (he says) prevailed at *Cottens a la Côte*; and some Peasants died under them, who had consulted the Conjurers and taken their heating Medicines; while of those, who pursued a directly opposite Method, almost every one recovered."

§ 573. But I shall employ myself no longer on this Topic, on which the Love of my Species alone has prompted me to say thus much; though it deserves to be considered more in Detail, and is, in Reality, of the greatest Consequence. None methinks could make themselves easy with Respect to it so much as Physicians, if they were conducted only by lucrative Views, since these Conjurers diminish the Number of those poor People, who sometimes consult the real Physicians, and with some Care and Trouble, but without the least Profit, to those Gentlemen. But what good Physician is mean and vile

vile enough to purchase a few Hours of Ease and Tranquillity at so high, so very odious a Price?

§ 574. Having thus clearly shewn the Evils attending this crying Nusance, I wish I were able to prescribe an effectual Remedy against it, which I acknowledge is far from being easy to do.

The first necessary Point probably was to have demonstrated the great and public Danger, and to dispose the State to employ their Attention on this fatal, this mortal Abuse; which, joined to the other Causes of Depopulation, has a manifest Tendency to render *Swisserland* a Desert.

§ 575. The second, and doubtless the most effectual Means, which I had already mentioned is, not to admit any travelling Mountebank to enter this Country; and to set a Mark on all the Conjurers: It may probably also be found convenient, to inflict corporal Punishment on them; as it has been already adjudged in different Countries by sovereign Edicts. At the very least they should be marked with public Infamy, according to the following Custom practised in a great City in *France*. " When any Mountebanks appeared in *Montpellier*, the Magistrates had a Power to mount each of them upon a meagre miserable Ass, with his Head to the Ass's Tail. In this Condition they were led throughout the whole City, attended with the Shouts and Hooting of the Children and the Mob, beating them, throwing Filth and Ordure at them, reviling them, and dragging them all about "

§ 576 A third conducive Means would be the Instructions and Admonition of the Clergy on this Subject, to the Peasants in their several Parishes. For this Conduct of the common People amounting, in Effect, to Suicide, to Self-murder, it must be important to convince them of it. But the little Efficacy of the strongest and repeated Exhortations on so many other Articles, may cause us to entertain a very reasonable Doubt of their Success on this. Custom seems to have determined, that there is nothing in our Day, which excludes a Person from the Title and Appellation of an honest or honourable Man, except it be meer and convicted Theft; and that for this simple and obvious Reason, that we attach ourselves more strongly to our Property, than to any Thing else. Even Homicide is esteemed and reputed honourable in many Cases. Can we reasonably then expect to convince the Multitude, that it is criminal to confide the Care of their Health to these Poisoners, in Hopes of a Cure of their Disorders? A much likelier Method of succeeding on this Point would certainly be, to convince the deluded People, that it will cost them less to be honestly and judiciously treated, than to suffer under the Hands of these Executioners. The Expectation of a good and cheap Health-market will be apt to influence them more, than their Dread of a Crime would.

§ 577. A fourth Means of removing or restraining this Nusance would be to expunge, from the Almanacs, all the astrological Rules relating

lating to Physick; as they continually conduce to preserve and increase some dangerous Prejudices and Notions in a Science, the smallest Errors in which are sometimes fatal. I had already reflected on the Multitude of Peasants that have been lost, from postponing, or mistiming a Bleeding, only because the sovereign Decision of an Almanac had directed it at some other Time. May it not also be dreaded, to mention it by the Way, that the same Cause, the Almanacs, may prove injurious to their rural Oeconomy and Management; and that by advising with the Moon, who has no Influence, and is of no Consequence in Vegetation or other Country Business, they may be wanting in a due Attention to such other Circumstances and Regulations, as are of real Importance in them?

§ 578. A fifth concurring Remedy against this popular Evil would be the Establishment of Hospitals, for the Reception of poor Patients, in the different Cities and Towns of *Swisserland*.

There may be a great many easy and concurring Means of erecting and endowing such, with very little new Expence; and immense Advantages might result from them: besides, however considerable the Expences might prove, is not the Object of them of the most interesting, the most important Nature? It is incontestably our serious Duty; and it would soon be manifest, that the Performance of it would be attended with more essential intrinsic Benefit to the Community, than any other Application of Money could produce. We must either admit, that the Multitude, the Body of the People is useless to the State, or agree, that Care should be taken to preserve and continue them. A very respectable *English* Man, who, after a previous and thorough Consideration of this Subject, had applied himself very assiduously and usefully on the Means of increasing the Riches and the Happiness of his Country-men, complains that in *England*, the very Country in which there are the most Hospitals, the Poor who are sick are not sufficiently assisted. What a deplorable Deficience of the necessary Assistance for such must then be in a Country, that is not provided with a single Hospital? That Aid from Surgery and Physic, which abounds in Cities, is not sufficiently diffused into Country-places: and the Peasants are liable to some simple and moderate Diseases, which, for Want of proper Care, degenerate into a State of Infirmity, that sinks them into premature Death.

§ 579. In fine, if it be found impossible to extinguish these Abuses (for those arising from Quacks are not the only ones, nor is that Title applied to as many as really deserve it) beyond all Doubt it would be for the Benefit and Safety of the Public, upon the whole, entirely to prohibit the Art, the Practice of Physic itself. When real and good Physicians cannot effect as much Good, as ignorant ones and Impostors can do Mischief, some real Advantage must accrue to the State, and to the whole Species, from employing

ploying none of either. I affirm it, after much Reflection, and from thorough Conviction, that **Anarchy** in Medicine is the moſt dangerous **Anarchy**. For this Profeſſion, when looſed from every Reſtraint, and ſubjected to no Regulations, no Laws, is the more cruel Scourge and Affliction, from the inceſſant Exerciſe of it; and ſhould its Anarchy, its Diſorders prove irremediable, the Practice of an Art, become ſo very noxious, ſhould be prohibited under the ſevereſt Penalties: Or, if the Conſtitution of any Goverment was inconſiſtent with the Application of ſo violent a Remedy, they ſhould order public Prayers againſt the Mortality of it, to be offered up in all the Churches; as the Cuſtom has been in other great and general Calamities.

§ 580. Another Abuſe, leſs fatal indeed than thoſe already mentioned (but which, however, has real ill Conſequences, and at the beſt, carries out a great deal of Money from us, though leſs at the Expence of the common People, than of thoſe of eaſy Circumſtances) is that Blindneſs and Facility, with which many ſuffer themſelves to be impoſed upon, by the pompous Advertiſements of ſome *Catholicon*, ſome univerſal Remedy, which they purchaſe at a high Rate, from ſome foreign Pretender to a mighty Secret or *Noſtrum*. Perſons of a Claſs or two above the Populace do not care to run after a Mountebank, from ſuppoſing they ſhould depretiate themſelves by mixing with the Herd. Yet if that very Quack, inſtead of coming among us, were to reside in some foreign City; if, instead of posting up his lying Puffs and Pretensions, at the Corners of the Streets, he would get them inserted in the Gazettes, and News-papers; if, instead of selling his boasted Remedies in Person, he should establish Shops or Offices for that Purpose in every City, and finally, if instead of selling them twenty times above their real Value, he would still double that Price, instead of having the common People for his Customers, he would take in the wealthy Citizen, Persons of all Ranks, and from almost every Country. For strange as it seems, it is certain, that a Person of such a Condition, who is sensible in every other Respect, and who will scruple to confide his Health to the Conduct of such Physicians as would be the justest Subjects of his Confidence, will venture to take, through a very unaccountable Infatuation, the most dangerous Medicine, upon the Credit of an imposing Advertisement, published by as worthless and ignorant a Fellow as the Mountebank whom he despises, because the latter blows a Horn under his Window; and yet who differs from the former in no other Respects except those I have just pointed out.

§ 581. Scarcely a Year passes, without one or another such advertized and vaunted Medicine's getting into high Credit; the Ravages of which are more or less, in Proportion to its being more or less in Vogue. Fortunately, for the human Species, but few of these *Nostrums* have attained an equal Reputation with *Ailhaud*'s Powders, an Inhabi-

Inhabitant of *Aix* in *Provence*, and unworthy the Name of a Physician; who has over-run *Europe* for some Years, with a violent Purge, the Remembrance of which will not be effaced before the Extinction of all its Victims. I attend now, and for a long time past, several Patients, whose Disorders I palliate without Hopes of ever curing them; and who owe their present melancholy State of Body to nothing but the manifest Consequences of these Powders; and I have actually seen, very lately, two Persons who have been cruelly poisoned by this boasted Remedy of his. A French Physician, as eminent for his Talents and his Science, as estimable from his personal Character in other Respects, has published some of the unhappy and tragical Consequences which the Use of them has occasioned; and were a Collection published of the same Events from them, in every Place where they have been introduced, the Size and the Contents of the Volume would make a very terrible one.

§ 582. It is some Comfort however, that all the other Medicines thus puffed and vended have not been altogether so fashionable, nor yet quite so dangerous. but all posted and advertized Medicines should be judged of upon this Principle (and I do not know a more infallible one in Physics, nor in the Practice of Physic), that whoever advertises any Medicine, as a universal Remedy for all Diseases, is an absolute Impostor, such a Remedy being impossible and contradictory. I shall not here offer to detail such Proofs as may be given of the Verity of this Proposition: but I freely appeal for it to every sensible Man, who will reflect a little on the different Causes of Diseases; on the Opposition of these Causes; and on the Absurdity of attempting to oppose such various Diseases, and their Causes, by one and the same Remedy.

As many as shall settle their Judgments properly on this Principle, will never be imposed upon by the superficial Gloss of these Sophisms contrived to prove, that all Diseases proceed from one Cause; and that this Cause is so very tractable, as to yield to one boasted Remedy. They will perceive at once, that such an Assertion must be founded in the utmost Knavery or Ignorance; and they will readily discover where the Fallacy lies. Can any one expect to cure a Dropsy, which arises from too great a Laxity of the Fibres, and too great an Attenuation or Thinness of the Blood, by the same Medicines that are used to cure an inflammatory Disease, in which the Fibres are too stiff and tense, and the Blood too thick and dense? Yet consult the News-papers and the Posts, and you will see published in and on all of them, Virtues just as contradictory; and certainly the Authors of such poisonous Contradictions ought to be legally punished for them.

§ 583. I heartily wish the Publick would attend here to a very natural and obvious Reflection. I have treated in this Book, but of a small Number of Diseases, most of them acute ones; and

and I am positive that no competent well qualified Physician has ever employed fewer Medicines, in the Treatment of the Diseases themselves. Nevertheless I have prescribed seventy-one, and I do not see which of them I could retrench, or dispense with the Want of, if I were obliged to use one less. Can it be supposed then, that any one single Medicine, compound or simple, shall cure thirty times as many Diseases as those I have treated of?

§ 584. I shall add another very important Observation, which doubtless may have occurred to many of my Readers; and it is this, that the different Causes of Diseases, their different Characters; the Differences which arise from the necessary Alterations that happen throughout their Progress and Duration; the Complications of which they are susceptible; the Varieties which result from the State of different Epidemics, of Seasons, of Sexes, and of many other Circumstances; that these Diversities, I say, oblige us very often to vary and change the Medicines; which proves how very ticklish and dangerous it is to have them directed by Persons, who have such an imperfect Knowledge of them, as those who are not Physicians must be supposed to have. And the Circumspection to be used in such Cases ought to be proportioned to the Interest the Assistant takes in the Preservation of the Patient, and that Love of his Neighbour with which he is animated.

§ 585.

§ 585. Must not the same Arguments and Reflections unavoidably suggest the Necessity of an entire Tractability on the Part of the Patient, and his Friends and Assistants? The History of Diseases which have their stated Times of Beginning, of manifesting and displaying themselves; of arriving at, and continuing in their Height, and of decreasing; do not all these demonstrate the Necessity of continuing the same Medicines, as long as the Character of the Distemper is the same; and the Danger of changing them often, only because what has been given has not afforded immediate Relief? Nothing can injure the Patient more than this Instability and Caprice. After the Indication which his Distemper suggests, appears to be well deduced, the Medicine must be chosen that is likeliest to resist the Cause of it; and it must be continued as long as no new Symptom or Circumstance supervenes, which requires an Alteration of it, except it should be evident, that an Error had been incurred in giving it. But to conclude that a Medicine is useless or insignificant, because it does not remove or abate the Distemper as speedily, as the Impatience of the Sick would naturally desire it, and to change it for another, is as unreasonable, as it would be for a Man to break his Watch, because the Hand takes twelve Hours, to make a Revolution round the Dial-plate.

§ 586. Physicians have some Regard to the State of the Urine of sick Persons, especially in inflammatory Fevers; as the Alterations occurring

ring in it help them to judge of the Changes that may have been made in the Character and Confiftence of the Humours in the Mafs of Blood; and thence may conduce to determine the Time, in which it will be proper to difpofe them to fome Evacution. But it is grofs Ignorance to imagine, and utter Knavery and Impofture to perfuade the Sick, that the meer Infpection of their Urine folely, fufficiently enables others to judge of the Symptoms and Caufe, of the Difeafe, and to direct the beft Remedies for it. This Infpection of the Urine can only be of Ufe when it is duly infpected; when we confider at the fame time the exact State and the very Looks of the Patient; when thefe are compared with the Degree of the Symptoms of the Malady; with the other Evacuations; and when the Phyfician is ftrictly informed of all external Circumftances, which may be confidered as foreign to the Malady; which may alter or affect the Evacuations, fuch as particular Articles of Food, particular Drinks, different Medicines, or the very Quantity of Drink. Where a Perfon is not furnifhed with an exact Account of thefe Circumftances, the meer Infpection of the Urine is of no Service, it fuggefts no Indication, nor any Expedient; and meer common Senfe fufficiently proves, and it may be boldly affirmed, that whoever orders any Medicine, without any other Knowledge of the Difeafe, than what an Infpection of the Urine affords, is a rank Knave, and the Patient who takes them is a Dupe.

§ 587.

§ 587. And here now any Reader may very naturally afk, whence can fuch a ridiculous Credulity proceed, upon a Subject fo effentially interefting to us as our own Health?

In Anfwer to this it fhould be obferved, that fome Sources, fome Caufes of it feem appropriated merely to the People, the Multitude. The firft of thefe is, the mechanical Impreffion of Parade and Shew upon the Senfes. 2, The Prejudice they have conceived, as I faid before, of the Conjurers curing by a fupernatural Gift. 3, The Notion the Country People entertain, that their Diftemper and Diforders are of a Character and Species peculiar to themfelves, and that the Phyficians, attending the Rich, know nothing concerning them. 4, The general Miftake that their employing the Conjurer is much cheaper. 5, Perhaps a fheepifh fhame-faced Timidity may be one Motive, at leaft with fome of them. 6, A Kind of Fear too, that Phyficians will confider their Cafes with lefs Care and Concern, and be likely to treat them more cavalierly, a Fear which increafes that Confidence which the Peafant, and which indeed every Man has in his Equal, being founded in Equality itfelf. And 7, the Difcourfe and Converfation of fuch illiterate Empirics being more to their Taft, and more adapted to their Apprehenfion.

But it is lefs eafy to account for this blind Confidence, which Perfons of a fuperior Clafs (whofe Education being confidered as much better

ter are regarded as better Reasoners) repose in these boasted Remedies; and even for some Conjurer in Vogue. Nevertheless even some of their Motives may be probably assigned.

The first is that great Principle of *Seity*, or *Selfness*, as it may be called, innate to Man, which attaching him to the Prolongation of his own Existence more than to any other thing in the Universe, keeps his Eyes, his utmost Attention, continually fixed upon this Object; and compels him to make it the very Point, the Purpose of all his Advances and Proceedings; notwithstanding it does not permit him to distinguish the safest Paths to it from the dangerous ones. This is the surest and shortest Way says some Collector at the Turnpike, he pays, passes, and perishes from the Precipices that occur in his Route.

This very Principle is the Source of another Error, which consists in reposing, involuntarily, a greater Degree of Confidence in those, who flatter and fall in the most with us in our favourite Opinions. The well apprised Physician, who foresees the Length and the Danger of a Disease; and who is a Man of too much Integrity to affirm what he does not think, must, from a necessary Construction of the human Frame and Mind, be listened to less favourably, than he who flatters us by saying what we wish. We endeavour to elongate, to absent ourselves, from the Sentiments, the Judgment of the first, we smile, from Self-complacency, at those of the last,

which

which in a very little time are sure of obtaining our Preference.

A third Cause, which results from the same Principle is, that we give ourselves up the most readily to his Conduct, whose Method seems the least disagreeable, and flatters our Inclinations the most. The Physician who enjoins a strict Regimen; who insists upon some Restraints and Self-denials, who intimates the Necessity of Time and Patience for the Accomplishment of the Cure, and who expects a thorough Regularity through the Course of it, disgusts a Patient who has been accustomed to indulge his own Tast and Humour; the Quack, who never hesitates at complying with it, charms him. The Idea of a long and somewhat distant Cure, to be obtained at the End of an unpleasant and unrelaxing Regimen, supposes a very perilous Disease; this Idea disposes the Patient to Disgust and Melancholy, he cannot submit to it without Pain; and he embraces, almost unconsciously, merely to avoid this, an opposite System which presents him only with the Idea of such a Distemper, as will give Way to a few Doses of Simples.

That Propensity to the New and Marvellous, which tyrannizes over so large a Proportion of our Species, and which has advanced so many absurd Persons and Things into Reputation, is a fourth and a very powerful Motive. An irksome Satiety, and a Tiresomeness, as it were, from the same Objects, is what our Nature is apt to be very apprehensive of, though we are incessantly

incessantly conducted towards it, by a Perception of some Void, some Emptiness in ourselves, and even in Society too: But new and extraordinary Sensations rousing us from this disagreeable State, more effectually than any Thing else, we unthinkingly abandon ourselves to them, without foreseeing their Consequences.

A fifth Cause arises from seven Eighths of Mankind being managed by, or following, the other Eighth; and, generally speaking, the Eighth that is so very forward to manage them, are the least fit and worthy to do it; whence all must go amiss, and absurd and embarrassing Consequences ensue from the Condition of Society. A Man of excellent Sense frequently sees only through the Eyes of a Fool, of an intriguing Fellow, or of a Cheat, in this he judges wrong, and his Conduct must be so too. A man of real Merit cannot connect himself with those who are addicted to caballing, and yet such are the Persons, who frequently conduct others.

Some other Causes might be annexed to these, but I shall mention only one of them, which I have already hinted, and the Truth of which I am confirmed in from several Years Experience; which is, that we generally love those who reason more absurdly than ourselves, better than those who convince us of our own weak Reasoning.

I hope the Reflexions every Reader will make on these Causes of our ill Conduct on this important Head, may contribute to correct or diminish it;

it; and to destroy those Prejudices whose fatal Effects we may continually observe.

[N. B. *The Multitude of* all *the Objects of this excellent Chapter in this Metropolis, and doubtless throughout* England, *were strong Inducements to have taken a little wholesome Notice of the Impostures of a few of the most pernicious. But on a second Perusal of this Part of the Original and its Translation, I thought it impossible (without descending to personal, nominal Anecdotes about the Vermin) to add any Thing material upon a Subject, which the Author has with such Energy exhausted. He even seems, by some of his Descriptions, to have taken Cognizance of a few of our most self-dignified itinerant Empirics, as these Genius's find it necessary sometimes to treat themselves with a little Transportation. In reality Dr.* TISSOT *has, in a very masterly Way, thoroughly dissected and displayed the whole* Genus, *every Species of Quacks. And when he comes to account for that Facility, with which Persons of very different Principles from them, and of better Intellects, first listen to, and finally countenance such Caitiffs, he penetrates into some of the most latent Weaknesses of the human Mind; even such as are often Secrets to their Owners. It is difficult, throughout this Disquisition, not to admire the Writer, but impossible not to love the Man, the ardent Philanthropist. His Sentiment that—*" *A Man of real Merit cannot connect himself with those who are addicted to cabalting,*"—*is exquisitely just, and so liberal, that it never entered into the Mind*

Mind of any disingenuous Man, however dignified, in any Profession. Persons of the simplest Hearts and purest Reflections must shrink at every Consciousness of Artifice; and secretly reproach themselves for each Success, that has redounded to them at the Expence of Truth] K.

Chapter XXXIV.

Containing Questions absolutely necessary to be answered exactly by the Patient, who consults a Physician.

Sect. 588.

GREAT Consideration and Experience are necessary to form a right Judgment of the State of a Patient, whom the Physician has not personally seen; even though he should receive the best Information it is possible to give him, at a Distance from the Patient. But this Difficulty is greatly augmented, or rather changed into an Impossibility, when his Information is not exact and sufficient. It has frequently happened to myself, that after having examined Peasants who came to get Advice for others, I did not venture to prescribe, because they were not able to give me a sufficient Information, in order to my being certain of the Distemper. To prevent this great Inconvenience, I subjoin a List of such Questions, as indispensably require clear and direct Answers.

General Questions.

What is the Patient's Age?
Is he generally a healthy Person?
What is his general Course of Life?
How long has he been sick?
In what Manner did his present Sickness begin, or appear?
Has he any Fever?
Is his Pulse hard or soft?
Has he still tolerable Strength, or is he weak?
Does he keep his Bed in the Day Time, or quit it?
Is he in the same Condition throughout the whole Day?
Is he still, or restless?
Is he hot, or cold?
Has he Pains in the Head, the Throat, the Breast, the Stomach, the Belly, the Loins, or in the Limbs, the Extremities of the Body?
Is his Tongue dry? does he complain of Thirst? of an ill Tast in his Mouth? of Reachings to vomit, or of an Aversion to Food?
Does he go to stool often or seldom?
What Appearance have his Stools, and what is their usual Quantity?

Does

Does he make much Urine? What Appearance has his Urine, as to Colour and Contents? Are they generally much alike, or do they change often?

Does he sweat?

Does he expectorate, or cough up?

Does he get Sleep?

Does he draw his Breath easily?

What Regimen does he observe in his Sickness?

What Medicines has he taken?

What Effects have they produced?

Has he never had the same Distemper before?

§ 589. The Diseases of Women and Children are attended with peculiar Circumstances; so that when Advice is asked for them, Answers must be given, not only to the preceding Questions, which relate to sick Persons in general; but also to the following, which regard these particularly.

Questions with Respect to Women.

Have they arrived at their monthly Discharges, and are these regular?

Are they pregnant? If so, how long since?

Are they in Child-bed?

Has their Delivery been happily accomplished?

Has the Mother cleansed sufficiently?

Has her Milk come in due Time and Quantity?

Does she suckle the Infant herself?
Is she subject to the Whites?

Questions relating to Children.

What is the Child's exact Age?
How many Teeth has he cut?
Does he cut them painfully?
Is he any-wise ricketty, or subject to Knots or Kernels?
Has he had the Small Pocks?
Does the Child void Worms, upwards or downwards?
Is his Belly large, swelled, or hard?
Is his Sleep quiet, or otherwise?

§ 590. Besides these general Questions, common in all the Diseases of the different Sexes and Ages, the Person consulting must also answer to those, which have a close and direct Relation to the Disease, at that very Time affecting the Sick.

For Example, in the Quinsey, the Condition of the Throat must be exactly inquired into. In Diseases of the Breast, an Account must be given of the Patient's Pains; of his Cough; of the Oppression, and of his Breathing, and Expectoration. I shall not enter upon a more particular Detail; common Sense will sufficiently extend this Plan or Specimen to other Diseases; and though these Questions may seem numerous, it will always be easy to write down their Answers
in

in as little Room, as the Queſtions take up here. It were even to be wiſhed that Perſons of every Rank, who occaſionally write for medical Advice and Directions, would obſerve ſuch a Plan or Succeſſion, in the Body of their Letters. By this Means they would frequently procure the moſt ſatisfactory Anſwers; and ſave themſelves the Trouble of writing ſecond Letters, to give a neceſſary Explanation of the firſt.

The Succeſs of Remedies depends, in a very great Meaſure, on a very exact Knowledge of the Diſeaſe; and that Knowledge on the preciſe Information of it, which is laid before the Phyſician.

F I N I S.

TABLE

Of the Prescriptions and Medicines, referred to in the foregoing Treatise: Which, with the Notes beneath them, are to be read before the taking, or Application, of any of the said Medicines.

AS in Order to ascertain the Doses of Medicines, I have generally done it by Pounds, Ounces, Half-Ounces, &c. &c. and as this Method, especially to the common People, might prove a little too obscure and embarrassing, I have specified here the exact Weight of Water, contained in such Vessels or liquid Measures, as are most commonly used in the Country.

The Pound which I mean, throughout all these Prescriptions, is that consisting of sixteen Ounces. These Ounces contain eight Drachms, each Drachm consisting of three Scruples, and each Scruple of twenty Grains, the medical Scruple of *Paris* solely containing twenty-four Grains.

The liquid Measure, the *Pot* used at *Berne*, being that I always speak of, may be estimated, without any material Error, to contain three Pounds and a Quarter, which is equal to three Pints, and eight common Spoonfuls English Measure.

Measure. But the exact Weight of the Water, contained in the Pot of *Berne*, being fifty-one Ounces and a Quarter only, it is strictly equal but to three Pints and six common Spoonfuls *English*. This however is a Difference of no Importance, in the usual Drinks or Aliments of the Sick.

The small drinking Glass we talk of, filled so as not to run over, contains three Ounces and three Quarters. But filled, as we propose it should for the Sick, it is to be estimated only at three Ounces.

The common middle sized Cup, though rather large than little, contains three Ounces and a Quarter. But as dealt out to the Sick, it should not be estimated, at the utmost, above three Ounces.

The small Glass contains seven common Spoonfuls; so that a Spoonful is supposed to contain half an Ounce.

The small Spoon, or Coffee Spoon, when of its usual Size and Cavity, may contain thirty Drops, or a few more; but, in the Exhibition of Medicines, it may be reckoned at thirty Drops. Five or six of these are deemed equal in Measure, to a common Soup-Spoon.

The Bason or Porrenger, mentioned in the present Treatise, holds, without running over, the Quantity of five Glasses, which is equivalent to eighteen Ounces and three Quarters. It may be estimated however, without a Fraction, at eighteen Ounces: and a sick Person should

never

never be allowed to take more than a third Part of this Quantity of Nourishment, at any one Time.

The Doses in all the following Prescriptions are adjusted to the Age of an Adult or grown Man, from the Age of eighteen to that of sixty Years. From the Age of twelve to eighteen, two thirds of that Dose will generally be sufficient: and from twelve down to seven Years one half, diminishing this still lower, in Proportion to the greater Youth of the Patient: so that not more than one eighth of the Dose prescribed should be given to an Infant of some Months old, or under one Year. But it must also be considered, that their different Constitutions will make a considerable Difference in adjusting their different Doses. It were to be wished, on this Account, that every Person would carefully observe whether a strong Dose is necessary to purge him, or if a small one is sufficient; as Exactness is most important in adjusting the Doses of such Medicines, as are intended to purge, or to evacuate in any other Manner.

N°. 1.

Take a Pugil or large Pinch between the Thumb and Fingers of Elder Flowers; put them into an earthen-ware Mug or Porrenger, with two Ounces of Honey, and an Ounce and a half of good Vinegar. Pour upon them three Pints and one Quarter of boiling Water. Stir it about a little with a Spoon to mix and dissolve the Honey; then cover up the Mug; and, when the

the Liquor is cold, strain it through a Linen Cloth.

N°. 2.

Take two Ounces of whole Barley, cleanse and wash it well in hot Water, throwing away this Water afterwards. Then boil it in five Chopins or *English* Pints of Water, till the Barley bursts and opens. Towards the End of the boiling, throw in one Drachm and a half of Nitre [Salt Petre] strain it through a Linen Cloth, and then add to it one Ounce and a half of Honey, and one Ounce of Vinegar.*

N°. 3.

Take the same Quantity of Barley as before, and instead of Nitre, boil in it, as soon as the Barley is put in to boil, a Quarter of an Ounce of Cream of Tartar. Strain it, and add nothing else † to it.

N°. 4.

Take three Ounces of the freshest sweet Almonds, and one Ounce of Gourd or Melon Seed; bruise them in a Mortar, adding to them by a little at a time, one Pint of Water, then strain it through Linen. Bruise what remains again, adding gradually to it another Pint of Water, then straining; and adding Water to the

---

* This makes an agreeable Drink; and the Notion of its being windy is idle, since it is so only to those, with whom Barley does not agree. It may, where Barley is not procurable, be made from Oats.

† In those Cases mentioned § 241, 262, 280, instead of the Barley, four Ounces of Grass Roots may be boiled in the same Quantity of Water for half an Hour, with the Cream of Tartar.

Residue, till full three Pints at least of Water are thus used: after which it may again be poured upon the bruised Mass, stirred well about, and then be finally strained off. Half an Ounce of Sugar may safely be bruised with the Almonds and Seeds at first, though some weakly imagine it too heating; and delicate Persons may be allowed a little Orange Flower Water with it.

N°. 5.

Take two Pugils of Mallow Leaves and Flowers, cut them small, and pour a Pint of boiling Water upon them. After standing some time strain it, adding one Ounce of Honey to it. For Want of Mallows, which is preferable, a similar Glyster may be made of the Leaves of Mercury, Pellitory of the Wall, the Marsh-Mallows, the greater Mallows, from Lettuce, or from Spinage. A few very particular Constitutions are not to be purged by any Glyster but warm Water alone, such should receive no other, and the Water should not be very hot.

N°. 6.

Boil a Pugil of Mallow Flowers, in a Pint of Barley Water for a Glyster.

N°. 7.

Take three Pints of simple Barley Water, add to it three Ounces of the Juice of Sow-thistle, or of Groundsel, or of the greater Houseleek, or of Borage.*

---

* These Juices are to be procured from the Herbs when fresh and very young, if possible, by beating them in a Marble

N°. 8.

To one Ounce of Oxymel of Squills, add five Ounces of a strong Infusion of Elder Flowers.

N°. 9.

There are many different emollient Applications, which have very nearly the same Virtues. The following are the most efficacious.

1, Flanels wrung out of a hot Decoction of Mallow Flowers.

2, Small Bags filled with Mallow Flowers, or with those of Mullein, of Elder, of Camomile, of wild Corn Poppy, and boiled either in Milk or Water.

3, Pultices of the same Flowers boiled in Milk and Water.

4, Bladders half filled with hot Milk and Water, or with some emollient Decoction.

5, A Pultice of boiled Bread and Milk, or of Barley or Rice boiled till thoroughly soft and tender.

6, In the Pleurisy (See § 89) the affected Part may be rubbed sometimes with Ointment of Marsh-mallows.

N°. 10.

To one Ounce of Spirit of Sulphur, add six Ounces of Syrup of Violets, or for want of

the

---

ble Mortar, or for Want of such [or a wooden Mortar] in an Iron one, and then squeezing out the Juice through a Linen Bag. It must be left to settle a little in an earthen Vessel, after which the clear Juice must be decanted gently off, and the Sediment be left behind.

the latter, as much Barley Water, of a thicker Confiftence than ordinary.*

N°. 11.

Take two Ounces of Manna, and half an Ounce of Sedlitz Salt, or for want of it, as much Epfom Salt; diffolving them in four Ounces of hot Water, and ftraining them.

N°. 12.

Take of Elder Flowers one Pugil, of Hyffop Leaves half as much. Pour three Pints of boiling Water upon them. After infufing fome time, ftrain, and diffolve three Ounces of Honey in the Infufion.

N°. 13.

---

* Some Friends, fays Dr. TISSOT, whofe Judgment I greatly refpect, have thought the Dofes of acid Spirit which I direct extremely ftrong, and doubtlefs they are fo, if compared with the Dofes generally prefcribed, and to which I fhould have limited myfelf, if I had not frequently feen their Infufficience. Experience has taught me to increafe them confiderably, and, augmenting the Dofe gradually, I now venture to give larger Dofes of them than have ever been done before, and always with much Succefs; the fame Dofes which I have advifed in this Work not being fo large as thofe I frequently prefcribe. For this Reafon I intreat thofe Phyficians, who have thought them exceffive, to try the acid Spirits in larger Dofes than thofe commonly ordered, and I am perfuaded they will fee Reafon to congratulate themfelves upon the Effect †

† Our Author's *French* Annotator has a Note againft this Acid, which I have omitted, for though I have given his Note Page 84 [with the Subftance of the immediately preceding one] to which I have alfo added fome Doubts of my own, from Facts, concerning the Benefit of Acids in inflammatory Diforders of the Breaft, yet with Regard to the ardent, the putrid, the malignant Fever, and *Eryfipelas*, in which Dr TISSOT directs this, I have no Doubt of its Propriety (fuppofing no infuperable Difagreement to Acids in the Conftitution) and with Refpect to their Dofes, I think we may fafely rely on our honeft Author's Veracity. Dr FULLER affures us, a Gentleman's Coachman was recovered from the Bleeding Small Pocks, by large and repeated Dofes of the Oil of Vitriol, in confiderable Draughts of cold Water. K.

N°. 13.

Is only the same Kind of Drink made by omitting the Hyssop, and adding instead of it as much more Elder Flowers.

N°. 14.

Let one Ounce of the best Jesuits Bark in fine Powder be divided into sixteen equal Portions.

N°. 15.

Take of the Flowers of St *John*'s Wort, of Elder, and of Melilot, of each a few Pinches; put them into the Bottom of an Ewer or Vessel containing five or six *English* Pints, with half an Ounce of Oil of Turpentine, and fill it up with boiling Water.

N°. 16.

Is only the Syrup of the Flowers of the wild red Corn Poppy.

N°. 17.

Is only very clear sweet Whey, in every Pint of which one Ounce of Honey is to be dissolved.

N°. 18.

Take of Castile or hard white Soap six Drachms; of Extract of Dandelion one Drachm and a half, of Gum Ammoniacum half a Drachm, and with Syrup of Maidenhair make a Mass of Pills, to be formed into Pills, weighing three Grains each.

N° 19.

Gargarisms may be prepared from a Decoction, or rather an Infusion, of the Leaves of Periwinkle, or of Red Rose-Leaves, or of Mallows. Two Ounces of Vinegar and as much Honey must be
added

added to every Pint of it, and the Patient should gargle with it pretty hot. The deterging, cleansing Gargarism referred to § 112, is a light Infusion of the Tops of Sage, adding two Ounces of Honey to each Pint of it.

N° 20.

Is only one Ounce of powdered Nitre, divided into sixteen equal Doses.

N°. 21.

Take of Jalap, of Senna, and of Cream of Tartar of each thirty Grains finely powdered, and let them be very well mixed.*

N° 22.

Take of *China* Root, and of Sarsaparilla of each one Ounce and a half, of Sassafras Root, and of the Shavings of Guiacum, otherwise called *Lignum vitæ*, of each one Ounce. Let the whole be cut very fine. Then put them into a glazed earthen Vessel, pouring upon them about five pints of boiling Water. Let them boil gently for an Hour; then take it from the Fire, and strain it off through Linen. This is called the Decoction of the Woods, and is often of different Proportions of these Ingredients, or with the Addition of a few others. More Water may, after the first boiling, be poured on the same Ingredients, and be boiled up into a small Decoction for common Drink.

N°. 23.

---

* This, our Author observes, will work a strong Countryman very well, by which however he does not seem to mean an Inhabitant of the Mountains in *Wales*. See P. 547

N°. 23.

Take one Ounce of the Pulp of Tamarinds, half a Drachm of Nitre, and four Ounces of Water; let them boil not more than one Minute, then add two Ounces of Manna, and when diffolved ftrain the Mixture off.

N°. 24.

Is only an Ounce of Cream of Tartar, divided into eight equal Parts

N°. 25.

This Prefcription is only the Preparation of Kermes mineral, otherwife called the Chartreufian Powder. Dr. Tissot orders but one Grain for a Dofe. It has been directed from one to three.

N° 26.

Take three Ounces of the common Burdock Root; boil it for half an Hour, with half a Drachm of Nitre, in three full Pints of Water.

N°. 27.

Take half a Pinch of the Herbs prefcribed N°. 9, Article 2, and half an Ounce of hard white Soap fhaved thin. Pour on thefe one Pint and a half of boiling Water, and one Glafs of Wine. Strain the Liquor and fqueeze it ftrongly out.

N°. 28.

Take of the pureft Quickfilver one Ounce; of Venice Turpentine half a Drachm, of the frefheft Hog's Lard two Ounces, and let the whole be very well rubbed together into an Ointment.*

---

* This Ointment fhould be prepared at the Apothecaries; the Receipt of it being given here, only becaufe the Proportions of

N°. 29.

This Prescription is nothing but the yellow Basilicon.

N°. 30.

Take of natural and factitious, or artificial Cinnabar, twenty-four Grains each; of Musk sixteen Grains, and let the whole be reduced into fine Powder, and very well mixed.†

N°. 31.

Take one Drachm of *Virginia* Snake Root in Powder; of Camphor and of Assa-foetida ten Grains each; of Opium one Grain, and with a sufficient Quantity of Conserve, or Rob of Elder, make a Bolus.‡

N°. 32.

---

the Quicksilver and the Lard are not always the same in different Places

† This Medicine is known by the Name of *Cob*'s Powder; and as its Reputation is very considerable, I did not chuse to omit it, though I must repeat here what I have said § 195— That the Cinnabar is probably of little or no Efficacy, and there are other Medicines that have also much more than the Musk, which besides is extremely dear for poor People, as the requisite Doses of it, in very dangerous Cases, would cost ten or twelve Shillings daily. The Prescription, N° 31, is more effectual than the Musk, and instead of the useless Cinnabar the powerful Quicksilver may be given to the Quantity of forty five Grains. I have said nothing hitherto in this Work of the red blossomed Mulberry Tree, which passes for a real Specific among some Persons, in this dreadful Malady. An account of it may be seen in the first Volume of the Oeconomical Journal of *Bern*. It is my Opinion however, that none of the Instances related here are satisfactory and decisive, its Efficacy now appearing to me very doubtful

‡ When this is preferred to N° 30, of which Musk is an Ingredient, the Grain of Opium should be omitted, except once or at most twice in the twenty-four Hours. Two Doses of Quicksilver, of fifteen Grains each, should be given daily in the Morning in the Intervals between the other Boluses

Nº 32.

Take three Ounces of Tamarinds. Pour on them one Pint of boiling Water, and after letting them boil a Minute or two, strain the Liquor through a Linen Cloth.

Nº. 33.

Take seven Grains of Turbith Mineral; and make it into a Pill or Bolus with a little Crumb of Bread.‖

Nº 34.

This is nothing but a Prescription of six Grains of Tartar * emetic

Nº 35.

Take thirty-five Grains of Ipecacuanna, which, in the very strongest Constitutions, may be augmented to forty-five, or even to fifty Grains.

Nº. 36.

Prescribes only the common blistering Plaister; and the Note observes that very young Infants who have delicate Skins may have Sinapisms applied instead of Blisters; and made of a little old Leaven, kneaded up with a few Drops of sharp Vinegar.

‖ This Medicine makes the Dogs vomit and slaver abundantly. It has effected many Cures after the *Hydrophobia*, the Dread of Water, was manifest. It must be given three Days successively, and afterwards twice a Week, for fifteen Days

* When People are ignorant of the Strength of the Tartar emetic (which is often various) or of the Patient's being easy or hard to vomit, a Dose and a half may be dissolved in a Quart of warm Water, of which he may take a Glass every Quarter of an Hour, whence the Operation may be forwarded, or otherwise regulated, according to the Number of Vomits or Stools. This Method, much used in *Paris*, seems a safe and eligible one

N°. 37.

Take of the Tops of *Chamaedrys* or Ground Oak, of the lesser Centaury, of Wormwood and of Camomile, of each one Pugil. Pour on them three Pints of boiling Water; and suffering them to infuse until it is cold, strain the Liquor through a Linen Cloth, pressing it out strongly.

N°. 38.

Take forty Grains of Rhubarb, and as much Cream of Tartar in Powder, mixing them well together.

N°. 39.

Take three Drachms of Cream of Tartar, and one Drachm of Ipecacuanna finely powdered. Rub them well together, and divide them into six equal Parts.

N° 40.

Take of the simple Mixture one Ounce, of Spirit of Vitriol half an Ounce, and mix them. The Dose is one or two Tea Spoonfuls in a Cup of the Patient's common Drink. The simple Mixture is composed of five Ounces of Treacle Water camphorated, of three Ounces of Spirit of Tartar rectified, and one Ounce of Spirit of Vitriol. If the Patient has an insuperable Aversion to the Camphor, it must be omitted; though the Medicine is less efficacious without it. And if his Thirst is not very considerable, the simple Mixture may be given alone, without any further Addition of Spirit of Vitriol.

N°. 41.

Take half a Drachm of *Virginia* Snake-root, ten

ten Grains of Camphor, and make them into a Bolus with Rob of Elder-Berries. If the Patient's Stomach cannot bear so large a Dose of Camphor, he may take it in smaller Doses and oftner, *viz.* three Grains, every two Hours. If there is a violent Looseness, Diascordium must be substituted instead of the Rob of Elder-berries.

N° 42

Prescribes only the *Theriaca pauperum*, or poor Man's Treacle, in the Dose of a Quarter of an Ounce. The following Composition of it is that chiefly preferred by our Author. Take equal Parts of round Birthwort Roots, of Elecampane, of Myrrh, and of Rob or Conserve of Juniper-berries, and make them into an Electuary of a rather thin, than very stiff Consistence, with Syrup of Orange-peel.

N°. 43

The first of the three Medicines referred to in this Number, is that already directed, N°. 37. The second is as follows.

Take equal Parts of the lesser Centaury, of Wormwood, of Myrrh, all powdered, and of Conserve of Juniper-berries, making them up into a pretty thick Consistence with Syrup of Wormwood. The Dose is a Quarter of an Ounce; to be taken at the same Intervals as the Bark.

For the third Composition—Take of the Roots of Calamus Aromaticus and Elecampane well bruised, two Ounces, of the Tops of the lesser Centaury cut small, a Pugil; of Filings of unrusted Iron two Ounces, of old white Wine, three Pints. Put them all into a wide necked Bottle, and set it upon Embers, or on a Stove, or by the Chimney, that it may be always kept hot. Let them infuse twenty-four Hours, shaking them well five or six Times; then let the Infusion settle, and strain it. The Dose is a common Cup every four Hours, four Times daily, and timing it one Hour before Dinner.

N°. 44.

Take a Quarter of an Ounce of Cream of Tartar, a Pugil of common Camomile; boil them in twelve Ounces of Water for half an Hour, and strain it off.

N°. 45.

Directs only the common Sal Ammoniac, from two Scruples to one Drachm for a Dose. The Note to it adds, that it may be made into a Bolus with Rob of Elder; and observes, that those feverish Patients, who have a weak delicate Stomach, do not well admit of this Salt, no more than of several others, which affect them with great Disorder and Anxiety.

N°. 46.

The Powder. Take one Pugil of Camomile Flowers, and as much Elder Flowers, bruising them well; of fine Flour or Starch three Ounces; of Ceruss and of blue Smalt each half an Ounce. Rub the whole, and mix them well. This Powder may be applied immediately to the Part.

The Plaister. Take of the Ointment called *Nutritum*, made with the newest sweet Oil, two Ounces,

Ounces; of white Wax three Quarters of an Ounce, and one Quarter of an Ounce of blue Smalt. Melt the Wax, then add the *Nutritum* to it, after the Smalt finely powdered has been exactly incorporated with it; stirring it about with an Iron Spatula or Rod, till the whole is well mixed and cold. This is to be smoothly spread on Linen Cloth.

A Quarter of an Ounce of Smalt may also be mixed exactly with two Ounces of Butter or Ointment of Lead, to be used occasionally instead of the Plaister.

N°. 47.

Take one Ounce of Sedlitz, or for want of that, as much Epsom Salt, and two Ounces of Tamarinds: pour upon them eight Ounces of boiling Water, stirring them about to dissolve the Tamarinds. Strain it off, and divide it into two equal Draughts, to be given at the Interval of Half an Hour between the first and last.

N°. 48.

Take of *Sydenham*'s Liquid Laudanum eighty Drops; of Bawm Water two Ounces and a-half. If the first, or the second, Dose stops or considerably lessens the Vomiting, this † Medicine should not be further repeated.

---

† The medical Editor at *Lyons* justly notes here, that these eighty Drops are a very strong Dose of liquid Laudanum, adding that it is scarcely ever given at *Lyons* in a greater Dose than thirty Drops, and recommending a Spoonful of Syrup of Lemon-peel to be given with it—But we must observe here in answer to this Note, that when Dr *Tissot* directs his Mixture

N°. 49.

Dissolve three Ounces of Manna and twenty Grains of Nitre in twenty Ounces, or six Glasses, of sweet Whey.

N°. 50.

To two Ounces of Syrup of Diacodium, or white Poppy Heads, add an equal Weight of Elder Flower Water, or, for want of it, of Spring-Water.

N°. 51.

Directs nothing but a Drachm of Rhubarb in Powder. †

N°. 52.

Take of *Sulphur vivum*, or of Flower of Brimstone, one Ounce; of Sal Ammoniac, one Drachm, of fresh Hogs Lard, two Ounces; and mix the whole very well in a Mortar.

N°. 53.

Take two Drachms of crude Antimony and as much Nitre, both finely powdered and very well mixed; dividing the whole into eight equal Doses ‡

N°. 54.

---

ture in the Iliac Passion § 318, to appease the Vomitings, Art 3, he orders but one spoonful of this Mixture to be taken at once, and an Interval of two Hours to be observed between the first and second Repetition, which reduces each Dose to sixteen Drops, and which is not to be repeated without Necessity.

‡ This Medicine, which often occasions Cholics in some Persons of a weakly Stomach, is attended with no such Inconvenience in strong Country People, and has been effectual in some Disorders of the Skin, which have baffled other Medicines—The Remainder of this Note observes the great Efficacy of Antimony in promoting Perspiration, and the extraordinary Benefit it is of to Horses in different Cases

Table of Remedies.

N°. 54.

† Take of Filings of Iron, not the least rusty, and of Sugar, each one Ounce; of Aniseeds powdered, half an Ounce. After rubbing them very well together, divide the Powder into twenty-four equal Portions; one of which is to be taken three times a Day an Hour before eating.

N°. 55.

Take of Filings of sound Iron two Ounces; of Leaves of Rue, and of white Hoar-hound one Pugil each, of black Hellebore Root, one Quarter of an Ounce, and infuse the whole in three Pints of Wine in the Manner already directed, N°. 43. The Dose of this is one small Cup three times a Day, an Hour before eating.*

N°. 56.

Take two Ounces of Filings of Iron; of Rue Leaves and Aniseed powdered, each half an Ounce.

---

† The Prescriptions N° 54. 55. 56. are calculated against Distempers which arise from Obstructions, and a Stoppage of the monthly Discharges, which N° 55 is more particularly intended to remove, those of 54 and 56 are most convenient, either when the Suppression does not exist, or is not to be much regarded, if it does. This Medicine may be rendered less unpalatable for Persons in easy Circumstances, by adding as much Cinamon instead of Aniseeds; and though the Quantity of Iron be small, it may be sufficient, if given early in the Complaint, one, or at the most, two of these Doses daily, being sufficient for a very young Maiden.

* I chuse to repeat here, the more strongly to inculcate so important a Point, that in Women who have long been ill and languid, our Endeavours must be directed towards the restoring of the Patient's Health and Strength, and not to forcing down the monthly Discharges, which is a very pernicious Practice. These will return of Course, if the Patient is of a proper Age, as she grows better. Their Return succeeds the Return of her Health, and should not, very often cannot, precede it.

Ounce. Add to them a sufficient Quantity of Honey to make an Electuary of a good Consistence. The Dose is a Quarter of an Ounce three times daily.

N°. 57.

Take of the Extract of the stinking Hemlock, with the purple spotted Stalk, one Ounce. Form it into Pills weighing two Grains each; adding as much of the Powder of dry Hemlock Leaves, as the Pills will easily take up. Begin the Use of this Medicine by giving one Pill Night and Morning. Some Patients have been so familiarized to it, as to take at length Half an Ounce daily.†

N°. 58.

† Our learned and candid Author has a very long Note in this Place, strongly in Favour of Storck's Extract of Hemlock, in which it is evident he credits the greater Part of the Cures affirmed by Dr Storck to have been effected by it. He says he made some himself, but not of the right Hemlock, which we think it very difficult to mistake, from its peculiar rank fetid Smell, and its purple spotted Stalk. After first taking this himself, he found it mitigated the Pain of Cancers, but did not cure them. But then addressing himself to Dr *Storck*, and exactly following his Directions in making it, he took of Dr *Storck*'s Extract, and of his own, which exactly resembled each other, to the Quantity of a Drachm and a half daily, and finding his Health not in the least impaired by it, he then gave it to several Patients, curing many scrophulous and cancerous Cases, and mitigating others, which he supposes were incurable. So that he seems fully persuaded Dr. Storck's Extract is always innocent [which in Fact, except in a very few Instances, none of which were fatal, it has been] and he thinks it a Specific in many Cases, to which nothing can be substituted as an equivalent Remedy, that it should be taken with entire Confidence, and that it would be absurd to neglect its Continuance.

The Translator of this Work of Dr Tissot's has thought it but fair to give all the Force of this Note here, which must be

Nº. 58.

Take of the Roots of Grass and of Succory well washed, each one Ounce. Boil them a Quarter of an Hour in a Pint of Water. Then dissolve in it Half an Ounce of Sedlitz, or of *Epsom* Salt, and two Ounces of Manna; and strain it off to drink one Glass of it from Half Hour, to Half Hour, till its Effects are sufficient. It is to be repeated at the Interval of two or three Days.

Nº. 59.

Is a Cataplasm or Pultice made of Crumb of Bread, with Camomile Flowers boiled in Milk; with the Addition of some Soap, so that each Pultice may contain half a Quarter of an Ounce of this last Ingredient. And when the Circumstances of female Patients have not afforded them that regular Attendance, which the Repetition of the Pultice requires, as it should be renewed every three Hours, I have successfully directed the Hemlock Plaister of the Shops.

Nº. 60.

Take a sufficient Quantity of dry Hemlock Leaves. Secure them properly between two Pieces of thin Linen Cloth, so as to make a very flexible Sort of small Matrass, letting it boil a few Moments in Water, then squeeze it out and apply it to the affected Part. It must thus be moistened

---

be his own, as his Editor at *Lyons* seems to entertain a very different Opinion of the Efficacy of this Medicine; for which Opinion we refer back to his Note, § 375, of this Treatise, which the Reader may compare with this of our Author's. *K.*

moistened and heated afresh, and re-applied every two Hours.

N°. 61.

Take of the Eyes of the Craw-fish, or of the true white Magnesia, two Drachms; of Cinnamon powdered four Grains. Rub them very well together, and divide the whole into eight Doses. One of these is to be given in a Spoonful of Milk, or of Water, before the Infant sucks.

N°. 62.

Take of an Extract of Walnuts, made in Water, two Drachms, and dissolve it in half an Ounce of Cinnamon Water. Fifty Drops a Day of this Solution is to be given to a Child of two Years old; and after the whole has been taken, the Child should be purged. This Extract is to be made of the unripe Nuts, when they are of a proper Growth and Consistence for pickling

N° 63.

Take of Rezin of Jalap two Grains. Rub it a considerable time with twelve or fifteen Grains of Sugar, and afterwards with three or four sweet Almonds; adding, very gradually, two common Spoonfuls of Water. Then strain it through clear thin Linen, as the Emulsion of Almonds was ordered to be. Lastly, add a Tea Spoonful of Syrup of Capillaire to it. This is no disagreeable Draught, and may be given to a Child of two Years old: and if they are older, a Grain or two more of the Rezin may be allowed. But under two

two Years old, it is prudent to purge Children rather with Syrup of Succory, or with Manna.

N°. 64.

Take of the Ointment called *Nutritum* one Ounce; the entire Yolk of one small Egg, or the Half of a large one, and mix them well together. This *Nutritum* may be readily made by rubbing very well together, and for some time, two Drachms of Cerufs [white Lead] half an Ounce of Vinegar, and three Ounces of common Oil.

N°. 65.

Melt four Ounces of white Wax; add to it, if made in Winter two Spoonfuls of Oil; if in Summer none at all, or at moft, not above a Spoonful. Dip in this Slips of Linen Cloth not worn too thin, and let them dry: or spread it thin and evenly over them.

N°. 66.

Take of Oil of Rofes one Pound; of red Lead half a Pound; of Vinegar four Ounces. Boil them together nearly to the Confiftence of a Plaifter; then diffolve in the liquid Mafs an Ounce and a Half of yellow Wax, and two Drachms of Camphor, ftirring the whole about well. Remove it then from the Fire, and fpread it on Sheets or Slips of Paper, of what Size you think moft convenient. The Ointment of *Chambauderie*, fo famous in many Families on the Continent, is made of a Quarter of a Pound of yellow Wax, of the Plaifter of three Ingredients (very nearly the fame with N°. 66) of compound Diachylon

and

and of common Oil, of each the same Quantity; all melted together, and then stirred about well, after it is removed from the Fire, till it grows cold. To make a Sparadrap, or Oil Cloth, which is Linen, covered with, or dipt in an emplastic Substance or Ointment, it must be melted over again with the Addition of a little Oil, and applied to the Linen as directed at N°. 65.

N°. 67.

Gather in Autumn, while the fine Weather lasts, the Agaric of the Oak, which is a Kind of *Fungus* or Excrescence, issuing from the Wood of that Tree.

It consists at first of four Parts, which present themselves successively, 1, The outward Rind or Skin, which may be thrown away. 2, That Part immediately under this Rind, which is the best of all. This is to be beat well with a Hammer, till it becomes soft and very pliable. This is the only Preparation it requires, and a Slice of it of a proper Size is to be applied directly over the bursting, open Blood-vessels. It constringes and brings them close together, stops the Bleedings; and generally falls off at the End of two Days. 3, The third Part, adhering to the second may serve to stop the Bleeding from the smaller Vessels, and the fourth and last Part may be reduced to Powder, as conducing to the same Purpose †

N°. 68.

† Our Author attests his seeing the happiest Consequences from this Application which M Brossard, a very eminent French

N°. 68.

Take four Ounces of Crumbs of Bread, a Pugil of Elder Flowers, and the same Quantity of those of Camomile, and of St. *John's* Wort. Boil them into a Pultice in equal Quantities of Vinegar and Water.

If Fomentations should be thought preferable, take the same Herbs, or some Pugils of the Ingredients for *Faltrank*: throw them into a Pint and a Half of boiling Water: and let them infuse some Minutes. Then a Pint of Vinegar is to be added, and Flanels or other woollen Cloths dipt in the Fomentation, and wrung out, are to be applied to the Part affected.

For the aromatic Fomentations recommended § 449, take Leaves of Betony and of Rue, Flowers of Rosemary or Lavender, and red Roses, of each a Pugil and a Half. Boil them for a Quarter of an Hour in a Pot with a Cover, with three Pints of old white Wine. Then strain off, squeezing the Liquor strongly from the Herbs, and apply it as already directed.

N° 69.

Directs only the Plaister of Diapalma.*

N°. 70.

Directs only a Mixture of two Parts Water, and one Part of Vinegar of Litharge.

N°. 71.

French Surgeon, first published, and declared his Preference of that Agaric which sprung from those Parts of the Tree, from whence large Boughs had been lopped

* To spread this upon Lint as directed, § 456, it must be melted down again with a little Oil.

N°. 71.

Take of the Leaves of Sow-bread, and of Camomile Tops, of each one Pugil. Put them into an earthen Vessel with half an Ounce of Soap, and as much Sal Ammoniac, and pour upon them three Pints of boiling Water.

N. B. I conceive all the Notes to this Table, in which I have not mentioned the Editor at *Lyons*, nor subscribed with my initial Letter *K*, to come from the Author, having omitted nothing of them, but the Prices.

TABLE

ERRATA.

Page 4, Line 6, for *of* read *ef*. p. 16, l. 16, for *be* read *me*. p. 29, l. 12, after *it* add . p. 48, l. 12, dele *and* at the End of it. p. 51, in the running Title, for *Causs* read *Causes*. ib. l. 2, dele *ard*. ib. l. 7, dele *and*. p. 57, last line, for *hurtsul* read *hurtful*. p. 67, l. 17, after *Water*, add, *may be placed within the Room*. p. 74, line last but two, after *never*, dele , p. 96, l. 11, for *Ailment* read *Ailment*. p. 106, l. 23, for the second *is* read *bas*. p. 126, l. 21, for *breato* read *breathe*. p. 137, l. 13, for *Efflorescene* read *Efflorescence*. p. 145, L. 1, for *Water* read *Tea*. p. 148, l. 19, for *becomes* read *becomes*. p 163, l. 30, in the Note, for *accured* read *occurred*. p. 171, l. 20, dele *and* p. 189, l. 28, dele *of*. p. 199, l. 6, for *Paulmier* read *Palmarius*, being the Lat. nized Name of that *Physician*, as we say for *Fernel Fernelius*, *Hotler Hollerius*, &c. N. B. His Powder for the Bite of a mad Dog consisted of equal Parts of Rue, Vervain, Plantain, Polypody, common Wormwood, Mugwort, Bastard Baum, Betony, St. *John*'s Wort, and lesser Centaury Tops, to which *Desault* adds *Corahne*.——p 237, L 2, for *Streakes* read *Streaks*. p 256, first line of the Note * de'e the first *ofteh*. p. 261, l. 15, for *happens* read *happen*. p. 270, l. 12, dele *t* in *Swo ferland*. p. 282, l. 23, for *enters* read *enter*. p. 283, l 23, for *Strmach* read *Stomachs*. p 284, L. 12, for *it* read *them*. p 287, Note* L 25, for *here* read *there*. p 303, l. 14, for *doubtful* read *doubtful*. p. 318, L. 18, for *abate* read *abates*. p 337, l 7, for *glary* read *glairy*. N. B. In the first Page that is folio'd 445 read 345. p. 346, l 19, for *two* read *to*. p. 351, l 25, after *Waters* add, *such as Infusion of Tea*, &c. p. 375, l 7, for *too* read *too*. p 392, last line, for *Leaves* read *Flowers*. p 393, l 26, after *them*, insert *ard*. p. 397, l 1 and 2, for *Temparrament* read *Temperament*. p. 422, l 6, between *several* and *Consequences* insert *bad*. p 454, l 5, for *Dissectors* read *Dissectors*. p 450, l 17, in *Ice-thaws* dele - . p 466, l 10, to *Cerastes* add -- . p. 486, l 29, after *or* add *if*. p 487, l 12, for *Parts* read *Part*. p 511, l. 12, for *not* read *nor*. p 533, l 12, for *arrives* read *arises*. p. 542, l. 22, for *Patent* read *Patents*. p. 562, l. 14, for *says* read *say*. p. 573, L 10, after *Causs*, dele *Comma*.

TABLE *of the several Chapters, and their principal Contents.*

Introduction — Page 1
The first Cause of Depopulation, Emigrations *ib.*
The second Cause, Luxury — 6
Third Cause, Decay of Agriculture — 10
Fourth Cause, the pernicious Treatment of Diseases — 12
Means for rendering this Treatise useful — 15
Explanation of certain physical Terms, and Phrases — 26

CHAPTER I

The most common Causes of popular Sickness — 31
First Cause, excessive Labour *ib.*
Second Cause, the Effect of cold Air, when a Person is hot — 33
Third Cause, taking cold Drink, when in a Heat *ib. & 34*
Fourth Cause, the Inconstancy and sudden Change of the Weather — 35
Fifth Cause, the Situation of Dunghills, and Marshes, near inhabited Houses, and the bad confined Air in the Houses — 37
Sixth Cause, Drunkenness — 38
Seventh Cause, the Food of Country People — 39
Eighth Cause, the Situation, or Exposure of Houses — 42
Concerning the Drink of Country People — 43

CHAP. II.

Of Causes which increase the Diseases of the People, with general Considerations — 47
First Cause, the great Care employed to force the Sick to sweat, and the Methods taken for that Purpose *ib. & 48*
The Danger of hot Chambers — 49
The Danger of hot Drinks and heating Medicines — 50
Second Cause, the Quantity and Quality of the Food given sick Persons — 53
Third Cause, the giving Vomits and Purges at the Beginning of the Disease — 57

CHAP III

Concerning what should be done in the Beginning of Diseases, and the Diet in acute Diseases — 61
Signs which indicate approaching Diseases, with Means to prevent them — 62
The common Regimen, or Regulations, for the Sick — 64
The Benefits of ripe sound Fruits — 68
Cautions and Means to be used, on Recovery — 73, 74

CHAP IV

Of the Inflammation of the Breast — 77
The Signs of this Disease *ib. & 78*
The Advantage of Bleeding — 81
Signs of Recovery — 85
Of *Crises*, and the Symptoms that precede them — 86
The Danger of Vomits, of Purges, and of Anodynes — 88
Of the Suppression of Expectoration, and the Means to restore it. — 89
Of the Formation of *Vomicas*, or Imposthumes in the Lungs, and the Treatment of them — 90
Of the Danger of Remedies, termed Balsamics — 103
The Inefficacy of the Antihectic of *Poterius* — 104

CONTENTS.

Of an *Empyema* 105
Of a Gangrene of the Lungs 106
Of a *Scirrhus* of the Lungs *ib.*

Chap V
Of the *Pleurisy* 108
The Danger of heating Remedies 112 to 115
Of frequent, or habitual, Pleurisies 116
Of Goats Blood; the Soot of a stale Egg, and of the Wormwood of the Alps, in Pleurisies 117, 118

Chap VI
Of *Diseases of the Throat* 119
Of their proper Treatment 124
Of the Formation of an Abscess there 127
Of swelled Ears, from the Obstruction of the parotid and maxillary Glands 131
Of the epidemic and putrid Diseases of the Throat, which prevailed in 1761 at Lausanne 132

Chap VII
Of C 139
Different Prejudices concerning Colds 140
The Danger of drinking much hot Water, and of strong spirituous Liquors, &c 146
Means for strengthening and curing Persons very subject to Colds 148

Chap VIII
Of *Diseases of the Teeth* 150

Chap IX
Of the *Apoplexy* 158
Of sanguine Apoplexy *ib. &* 159
Of a serous, or watery, Apoplexy 162
Means to prevent relapsing into them 164 &c

Chap X
Of *morbid Strokes of the Sun* 167

Chap XI
Of *the Rheumatism* 177
Of the acute Rheumatism, attended with a Fever *ib*
Of the slow, or chronical, without a Fever 186
The Danger of spirituous and greasy Remedies 191, 192

Chap XII
Of the *Bite of a mad Dog* 194

Chap XIII
Of the *Small Pocks* 207
Of the preceding Symptoms of this Disease 209
—The Danger of sweating Medicines 217
—The Treatment of the benign distinct Small Pocks 220
—The Use of Bleeding 222
—The Fever of Suppuration 223
—The Necessity of opening the ripe Pustules 226
—The Danger of Anodynes 228
Of the striking in of the Eruptions 229
Preparations for receiving it favorably 230

Chap XIV
Of the *Measles* 235
Of their Treatment and the Means to prevent any of their bad Consequences, to 243

Chap XV
Of *the hot, or burning, Fever* 245

Chap XVI
Of *putrid Fevers* 248

Chap XVII
Of *malignant Fevers* 257
The Danger of applying living Animals in them 267

Chap XVIII
Of *intermitting Fevers* 269
—Spring

CONTENTS.

—Spring and Autumn Intermittents — 272
Method of Cure by the Bark 275
Method of treating the Patient in the Fit — 277
Of other Febrifuges, besides the Bark — 278
The Treatment of long and obstinate Intermittents 279
Of some very dangerous Intermittents — 284
Of some periodical Disorders, which may be termed, Fevers disguised — 285
Of Preservatives from unwholesome Air 286

CHAP. XIX

Of an Erisipelas, or St Anthony's Fire — 288
Of a frequent or habitual Erisipelas — 295
Of the Stings or Bites of Animals — 296

CHAP XX.

Of Inflammations of the Breast, and of Bastard and bilious Pleurisies — 298
—Of the false Inflammation of the Breast — 300
—The false Pleurisy 303

CHAP. XXI.

Of Cholics — 306
Of the inflammatory Cholic 307
—the bilious Cholic 312
—the Cholic from Indigestion, and of Indigestions 314
—the flatulent, or windy, Cholic — 317
—the Cholic, from taking Cold — 319

CHAP. XXII.

Of the Miserere, or Iliac Passion, and of the Cholera Morbus — 322
The *Miserere* ib. & 323
The *Cholera Morbus* 327

CHAP. XXIII.

Of a Diarrhæa, or Looseness 332

CHAP XXIV.

Of a Dysentery, or Bloody-Flux 335
The Symptoms of the Disease 336
The Remedies against it 338
Of the beneficial Use of ripe Fruits — 341
Of the Danger of taking a great Number of popular Remedies in it — 345

CHAP. XXV.

Of the Itch — 347

CHAP. XXVI.

Directions peculiar to the Sex 352
Of the monthly Customs 353
Of Gravidation, or going with Child — 365
Of Labours or Deliveries, 367
Of their Consequences 371
Of a Cancer — 373

CHAP XXVII

Directions with Regard to Children — 375
Of the first Cause of their Disorders, the *Meconium* 377
—the second, the souring of their Milk — 379
—the Danger of giving them Oil — ib.
—Disorders from their Want of Perspiration, the Means of keeping it up, and of washing them in cold Water 381 & 382
—the third Cause, the cutting of their Teeth 386
—the fourth Cause, Worms 387
Of Convulsions — 91
Methods necessary to make them strong and hardy, with general

CONTENTS.

general Directions about
them ——— 396 & seq.

CHAP XXVIII
Of Assistances for drowned Persons
403

CHAP XXIX
Of Substances fast bitten in the
Mouth and the Stomach 411

CHAP XXX
Of Disorders requiring the Assistance of a Surgeon — 435
Of Burns ——— 436
Of Wounds ——— 437
Of Bruises, and of Falls 444
Of Ulcers ——— 454
Of frozen Limbs, or Joints 458
Of Chilblains — — 462
Of Ruptures — — 474
Of Phlegmons, or Boils 480
Of Felons, or Whitlows 481
Of Thorns, Splinters, &c. in the Skin or Flesh 486
Of Warts ——— 488
Of Corns ——— 490

CHAP XXXI
Of some Cases, which require immediate Assistance 491
Of Swoonings, from Excess of Blood — — 492
Of Swoonings, from great Weakness — — 494
Of Swoonings occasioned by a Load on the Stomach 497
Of Swoonings, resulting from Disorders of the Nerves 500

Of Swoonings, occasioned by the Passions 504
Of the Swoonings, which occur in Diseases — 506
Of Hæmorrhages, or Fluxes of Blood ——— 508
Of Convulsion Fits — 512
Of suffocating, or strangling Fits ——— 514
Of the violent Effects of great Fear ——— 516
Of Accidents produced by the Vapours of Charcoal, and of Wine — — — 519
Of Poisons — 526
Of acute and violent Pains 529

CHAP XXXII
Of giving Remedies by Way of Precaution ——— 531
Of Bleeding — — 532
Of Purges — — 540
Remedies to be used after excessive Purging — 544
Reflections on some other Remedies ——— 546, &c.

CHAP XXXIII
Of Quacks, Mountebanks, and Conjurers ——— 551

CHAP XXXIV.
Questions necessary to be answered by any Person, who goes to consult a Physician. — 579
The Table of Remedies 584

Lightning Source UK Ltd.
Milton Keynes UK
UKHW030610220519
343122UK00007B/736/P